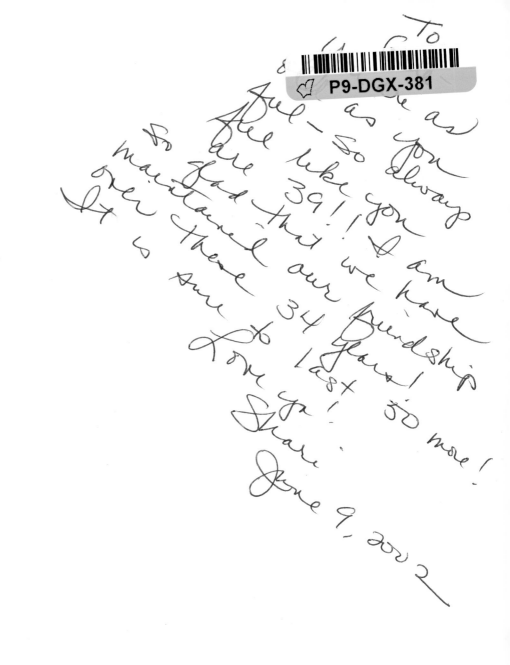

To [...]
as you
ful — So always
feel like you
are 39!! I am
so glad that we have
maintained our friendship
over these 34 years!
It is sure to last 50 more!
Love ya
Sheri
June 9, 2002

Growing Younger

Growing Younger

Breakthrough Age-Defying Secrets for Women

By Bridget Doherty, Julia VanTine, and the Editors of

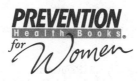

RODALE

NOTICE

This book is intended as a reference volume only, not as a medical manual. The information given here is designed to help you make informed decisions about your health. It is not intended as a substitute for any treatment that may have been prescribed by your doctor. If you suspect that you have a medical problem, we urge you to seek competent medical help.

Mention of specific companies, organizations, or authorities in this book does not imply endorsement by the publisher, nor does mention of specific companies, organizations, or authorities in the book imply that they endorse the book.

Internet addresses and telephone numbers given in this book were accurate at the time this book went to press.

Portions of this book were previously published as *Growing Younger*, *Natural Remedies*, and *Get Well, Stay Well* from the series Women's Edge Health Enhancement Guides (a trademark of Rodale Inc.).

Prevention Health Books is a registered trademark of Rodale Inc.

Printed in the United States of America

Rodale Inc. makes every effort to use acid-free ∞, recycled paper ♲ .

Illustrations by Shawn Banner, Nardo Lebo, Judy Newhouse, Laura Stutzman, and Tom Ward

Cover photographs by Amy Neunsinger/Stone and Tony Hutchings/Stone

Library of Congress Cataloging-in-Publication Data

Doherty, Bridget.
    Growing younger : breakthrough age-defying secrets for women / by
Bridget Doherty, Julia VanTine, and the the editors of Prevention Health
Books for Women.
        p.   cm.
    Portions of this book were formerly published as part of the Women's edge
health enhancement guides series.
    ISBN 1–57954–563–7 hardcover
    1. Women—Care and hygiene. 2. Longevity. 3. Rejuvenation.
4.Youthfulness.   I. VanTine, Julia.   II. Prevention Health Books for Women.
III. Title.
RA778 .D654 2001
613'.04244—dc21   2001048517

Distributed to the book trade by St. Martin's Press

2 4 6 8 10 9 7 5 3 1 hardcover

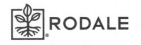

RODALE

WE **INSPIRE** AND **ENABLE** PEOPLE TO IMPROVE
THEIR LIVES AND THE WORLD AROUND THEM

FOR PRODUCTS & INFORMATION

WWW.RODALESTORE.COM
WWW.PREVENTION.COM

(800) 848-4735

SENIOR EDITOR: Sharon Faelten

EDITORS: Debra L. Gordon, E. A. Tremblay

WRITERS: Susan G. Berg, Bridget Doherty, Gale Maleskey, Arden Moore, Deanna Portz, Julia VanTine

CONTRIBUTING WRITERS: Sara Altshul, Jennifer Bright, Julie Knipe Brown, Leah Flickinger, Grete Haentjens, Sarí Harrar, Lois Guarino Hazel, Joely Johnson, Mary Kittel, Nanci Kulig, Sandra Salera Lloyd, Holly McCord, Deanna Moyer, Deborah Pedron, Kathryn Piff, Judith Springer Riddle, Cheryl A. Romano, Elizabeth Shimer, Marie Elaina Suszynski, Carla Thomas, Shea Zukowski

INTERIOR DESIGNER: Leanne Coppola

COVER DESIGNER: Maia Ranieri

ASSISTANT RESEARCH MANAGER: Shea Zukowski

PRIMARY RESEARCH EDITOR: Anita C. Small

RESEARCH EDITOR: Carol J. Gilmore

LEAD RESEARCHER: Grete Haentjens

EDITORIAL RESEARCHERS: Jennifer Bright, Molly Donaldson Brown, Lori Davis, Adrien Drozdowski, Jan Eickmeier, Bella Hebrew, Jennifer S. Kushnier, Mary S. Mesaros, Paris Muchanic, Elizabeth B. Price, Paula Rasich, Valerie Rowe, Staci Ann Sander, Amy Seirer, Elizabeth Shimer, Lucille Uhlman, Teresa A. Yeykal, Nancy Zelko

SENIOR COPY EDITORS: Amy Fisher Kovalski, Kathryn C. LeSage, Karen Neely

EDITORIAL PRODUCTION MANAGER: Marilyn Hauptly

LAYOUT DESIGNER: Keith Biery

PRODUCT SPECIALIST: Jodi Schaffer

Rodale Women's Health Books

VICE PRESIDENT, EDITORIAL DIRECTOR: Elizabeth Crow

EDITOR-IN-CHIEF: Tammerly Booth

PRODUCT MARKETING MANAGER: Stephanie Hammerstone

WRITING DIRECTOR: Jack Croft

RESEARCH DIRECTOR: Ann Gossy Yermish

MANAGING EDITOR: Madeleine Adams

ART DIRECTOR: Darlene Schneck

OFFICE STAFF: Julie Kehs Minnix, Catherine E. Strouse

JEFFREY R. LISSE, M.D.

Head of clinical osteoporosis research, associate chief of the Arizona Arthritis Center, and professor of medicine at the University of Arizona College of Medicine in Tucson

JoANN E. MANSON, M.D., DR.P.H.

Professor of medicine at Harvard Medical School and chief of preventive medicine at Brigham and Women's Hospital in Boston

DAVID MOLONY, L.Ac., DIPL.C.H.

Executive director of the American Association of Oriental Medicine, diplomate in Chinese herbology of the National Certification Commission for Acupuncture and Oriental Medicine, and licensed acupuncturist in Catasauqua, Pennsylvania

TERRY L. MURPHY, PSY.D.

Assistant clinical professor in the department of community health and aging at Temple University and licensed clinical psychologist in Philadelphia

DAVID J. NICKEL, O.M.D., L.Ac., DIPL.C.H.

Doctor of Oriental medicine, licensed acupuncturist, diplomate in Chinese herbology of the National Certification Commission for Acupuncture and Oriental Medicine, chairman and CEO of PrimeZyme, and nutritionist in Santa Monica, California

SUSAN C. OLSON, PH.D.

Clinical psychologist, life transition/psychospiritual therapist, and weight-management consultant in Seattle

MARY LAKE POLAN, M.D., PH.D.

Professor and chair of the department of gynecology and obstetrics at Stanford University School of Medicine

DAVID P. ROSE, M.D., PH.D., D.Sc.

Chief of the division of nutrition and endocrinology at Naylor Dana Institute, part of the American Health Foundation in Valhalla, New York, and an expert on nutrition and cancer for the National Cancer Institute and the American Cancer Society

MARK STENGLER, N.D.

Naturopathic and homeopathic doctor, director of natural medicine at Personal Physicians clinic in La Jolla, California, and associate clinical professor at the National College of Naturopathic Medicine in Portland, Oregon

SHAWN M. TALBOTT, PH.D.

Executive editor for SupplementWatch in Provo, Utah

LILA AMDURSKA WALLIS, M.D., M.A.C.P.

Clinical professor of medicine at Weill Medical College of Cornell University in New York City, past president of the American Medical Women's Association (AMWA), founding president of the National Council on Women's Health, director of continuing medical education programs for physicians, and master and laureate of the American College of Physicians

ANDREW T. WEIL, M.D.

Director of the program in integrative medicine and clinical professor of medicine at the University of Arizona College of Medicine in Tucson

E. DOUGLAS WHITEHEAD, M.D.

Associate attending physician in urology at Beth Israel Medical Center and New York University Downtown Hospital and cofounder and director of the Association for Male Sexual Dysfunction, all in New York City, and associate clinical professor of urology at Albert Einstein College of Medicine in the Bronx

ROBERT E. C. WILDMAN, R.D., PH.D.

Assistant professor of nutrition at the University of Louisiana at Lafayette

DAVID WINSTON

Herbalist; founding and professional member of the American Herbalists Guild; and president of Herbalist and Alchemist and dean of the Herbal Therapeutics School of Botanical Medicine, both in Washington, New Jersey

CARLA WOLPER, R.D.

Nutritionist and clinical coordinator at the obesity research center at St. Luke's–Roosevelt Hospital Center and nutritionist at the center for women's health at Columbia-Presbyterian/Eastside, both in New York City

Contents

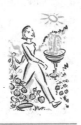
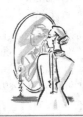

PART THREE
Think Sharp, Feel Young

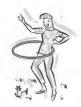

PART FOUR
Get Well, Stay Well

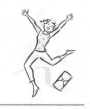

PART FIVE
Doctors' Best Disease Fighters

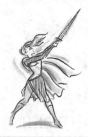

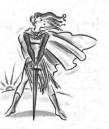

You *Can* Stop the Clock

Y ou haven't aged a bit."

"How do you stay so young?"

"You certainly don't look your age!"

How often do you find yourself paying others compliments like those when you run into old friends, former coworkers, or high school classmates? We all know women who look younger than their years, carry themselves youthfully, or have an energetic, adventurous outlook on life.

How do they do it?

Certainly, good genes play a role. But increasingly, science is finding that diet and lifestyle factors—like exercise—also play a role in determining who looks their age and who does not.

Consider what exercise did for Filomena Warihay, featured on page 57. At age 40, this mother of four was so out of shape that she couldn't run a mile.

After she began exercising, the pounds and the years melted away. Now in her sixties, she's often mistaken for a woman in her forties, and she feels as good as she did in her thirties. Not only does Warihay not dread going to the beach, she sometimes has trouble deciding which of her six bikinis to wear!

In the following pages, you'll meet dozens of women who look years or even decades younger than their chronological ages. And you'll read expert advice, based on solid anti-aging science, showing how you, too, can turn back your biological clock. You'll find out how to avoid not only outward signs of aging, such as wrinkles and sagging skin, but also less visible problems like declining energy or life-threatening problems, such as heart disease and cancer.

Here's a glimpse of what you'll find.

- Discover how scrumptious foods—like cherries—produce "youth hormones" that increase energy, strengthen immunity, promote stronger muscles and denser bones, and improve hearing, vision, and memory.
- Learn how phytochemical-rich soy foods decrease the risk of heart attack while reducing your risk of developing breast cancer, osteoporosis, and hot flashes.
- Find out why just 30 minutes of exercise a day boosts metabolism, increases energy, reduces stress, promotes sleep, liberates your sex drive, and lowers the risk of common age-related diseases.
- Read about the hottest new anti-aging supplements. Many times more potent than vitamins C and E, the next generation of antioxidants includes phosphatidylserine, alpha-lipoic acid, and Pycnogenol.
- Learn from cosmetologists, fashion experts, and wardrobe consultants how actresses, models, and other celebrities pull themselves together in a hurry.
- Discover why a sizzling sex life can make you look up to 7 years younger.

Trust me: After using tips and secrets in this book, you will be receiving compliments on your youthfulness!

Sharon Faelten

Sharon Faelten
Senior Editor

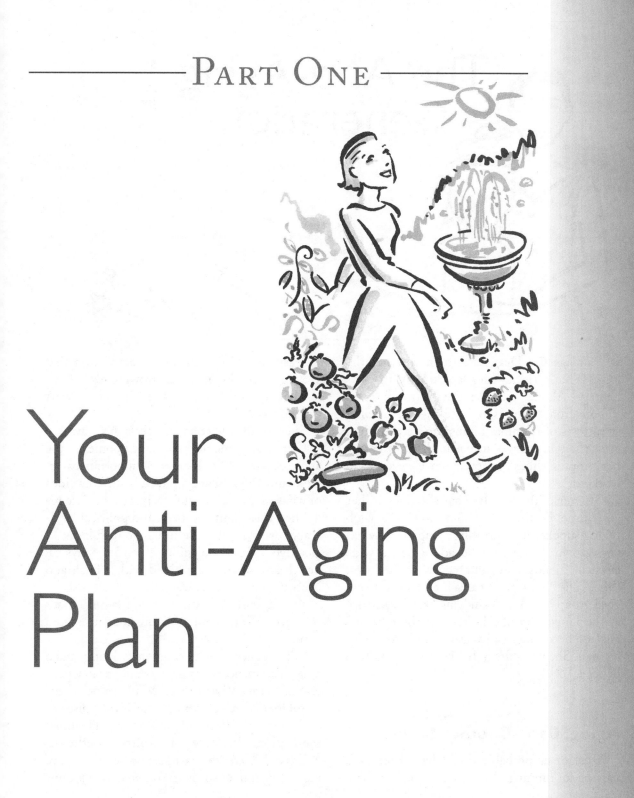

PART ONE

Your Anti-Aging Plan

The Anti-Aging Generation

At age 62, Deane Feetham wins triathlons. That's right. Her apartment in Anchorage, Alaska, is cluttered with trophies and ribbons from victories in those all-day, grueling sweatfests of running, biking, and swimming, even though she was in her midforties before her running shoes or bicycle wheels ever got a workout.

Of course, that's only what she does in her *spare* time. Feetham also holds down a day job selling supplies for a printing company. She has two grown daughters who adore her, a wide circle of friends, and volunteer work she loves. (She's a facilitator for an area breast-cancer survival group.) And she's studying exercise science at the University of Alaska with the eventual goal of becoming a physical trainer for older women. She has a fire in her belly and a light in her eye.

Aging, Baby-Boomer Style

Most of us probably don't share Feetham's passion for running. But it's likely that we share at least one thing with her: a conviction that growing older doesn't mean growing *old*.

"The idea of getting old just kind of doesn't exist for me," she says.

She isn't the only one who feels this way.

Our entire generation of baby boomers—the approximately 39 million women born between 1946 and 1964—have a radically different idea of what *old* is, and we ain't it. Just as we once redefined this country's social and political landscape, we're now redefining youthfulness as 'positive aging,' meaning extended physical health and vitality combined with a fresh and lively mental attitude.

But it isn't just our idea of aging that's changed. We're actually living longer . . . and better.

"This generation of women is living much longer past menopause than those of previous generations," says Vivian Pinn, M.D., associate director for research on women's health and director of the Office of Research on Women's Health at the National Institutes of Health in Bethesda, Maryland. "Over the past 10-plus years, we have made tremendous strides. Women now enjoy unprecedented opportunities for preserving and improving their health."

Why We Can Live Longer and Better

From the civil-rights movement to the Vietnam War, our generation experienced a unique time in American history. We were also fortunate enough to be born in an era of constant medical discoveries and advances.

In this century alone, a woman's life expectancy has increased by 31 years (a man's, by 28 years). The average woman now lives to be 79, the average man, 74. Moreover, the rate of disabilities among older people has dropped dramatically, most likely because of medical breakthroughs, better nutrition, and a decline in cigarette smoking.

We also stand to benefit from the recent explosion of research into women's health, particularly the health of women at midlife and beyond.

The Women's Health Initiative (WHI), a long-term national health study of heart disease, cancer, stroke, and osteoporosis in some 160,000 women ages 50 and over, is one of the largest prevention studies of its kind. It is examining the effect of hormone-replacement therapy (HRT) on the prevention of heart disease, osteoporosis, and breast and endometrial cancers; the effect of a healthy diet on the prevention of heart disease and breast and colo-

THE GIFTS OF AGING

Maybe we don't have the body we had when we were 20, but growing older isn't without its perks, says Sue Patton Thoele, a licensed psychotherapist in Boulder, Colorado, and author of *Freedoms after 50*. Below is her top-10 list of aging's more subtle gifts.

We can act "disgracefully." "To me, that's laughing uproariously in public, throwing your arms around a dear friend you haven't seen in a long time, using some spicy words to make your point. We're free to ignite the fiery part of ourselves."

We can take care of ourselves—and we know it. "For me, one of the benefits of aging is a deep, hard-earned trust in my ability to regain my equilibrium when I'm knocked off-kilter."

We can just say no. Period. "Being able to say that wonderfully assertive word without guilt, explanation, or remorse is to break free from the prison of obligation. At our age, we've certainly earned the privilege."

We have more time to let our creative juices flow. "Most of us have more leisure time as we get older, so we can develop our creativity more fully. And since we don't have to prove ourselves, we're more inclined to try anything."

Sex becomes more spiritual. "There's a depth of feeling between you and your mate that makes sex less about performance and more about tenderness and sharing."

We don't have to cook if we don't want to. "There are many times now when I grant myself the freedom to assert my noncooking credo of 'Forage, take out, or take me out.' "

We can snooze when we choose. "Pets are admirable nappers, able to doze off whenever the mood strikes. We now have the time to follow their example."

We can can the guilt. "There's a saying, 'Show me a woman without guilt, and I'll show you a man.' It's time that we kiss guilt goodbye."

We learn to accept things as they are. "One of the joys of maturity is realizing that it's perfectly all right to give up trying to control everything and accept what is. What a blessed relief."

Our "wisdom gland" kicks in. "With our wealth of experience, we gain perspective—a much deeper understanding of what's *really* important in our lives."

rectal cancers; and the effect of calcium and vitamin D supplementation on the prevention of osteoporosis and colorectal cancer.

The emerging field of gender-based biology, which examines the biological and physiological differences between women and men, has already made discoveries with potential long-term health implications. According to the Society for Women's Health Research, it is now known that women who smoke are 20 to 70 percent more likely to develop lung cancer than men who smoke the same number of cigarettes. They are more likely than men to suffer a second heart attack within a year of their first. And they can metabolize medications differently from the way men do.

We have access to a mind-boggling amount of health information, says Florence Haseltine, M.D., founder of the Society for Women's Health Research, now director of the Center for Population Research at the National Institutes of Health in Washington, D.C. From morning news shows to the Internet, never has there been so much coverage of women's health. With more information, we're in a better position to make informed health-related decisions that can affect the length and quality of our lives.

Finally, we boomer women are discriminating—and vocal—health-care consumers. In the 1970s, we took on the medical establishment over reproductive health issues such as access to birth control and abortion. As we enter menopause, we're still challenging conventional medical wisdom. In fact, our generation of women has been credited for fueling interest in alternative medicine in this country. One study found that 4 of every 10 Americans used alternative therapies in 1997, including more than half of people between 30 and 50 years old.

Our New Health Strategy: Defense

When our moms were young, people who ate more vegetables than meat, exercised regularly, and took vitamins were considered, well, a bit strange. The all-American way to age was to accept that you would get sick—"old" people always did—and that a kindly, wise Marcus Welby type would make all of your medical decisions for you.

Not anymore. Our generation has a new focus: preventing age-related diseases before they strike us. "Women are saying, 'Okay, we're living longer. We want to know more about how to prevent illnesses that can keep us from enjoying these longer years of life,'" says Dr. Pinn.

It's long been known that a healthy diet and regular exercise help prevent many of the illnesses associated with aging, such as cancer, diabetes, and especially cardiovascular disease, which kills more women than all forms of cancer combined.

What's new, however, is the growing evidence that antioxidants and plant chemicals (phytochemicals) in fruits and vegetables may also stave off age-related diseases, including diabetes, macular degeneration, and breast cancer. Found in our bodies as well as in fruits and vegetables, antioxidants neutralize free radicals, which are "crippled" oxygen molecules that steal electrons from our healthy cells and cause aging and illness.

For example, soy foods, such as tofu and soy milk, are rich in phytoestrogens, natural substances in soybeans that show great promise in preventing breast cancer, osteoporosis, and menopausal hot flashes. And one Swedish study of women over 50 found that women who consumed daily the amount of beta-carotene found in half a carrot had up to 68 percent less risk for breast cancer than women who ate the least.

As for exercise, "it's the best anti-aging medicine in the world," says Andrea Z. LaCroix, Ph.D., professor of epidemiology at Group Health Cooperative of Puget Sound in Seattle. Lifelong exercise may add as much as 7 years to our life span. Studies suggest that regular exercise may boost our bodies' levels of antioxidants, preventing the free-radical damage that gums up our works.

Free at Last

One of the most important "breakthroughs" in women's health is our generation's radically different take on menopause. "The women's health movement has brought menopause out of the closet," says Dr. Pinn. "Women don't fear it anymore. They understand that it's a natural part of our maturing and that it marks the beginning of the rest of our lives."

One poll of 750 women between the ages of 45 and 60 found that 52 percent viewed menopause as a new and fulfilling stage of life, 60 percent did not feel that menopause made them less attractive, and 80 percent said that they were actually relieved that their periods had stopped.

In our mothers' day, women may have whispered about "the change" behind closed doors, but now we form menopause support groups and actively seek information on menopause and hormone-replacement therapy. We play a far more active role in our midlife health care than our mothers did. "There's a well-educated group of women who visit their doctors with a checklist of things they want information about, particularly HRT," says Ruth C. Fretts, M.D., assistant professor of obstetrics, gynecology, and reproductive biology at Harvard Medical School.

We're Hot—And We Don't Mean Hot Flashes

Not all of us went in for the free-love, if-it-feels-good-do-it attitude toward sex that began in the late 1960s. But many of us maintain a healthy interest in sex. In fact, in a large national study, women in their forties and fifties reported more orgasms than women in their early twenties.

In part, this increased sexual satisfaction has to do with more leisure time. "As we get older, there's less hurry-hurry and rush-rush. That attitude translates beautifully into the sexual arena," says Sue Patton Thoele, a licensed psy-

WOMEN ASK WHY

Why do women live longer than men?

There is a multitude of possible explanations. But the available evidence suggests that biological, behavioral, social, and psychological differences between men and women all play a part. The three biggies seem to be related to behavior, cardiovascular disease risk, and chromosomes.

More men tend to die of factors caused by reckless behavior or violence, whatever their age. In men ages 55 to 64, for example, behavior-related fatalities—car accidents, falls, drownings, homicides, suicides—are among the most common causes of death and are much higher than in women.

Cardiovascular disease hits men earlier than it does women. Smoking is a huge risk factor in heart disease, and men still smoke more than women. A man's risk of heart disease skyrockets beginning in his forties. A woman's risk doesn't rise until she enters menopause. Sex hormones may play a role here. It's known that the male sex hormone testosterone raises levels of artery-clogging low-density lipoprotein (LDL) cholesterol and decreases levels of beneficial high-density lipoprotein (HDL) cholesterol. Estrogen, the primary female sex hormone, lowers LDL and increases HDL.

The fact that women have two X chromosomes, while men have only one, may also explain our longevity edge. Recent research suggests that the X chromosome may directly determine life span. One of a woman's two X chromosomes is inactivated early in life. But the second appears to kick in as she grows older, and so it compensates for lost or damaged genes on the first X. So from a genetic standpoint, women may just start out healthier.

Continuing research into the causes for the longevity gap will undoubtedly find clues to how both men and women can live longer, healthier lives.

Expert consulted
Ruth C. Fretts, M.D.
Assistant professor of obstetrics, gynecology,
*   and reproductive biology*
Harvard Medical School

chotherapist in Boulder, Colorado, and author of *Freedoms after 50*. It doesn't hurt that the kids are out of the house and that we don't have to worry about unplanned pregnancy, she adds.

Because we know more about our bodies than our mothers did, we also have a better understanding of how to cope with the natural physical changes that can affect our sexuality. Vaginal dryness, for example, is easily remedied with lubricants. And while we take longer to become physically aroused—about 5 minutes, compared to premenopausal women's 10 to 15 seconds—even this has its benefits. Our partners take longer to become aroused, too. And didn't we always want a guy to take his time?

It's Our Turn Now

Few of us burned our bras in the 1970s, but to a large extent, that first wave of feminism gained us freedoms and opportunities that are helping to keep us young.

In attitude, that is.

Studies of older women find that, to many, midlife and beyond mean more choices, more opportunities, more freedom—perks in short supply during our younger days. Instead of hitting the recliner, we're returning to school or to work, advancing in our careers, finding new interests, and discovering or rediscovering our talents.

"My research strongly supports the view that women are happier and more fulfilled as they age. Many feel that it's the best time in their lives," says Mary Guindon, Ph.D., associate professor of counseling in the department of graduate education at Rider University in Lawrenceville, New Jersey.

Released from the obligations of home and family, midlife women have incredible opportunities to develop themselves in any way they choose, says Dr. Guindon. Many women choose to go back to school.

Education is one predictor of successful aging. A study conducted at the California Public Health Foundation in Berkeley found that people with 12 years or more of education were healthier in their later years than those who had less schooling.

Many of us discover or rediscover our creative talents, which encompass everything from cooking to gardening to the arts. Others bring their creativity to volunteerism, another activity that research suggests increases our happiness and improves our health.

"One of my friends tapped her creativity by devising a plan to get food and supplies to an Indian reservation about 10 hours from where we live," says Thoele. "Last year, this woman was saying, 'I know I'm here for a reason. I just don't know what it is.' Now she does—and she's on fire."

There comes a point where women come into their own, says Dr. Guindon. "One 52-year-old woman from my study said, 'I used to think that 50 or 60 was old. But I'm energized. We're alive. We're out there. We need to plan for a long future because we're going to be out there for a very long time.'"

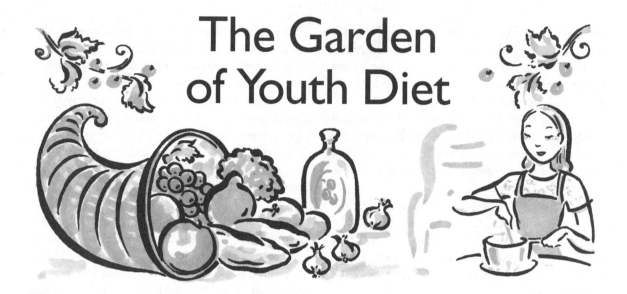

The Garden of Youth Diet

Pablo Picasso once said, "It takes a long time to become young." He could easily have added, "And a lot of food."

Yes, food.

There's no longer the slightest doubt that eating the right foods is one of the keys, if not *the* key, to preventing heart disease, cancer, and other age-related diseases. But now there's scientific evidence that a healthy diet can actually delay—or in some cases, even reverse—the aging process itself. Pretty cool, don't you think?

The right diet can encourage our bodies to produce "youth hormones" that control the ebb and flow of our bodies' anti-aging mechanisms, says Vincent C. Giampapa, M.D., president of the American Board of Anti-Aging Medicine and president of Longevity Institute International, a company based in Montclair, New Jersey, that provides personalized anti-aging programs through member physicians. The result: increased energy; stronger immunity; improvements in memory, vision, and hearing; more muscle; and denser bone.

Eating right can also help our cells repair and replace themselves more quickly, transport energy, and get rid of waste and toxins more efficiently. Just as important, diet can help protect our DNA, the genetic blueprint that tells our bodies' 50 to 60 trillion cells how to do their jobs.

Take a Bite Out of Aging

According to Dr. Giampapa, the goal of a "longevity diet" is to return our bodies to their youthful efficiency, which it can do in three ways.

Boost our youth hormones. The most important hormones for keeping us young are human growth hormone (hGH), which is released by the pituitary gland and converted in the liver to another anti-aging hormone called insulin growth factor (IGF-1), and dehydroepiandrosterone (DHEA), which is produced by the adrenal glands.

Starting in our twenties, our bodies slow down production of these hormones by about 10 percent every decade. By age 65, we are making only 15 to 20 percent of the hGH and 10 to 20 percent of the DHEA that we did when we were in our twenties.

With fewer youth hormones around, says Dr. Giampapa, chemical messages don't come and go as efficiently, which reduces the ability of our cells and organs to maintain and repair themselves. We experience loss of muscle and bone density, lowered immunity, and more illnesses, including diabetes and cancer.

Situation hopeless? Not quite.

"Increasing the body's production of these hormones can slow the aging process significantly," says Dr. Giampapa. "And it can be done primarily through diet."

Stem free-radical damage. Our cells use oxygen to produce energy. In the process, they generate free radicals—unstable oxygen molecules that damage cells and DNA. Free radicals are also produced by pollution, by the pesticides in our food supply, and by a diet high in chemical additives, refined starches and sugars, artery-clogging saturated fat found in meat, whole-milk dairy products, tropical oils, and foods like cookies and crackers that contain hydrogenated or partially hydrogenated oils.

Our bodies are good at fending off free radicals when we're young. But as we grow older, we start to lose some of that fight as the damage caused by years of exposure starts to take its toll. We begin to need help from antioxidant nutrients such as vitamins C and E, the minerals zinc and selenium, and the plant chemicals (phytochemicals) in many fruits and vegetables, which

LIFE EXTENDER
The Magic Mushroom

The Roman emperor Nero called mushrooms the food of the immortal gods. For thousands of years, healers in China and Japan have prized one particular variety, the maitake (pronounced "my-TAH-key"), believing it held the secret to longevity and immortality.

Is there truth in any of this?

According to modern science, there just may be. Research suggests that the succulent maitake may extend our lives by preventing or treating several age-related diseases.

Maitake D-fraction, an extract of the mushroom developed by Japanese researchers, seems to turn on certain cells in our immune systems (T cells), which then may help to fight cancer cells. Investigators have found evidence that maitake D-fraction may help prevent tumor growth, keep cancer from spreading from one part of the body to another, and prevent normal cells from mutating into cancer cells.

Maitake also contains compounds known as ES- and X-fractions, which, according to recent studies at Georgetown University, may help to lower levels of sugar and fats in the blood. In one Japanese laboratory study, maitake-enriched food significantly lowered levels of blood glucose and triglycerides after 8 weeks.

To get the most out of maitake, consume the D-fraction (available in capsules and tinctures), which is the most potent and active form, says Shari Lieberman, Ph.D., a nutrition scientist and exercise physiologist in New York City. Maitake is also sold in a tea. The various forms of maitake are available in gourmet markets and health food stores. Whole maitakes are considered to be the tastiest of the medicinal mushrooms.

Maitake D-fraction dissolves in hot water. If you steam or boil maitakes in their whole mushroom form, Dr. Lieberman suggests that you either consume the liquid in which they have been cooked or use it in soups, stews, or sauces. Also, don't stir-fry maitakes. The compounds responsible for lowering high blood sugar and high blood pressure levels will dissolve in the cooking oil.

join forces with our bodies' internal defense systems.

Replenish our "cellular soup." Each of our cells contains a substance called cytoplasm, which is made up of fluid, nutrients, and other materials that help make energy and fight free-radical damage, says Israel Kogan, M.D., director of the Anti-Aging Medical Center in Washington, D.C.

The typical American diet is loaded with chemical additives, pesticides and fertilizers, and other toxic substances, all of which encourage the formation of free radicals, says Dr. Kogan. When our diets are free of these toxins, we protect our cells from free-radical damage, give our cytoplasm the nutrients it needs, and help our cells to function at their peak.

A "clean" diet also helps return our bodies to the right level of acidity (pH), which is tremendously important in building up our cellular soup, says Dr. Giampapa. That's because our bodies make hormones, repair cells, and generally work most effectively at a neutral pH.

Check the Index

So how do we boost—or even hang on to—our youth hormones? One way is to skip the cherry-cheese Danish and enjoy the cherries straight. That's good advice for all the obvious reasons, but for a not-so-obvious one as well: Sugary pastries like that cherry-cheese Danish have what is known as a high glycemic index. The glycemic index measures how quickly a food raises our blood sugar levels after we eat it and how quickly our levels return to normal.

REAL-LIFE SCENARIO
A Vegetarian Who's Doing It All Wrong

Cheryl, a 42-year-old homemaker, had known for a long time that fast food, coffee, and playing supermom didn't exactly add up to a healthy lifestyle. But something she saw in the mirror one morning jolted her. Her skin and her eyes looked sallow and lifeless, which reflected exactly the way she felt: old. She made an instant decision to turn her life around. She knew where to start: cut out fatty foods and start an exercise program. Never one to do anything halfway, she became a vegetarian and began filling her plate with carbohydrates, such as macaroni and potatoes, to "boost her energy." She also started a vigorous weight-lifting program. But now, after weeks and weeks on her do-it-yourself rejuvenating program, she feels and looks more haggard than ever. And to make matters worse, she seems to have gained weight. What should she do?

While it may come as a surprise to Cheryl that she's feeling haggard and gaining weight, there may be two not-so-surprising culprits here: an unbalanced diet and, perhaps, a too-vigorous weight-training program.

First, Cheryl's diet. Vegetarian eating isn't automatically healthy eating. And, like many new vegetarians, Cheryl isn't consuming a balanced diet. While she may love macaroni, potatoes, and other starchy foods, they alone can't give her body the nutrients it needs to stay healthy, and they may even cause her to gain weight.

If Cheryl really wants to boost her energy—and improve her health—she needs to eat a wide variety of plant-based foods, including whole grains, legumes, and fresh fruits and vegetables. Legumes and whole grains should be the centerpiece of her diet. If Cheryl is a vegetarian who also eats dairy products (a lacto-vegetarian), she should choose low-fat milk and yogurt over their whole-fat counterparts.

Following these basic guidelines, Cheryl might breakfast on

Foods with a low glycemic index, like cherries, along with most fruits and vegetables and whole grains, encourage youthful levels of hGH and IGF-1, according to Dr. Giampapa.

a bowl of whole-grain cereal or oatmeal, topped with a sliced banana and a small amount of fat-free or soy milk. For lunch, she might opt for a vegetarian burger on a whole-grain bun with lettuce, tomato, and mustard or a bowl of hearty lentil soup with a slice of whole-grain bread. Dinner might be stir-fried vegetables over whole-grain brown rice or pasta.

Between meals, she might snack on fresh fruit, a piece of whole-grain bread spread with almond butter, or a cup of plain, low-fat yogurt with fresh fruit.

Consuming a wide variety of plant foods will also ensure that Cheryl gets adequate amounts of protein. Dried beans, such as chickpeas and black beans, are an excellent source of plant protein, as are grains, nuts, and seeds. If she's not crazy about seeds and grains, she can also get protein from more everyday foods, such as potatoes and broccoli.

Finally, Cheryl should consider taking a high-potency multivitamin/mineral supplement. It will be her "insurance" against missing out on essential vitamins and minerals.

Cheryl's weight gain is most likely caused by a combination of her vigorous weight-training program and her high-carbohydrate diet. Actually, a small weight gain from weight training is normal: Muscle weighs more than fat; so if she's putting on muscle, the needle on the scale will naturally go up. But again, her diet may be causing her to gain fat along with the muscle.

To lose the fat while keeping the muscle, Cheryl should watch her intake of sweets and other high-fat foods, even if they come from plant sources. She should also consider adding aerobic exercise to her program, which will burn calories and help her shed excess weight.

Expert consulted
Michael Janson, M.D.
President
American College for Advancement in Medicine
Barnstable, Massachusetts

They travel slowly through our digestive systems, so sugar enters our bloodstreams a little at a time, says Shari Lieberman, Ph.D., a nutrition scientist and exercise physiologist in New York City. This slow, steady rise in blood sugar promotes a stable release of insulin, the hormone that moves energy (glucose) from our blood to our cells.

When our insulin levels stay steady, our bodies produce less cortisol, often called the stress hormone, says Dr. Giampapa. That's good. Low cortisol levels encourage our bodies to produce DHEA as well as the hormones made from it.

By contrast, we digest high-glycemic foods, such as cornflakes, rice cakes, white potatoes, and white rice, more quickly. As a result, our blood sugar rises rapidly, triggering a flood of cortisol. High insulin and cortisol levels reduce our output of DHEA and the hormones made from it.

We can discourage these youth-stealing spikes in insulin and cortisol by eating mostly foods with a low to medium glycemic index, says Dr. Giampapa.

Aim Low

As you may have guessed by now, low-glycemic foods tend to be high in fiber and complex carbohydrates, while high-glycemic foods contain virtually none. Here's how to make your diet more "complex."

Eat heavyweight bread. Buy whole-grain bread that contains at least 3 grams of dietary fiber per slice, says Dr. Lieberman. It will have a much lower glycemic index than white bread or even low-calorie whole-wheat bread.

Rule of thumb: The heavier the loaf, the better. "The bread I eat? You can eat it or use it as a paperweight," says Dr. Lieberman. (While

LIFE EXTENDER
Eat Less, Live Longer

There's growing evidence that we may be able to extend our lives simply by eating less.

Studies of mice and rats have demonstrated that both live 30 percent longer when they consume 30 percent fewer calories. More recent laboratory studies conducted at Johns Hopkins University show that consuming a low-calorie, low-fat diet helps maintain higher levels of dehydroepiandrosterone (DHEA), a "youth hormone" produced by our bodies.

Experts aren't sure why eating less seems to slow aging. But a growing body of evidence suggests that reducing calories also reduces the body's production of age-accelerating free radicals.

dense bread contains more calories, it also fills you up, leaving you more satisfied.)

Pass on the lightweight cereal. Puffed wheat, puffed rice, and cornflakes may be light on calories, but as low-fiber, high-glycemic foods, they send blood sugar through the roof, says Dr. Lieberman. Choose an unsweetened cereal that contains at least 3 grams of fiber per serving, such as Nabisco Shredded Wheat.

Pick beans. Dried beans score low on the glycemic index and are an excellent source of protein, says Dr. Lieberman. While virtually all dried beans are also a good source of fiber, black-eyed peas, chickpeas, kidney beans, lima beans, and black beans are fiber champs, containing 6 to 8 grams of fiber in a ½-cup serving.

Yam it up. Sweet potatoes have a lower glycemic index than white potatoes, so enjoy them often, says Dr. Lieberman. They're great mashed, for example. Or, for mouthwatering "fries," slice sweet potatoes into thin strips, coat them with a tablespoon of olive oil and a sprinkling of paprika, and bake them at 400°F for 40 minutes.

Make mixed-up meals. Consume high-glycemic foods, such as white rice, with a high-protein food, such as chicken. The mix of carbohydrates and protein will keep your blood sugar from rising too quickly, which will slow your body's release of insulin.

The Fat Factor

Is there any woman who doesn't slow down when she wheels her shopping cart past a display of sticky buns?

If you need a good reason to keep walking, here it is: Eating less pastry and other foods high in saturated fat can help us maintain or increase our levels of youth hormones, according to Dr. Giampapa.

On the other hand, a steady diet of saturated fat switches off production of hGH, IGF-1, and DHEA. "We don't know why saturated fat has this effect, but it does," says Dr. Kogan.

We can encourage our bodies' production of youth hormones by getting no more than 10 percent of our daily calories from saturated fat, says Dr. Giampapa. In other words, if you consume 1,800 calories a day, no more than 180 of them (about 16 to 20 grams) should come from saturated fat.

As you trim the saturated fats from your diet, replace them with foods high in monounsaturated fats, such as nuts, avocados, and canola, olive, and peanut oils, says Dr. Giampapa.

Monounsaturated fats tend to reduce low-density lipoprotein (LDL) cholesterol and raise high-density lipoprotein (HDL) cholesterol. That's not only good for our hearts, it's good for our youth hormone levels, too. The higher our HDL levels, the better equipped our bodies are to make DHEA, estrogen, and testosterone, says Dr. Giampapa. (That's because these particular hormones are actually made from cholesterol.)

Olive oil is perhaps the best-known monounsaturated fat. And it can do more than lower LDL cholesterol. It contains several compounds, such as polyphenols, that are powerful antioxidants. These substances keep the LDL cholesterol in our bloodstream from being damaged by free radicals, making it less likely to stick to artery walls.

The Zorba Diet

Fish, nuts, olive oil . . . Zorba the Greek would have no problem getting 30 percent of his daily calories from monounsaturated fats, as Dr. Giampapa suggests. The tips below can help you eat like Zorba.

Go a little nutty. The people in Mediterranean countries eat a lot of nuts, a primo source of monounsaturated fats. Follow their example and toss a small handful of raw almonds, walnuts, or sunflower or pumpkin seeds on salads, rice dishes, or veggies, suggests Dr. Lieberman. In a 10-year study of 86,016 women ages 34 to 59 conducted by researchers at the Harvard School of Public Health, women who ate 5 ounces of nuts a week were 35 percent less likely to have heart disease, most likely because of the nuts' beneficial effects on cholesterol.

Get hooked on fish. Eat fish such as salmon, tuna, cod, haddock, herring, perch, or

WOMEN ASK WHY

If bean curd is so good for you, why does it sound so bad?

There's no denying it. Bean curd, more commonly called tofu, has a bad rep in this country. Perhaps the phrase *bean curd* conjures up a vision of curdled milk. But despite the negative impressions that this soy-derived food inspires, its health benefits are quite positive.

Research shows, for example, that soy is rich in antioxidants, specifically genistein and daidzein. Antioxidants help reduce the negative effects of free radicals—unstable oxygen molecules that damage cells and contribute to many age-related health problems in this country, such as heart disease and cancer. It's noteworthy that people in Japan and China, who tend to consume diets high in soy, are less likely to develop these serious diseases. And American women may be interested to know that Asian women going through menopause seem to experience fewer hot flashes.

Tofu is an excellent source of high-quality protein, and it is a good source of other beneficial nutrients, such as iron, calcium, and potassium. But unlike the protein in meat and dairy products, it contains no cholesterol and only a small amount of saturated fat.

People may believe that tofu has an unpleasant taste, but actually, tofu has virtually no taste at all. This blandness actually works in its favor, because it takes on the flavor of anything it's cooked with. For example, you can hide soft tofu in soups, sauces, and desserts. And firm tofu can be grilled, added to soups and stews, or fried in olive or canola oil.

Expert consulted
John H. Weisburger, M.D., Ph.D.
Senior member
American Health Foundation
Valhalla, New York

snapper once or twice a week, suggests Dr. Lieberman. These fish, caught in the deepest and coldest waters of the North Atlantic, are rich in omega-3 fatty acids, substances that

THE BULB OF LONG LIFE

Suddenly realizing that your breath smells of garlic ranks near the top of our Most Mortifying Moments index. But from a scientific standpoint, reeking of garlic is a *good* thing.

Why? Research suggests that the powerful chemicals that make our breath reek may also help us live longer.

"Garlic has so many anti-aging properties," says Alexander G. Schauss, Ph.D., director of natural and medical products research at the American Institute for Biosocial Research in Tacoma, Washington. "That's because it prevents or treats many illnesses that shorten life span, such as cardiovascular disease and cancer."

Garlic has been found to thin the blood and lower cholesterol, which can help prevent the blood vessel problems that can lead to high blood pressure, heart disease, and stroke, says Dr. Schauss.

While recent research has cast doubt on garlic's cholesterol-fighting abilities, critics say that the garlic powder and garlic oil used in those studies may not have contained the bulb's cholesterol-lowering compounds.

Garlic also seems to help prevent cancer. Population studies have found that people in garlic-loving countries such as Italy and China tend to develop less gastrointestinal cancers—those that affect the mouth, esophagus, stomach, colon, and rectum, says Dr. Schauss.

Consuming just two to four cloves a day can help prevent and treat disease, according to research conducted by Dr. Schauss.

Garlic is so versatile that you can throw a few cloves into virtually any dish, from spaghetti sauce, soups, and stews to stir-fried vegetables. Or roast it, which gives garlic a sweet, caramelized flavor. Simply cut the top from the garlic bulb to expose the tips of the cloves, rub with a little olive oil, wrap in foil, and bake for 45 minutes at 350°F.

Important: After you chop or crush garlic, let it stand for 15 to 20 minutes, says Dr. Schauss. According to recent studies, immediately cooking garlic after it has been chopped or crushed can reduce or eliminate its healing properties. Letting garlic sit allows enough time for oxygen to react with the chemicals in garlic to form the therapeutic substance allicin.

have been shown to raise HDL cholesterol. (Omega-3's also help make eicosanoids, hormonelike substances that encourage our bodies to make hGH, says Dr. Giampapa.)

Feast on a fatty fruit. Toss a few chunks of avocado into your salads, or add a few slices to a sandwich in place of cheese. Avocados are rich in oleic acid, the same monounsaturated fat found in olive oil. Since avocados are high in calories and contain about 30 grams of fat apiece, enjoy them in moderation, says Dr. Lieberman.

Protect olive oil. Buy small bottles of olive oil with long, narrow necks. And after you use the oil, cap the bottle tightly and refrigerate it. "These steps limit the oil's exposure to oxygen, which will keep it from turning rancid and discourage the formation of free radicals," says Robert Goldman, D.O., Ph.D., cofounder of the American Academy of Anti-Aging Medicine and coauthor of *Stopping the Clock*.

Refrigerated olive oil will solidify. When you're ready to use it, run the bottle under warm water for a few minutes, then pour off the reliquefied oil that forms at the top.

What about Meat?

Just like Mom always said, meat is an excellent source of protein. And what was good for you when you were growing up is still good for you now that you're growing older.

Our bodies use the protein in

meat and other high-protein foods to make amino acids. These substances help our bodies make their own proteins, which are used to regulate hormones, grow new tissue, and repair or replace worn-out tissue.

Unfortunately, meat tends to be high in saturated fat. So you may be wondering: If I cut back on meat, will I lose out on protein? No, says Dr. Giampapa. We can get the protein we need from food without consuming meat at all.

A wide array of plant foods, including beans and grains, are excellent sources of protein, says Dr. Lieberman. Some, such as soy and the grain quinoa (pronounced "KEEN-wah"), are considered "complete" proteins because they contain all of the nine essential amino acids we need to stay healthy. But our bodies will make their own complete proteins if we eat enough calories and a variety of plant foods, such as nuts and seeds, grains, and fruits and vegetables.

Get the Protein, Forgo the Fat

The bottom line? It's absolutely okay to eat meat as long as you don't eat Fred Flintstone–size portions every day and you get the majority of your protein from plant sources, says Dr. Lieberman. Here's how to get the protein you need without the saturated fat.

Toss back a soy cocktail. Soy foods such as soy milk and tofu are an excellent source of protein. But if you don't enjoy these foods, drink one of the great-tasting soy shakes available in health food stores, suggests Dr. Lieberman. "They're a great way to consume high-quality protein every day or a few times a week."

Before you select a soy shake, read its label, advises Gregory Burke, M.D., professor and interim chairperson in the department of public health sciences at Wake Forest University School of Medicine in Winston-Salem, North Carolina. While some brands are low in fat and contain natural sweeteners, others are loaded with sugar and fat.

Get keen on quinoa. The beadlike, ivory-colored seeds of this plant are usually eaten like rice. But you can also cook it in fruit juice and eat it for breakfast, use it as a substitute for rice in pudding, or make a cold salad of quinoa, beans, and chopped vegetables. Its soft texture and somewhat bland flavor make it easy to add to other foods, such as soups and pasta dishes. You'll find quinoa in health food stores.

Use the palm computer. To avoid eating too much meat at any one meal, use this simple guideline of Dr. Giampapa's: Don't eat more meat than you can fit in the palm of your hand. And aim to eat four handfuls of vegetables to every one handful of fish or lean meat.

Wok meat into your diet. Adding a small amount of steak or pork to a vegetable stir-fry lets you savor the flavor of meat for a fraction of its saturated fat and calories, says Dr. Lieberman.

The Toxic Avengers

Free radicals hit our bodies 10,000 times a day. Adding injury to injury, these little molecules actually burn holes through the membranes that surround cells, the better to penetrate and vanquish them.

Faced with this onslaught of malicious marauders, hell-bent on crippling our cells and mutating our cellular DNA, our bodies could use a little help. That's where antioxidants come in. These common vitamins such as C and E and minerals such as zinc and selenium neutralize free radicals.

So do phytochemicals, substances in common fruits, vegetables, and other plant foods. Phytochemicals also seem to fight a plethora of age-related diseases, from arthritis to cancer.

To give just a few examples, ellagic acid, a compound found in berries (with strawberries and blackberries containing the most), may help prevent cellular changes that can lead to cancer. Lutein, found in dark green vegetables like spinach and kale, has been found to cut the risk of macular degeneration nearly in half. Indole-3 carbinol, found in broccoli, cabbage, and other cruciferous vegetables, may help prevent breast and cervical cancer.

In short, every juicy berry, steamed broccoli floret, or spinach salad we consume helps sheath our bodies in nutritional armor to stem free-radical damage and help prevent age-related disease.

Great Ways to Ambush Radicals

The way we choose, store, and cook antioxidant-rich fruits and vegetables can boost their protective effect. Here's how to get the most from their anti-aging powers.

Choose the antioxidant all-stars. Wondering which vegetables will give you the most antioxidant bang for your buck? Wonder no more. Researchers at the Jean Mayer USDA Human Nutrition Research Center on Aging at Tufts University in Boston analyzed 22 common vegetables, then calculated the ability of each to neutralize free radicals. The winners included kale, beets, red bell peppers, brussels sprouts, broccoli florets, potatoes, sweet potatoes, and corn.

Follow Popeye's lead. Consider eating more spinach and strawberries, too. Their high levels of antioxidants may prevent or even re-

WOMAN TO WOMAN
Going Vegetarian Sparked Her Youth

For 13 years, Mary Jane Soares tried every conceivable type of diet to control the health conditions that were sapping her youthful energy. Now, at 48, this registered nurse in Emeryville, California, has found a way of eating that has improved her health and helped her regain her zest for life.

In 1982, I began getting sick when I ate certain foods, especially if they contained sugar or wheat. And I was exhausted all the time. It was a chore just to get up in the morning. I was 31 and feeling ancient.

I went to a doctor, who diagnosed me with a triple whammy—food allergies, yeast infection, and chronic fatigue syndrome. I was put on various elimination diets—no wheat or sugar, just fruits and vegetables, meat, and a few grains—to discover which foods I couldn't eat.

I ate this way and felt good until 1984, when I moved from Little Rock, Arkansas, to California. I thought I could continue the diet on my own. But I splurged too much on sugar and started getting sick again. Truthfully, I never really got well.

For the next 10 years, I tried a variety of treatments to control my health problems, from homeopathy to supplementation programs. Nothing helped much.

In 1997, I found a new doctor, who did some tests and found undigested protein in my blood, which meant that I was not digesting my food properly. He prescribed medication and supplements. In search of a more natural remedy, I then went to a nutritionist. She started me on an intensive detoxification program and encouraged me to become a vegetarian.

So I did.

verse the effects of free-radical damage to the brain, helping to keep it sharp as we age, according to another study conducted at the USDA Human Nutrition Research Center on Aging at Tufts University.

Since then, I've never felt better. I have fruit in the morning and a midmorning snack of organic raw almond butter on some flaxseed crackers. Lunch is usually vegetables—my favorites are broccoli, pea pods, and asparagus, when it's in season. Or I'll have potato-and-leek soup. Dinner is more vegetables and, occasionally, salmon.

As good as I feel, it's hard to not be able to eat everything I want, especially to a sugarholic like me. What saved me is my love for cooking. I wasn't going to eat steamed vegetables, baked potatoes, and salad all my life without at least trying to make them interesting and tasty. I learned to make things such as vegetarian sushi rolls, creamed curried squash soup made with almond milk, and sherbets made from fresh frozen fruit. To calm my sweet tooth, I mash up butternut squash and sprinkle it with cinnamon and an herbal sweetener called stevia.

Since I eat virtually no meat, I get the majority of my protein through nuts and seeds. I love almonds—sometimes I eat them like M&Ms, a handful at a time. Or I grind them and make a pâté that I put in my vegetarian sushi rolls. I get my calcium primarily through green vegetables and in my multivitamin/mineral supplement. I just had a bone-density scan this last year, and my bones are strong and healthy.

I feel strong and healthy, too. My candida is under control—so much so that once a month or so, I can splurge and have a piece of chocolate cake without feeling ill.

And I've got energy to burn. When I started this way of eating, I was able to jump on my mini-trampoline for 2 minutes. Now I can do it for 20 to 30 minutes at a clip. I've even started snowboarding. I just feel more alive and vibrant. And, yes, younger.

This way of eating allows me to live life the way it should be lived—to the fullest.

Researchers fed 344 test animals extracts of strawberry or spinach, vitamin E, or a control diet. After 8 months, they tested the rats' long- and short-term memories. The rats that consumed the daily equivalent of a large spinach salad performed better when made to run a maze than those fed a normal diet, strawberry extract, or vitamin E. However, the spinach and strawberry extracts and the vitamin E diet all slowed signs of aging in the rats in other tests. The spinach extract, in particular, is speculated to have protected different types of nerve cells in various parts of the brain against the effects of aging.

Choose high-octane olive oil. Cold-pressed, extra-virgin olive oil contains more antioxidants and phytochemicals than yellow olive oil, says Dr. Lieberman. That's because it is extracted by literally crushing the olives, rather than by using heat and chemicals.

Don't be put off by this oil's greenish hue. "Yellow olive oil is yellow because it's been processed and heated, which removes all the good stuff," says Dr. Lieberman. While you'll pay more for extra-virgin oil, it's healthier (and, according to many folks, tastier) than less expensive varieties.

Seek the color purple. If you see broccoli that's so dark it's almost purple, put it in your shopping cart. That purply color means it's packing a mother lode of beta-carotene. If it's yellow, don't buy it—it's lost its vital nutrients.

Quick-cook veggies. Steam rather than boil your vegetables, advises Dr. Lieberman. "Steaming locks in their antioxidants and phytonutrients," she says. When you boil them, you leave their protective substances in the water.

Simplify salad prep. No time to peel, slice, and dice salad fixings? Do it once a week, suggests Dr. Giampapa. Every Sunday, prepare a huge bowl of dark green lettuce, along with carrots, peppers, and other fixings. Store them separately in airtight plastic bags or containers to limit their exposure to oxygen.

Is That a Toxin in My "Soup"?

As we mentioned earlier, our cells are filled with a broth of nutrients and other substances called cytoplasm. It's where the action is—where cellular machinery makes energy, synthesizes proteins, and disarms free radicals.

It's hard for cells to get the fuel they need to perform these important jobs from the typical American diet, say anti-aging experts. Foods high in fat and sugar and processed foods containing additives and preservatives sic free radicals on our hapless bodies. These chemicals build up in our bodies, gradually weakening our cellular machinery.

What's more, sugary, fatty foods laced with preservatives and additives tend to turn to acid in our blood, upsetting our bodies' delicate pH balance, says Dr. Giampapa. A steady diet of them acidifies our cellular soup, causing cells and tissues to age before their time.

Just as cars run smoother and cleaner on high-octane fuel, we run best on foods that don't contain additives and preservatives and that keep our bodies close to a neutral pH, says Dr. Giampapa. These foods are—you guessed it—fruits, vegetables, legumes, and whole grains.

Put Your Diet into Rehab

The cleaner and more natural our diets, the more nutrients our cells get—and the more efficiently they are likely to work, says Dr. Giampapa. The strategies below can help put your diet into detox.

Eat naked produce. Make an effort to buy organic fruits and vegetables (those grown without these chemicals) whenever you can, says Dr. Goldman. It's easier to find organic produce than it used to be, he says. "Many supermarkets now carry organic fruits and vegetables alongside the commercially grown variety, and some food chains (such as Fresh Fields, Bread and Circus, and Whole Food Markets) carry only organic food." Make sure that you wash organic produce to remove as much bacteria and dirt as possible.

Buy boxed organics. If you can't find organic fruits and vegetables, consider buying other organic products, says Dr. Lieberman. "I buy organic cereal, organic milk, and organic juice and eggs," she says. "If you can get even 20 percent of your diet organic, that's 20 percent less of a toxic burden on your immune system."

Waylay white-sugar cravings. When a craving for a slice of coffee ring or another sugary, fatty food strikes, "eat a cold sweet potato," says Dr. Lieberman. "Its natural sweetness may be enough to satisfy your craving for white sugar." If this trick works for you, bake up a mess of them and have them on hand for those times when you get the "craves."

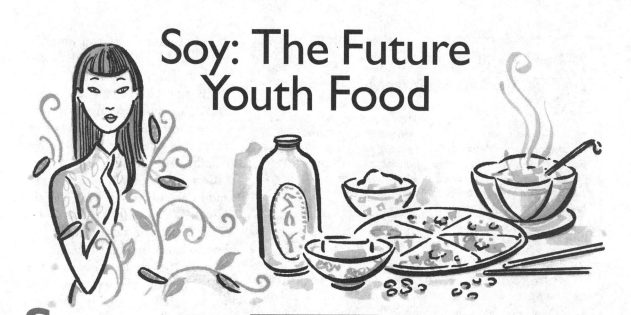

Soy: The Future Youth Food

"Soy is a superfood," says Shari Lieberman, Ph.D., a nutrition scientist and exercise physiologist in New York City. "You might even call it a youth food because it has such potential to stave off age-related conditions from menopausal symptoms to osteoporosis to breast cancer."

Skeptical? Think about the robust health and super-longevity of people in Asian countries, where soy is a dietary staple. Compared to Americans, Asians who eat a traditional soy-rich diet have fewer heart attacks; are less likely to develop breast, colon, and prostate cancers; and suffer fewer hip fractures. Asian women going through menopause don't have as many hot flashes. And the Japanese, as a population, have the longest life expectancies in the world.

Adding soy to your diet is easy. The new generation of soy foods actually tastes good, with none of the beany flavor or unpleasant aftertaste that characterized soy products of the past. Your family will never suspect that you're serving them soy in those delicious new burgers, hot dogs, or sausage or that you're sneaking tofu or soy milk into their favorite dishes. And afterward, you'll feel great for having treated yourself—and your family—to a delectable serving of good health.

Little Bean, Big Benefits

Soy is an excellent source of low-calorie, high-quality protein, a nutrient we need more of as we grow older. Protein builds and repairs tissue and makes infection-fighting antibodies. But unlike the protein in animal foods, such as meat, eggs, and milk, soy protein contains zero heart-damaging saturated fat and cholesterol. Soy is packed with other nutrients that older bodies need, such as iron, calcium, and B vitamins like thiamin, riboflavin, and niacin.

But that's not all. Nestled in the heart of soybeans are substances called isoflavones, which are part of a group of plant substances known as phytochemicals. The isoflavones in soy, called phytoestrogens, may be the key to soy's disease-fighting powers, says Gregory Burke, M.D., professor and interim chairperson in the department of public health sciences at Wake Forest University School of Medicine in Winston-Salem, North Carolina.

WOMAN TO WOMAN

Thanks to Soy, Menopause Is a Breeze

Linda Townsend, 46, was getting hot under the collar about her menopausal symptoms—literally. As a controller for a construction company in Titusville, Florida, she'd often find herself in an important meeting when she'd suddenly experience a debilitating hot flash. Her hot flashes were so noticeable and frequent that people would stop and stare. Her night sweats were so bad that she'd get up two and three times a night to change clothes. Then she found an answer. Here is her story.

I would be sitting there, and out of nowhere I would be flushed.

The hot feeling would start in my chest and work its way up to my neck, then my face. My face would turn red, and I'd sweat like crazy. Not only did the flashes come fast and furious, but they happened all the time. It got to the point where I'd bring an extra shirt to work every day because I'd sweat so bad that the shirt I'd have on would get soaked. The flashes became so noticeable that my boss would sometimes walk in and say, "You're having another one."

For 4 months, I didn't get a good night's sleep. At least twice a night, I'd have to get up and change my nightgown, then try to find a dry spot on the bed.

I didn't get any relief from what my doctor gave me. But I had been reading Dr. Andrew Weil's Web site, and he had recommended soy for hot flashes. I thought about using soy, but for the longest time I couldn't bring myself to do it. To me, even the word *soy* didn't sound good. After reading hundreds of testimonials, though, I finally gave in. I started with a glass of soy milk every day and ate a soy burger every other day or so.

Within 2 weeks, the hot flashes stopped. I couldn't believe it. I thought maybe it wasn't the soy. Maybe they'd stopped on their own. But when I went on a 2-week vacation in Europe where there was no soy available, my flashes came back. The first thing I did when I got home was pour myself a glass of soy milk.

I feel empowered now. I used to think hot flashes were just something I was stuck with, but I was wrong. I've learned how to take control of them.

The average Asian consumes 50 milligrams of isoflavones a day—the amount in 2 to 3 ounces of soy, says Dr. Burke. Consuming these minuscule amounts may afford you the protection that many Asians enjoy from many of the illnesses of aging, including the ones below.

Cancer. In animal and test-tube studies, the phytoestrogen genistein slows the growth of cancer cells. How? Researchers don't know. But they do know that genistein and another phytoestrogen, daidzein, act as weaker versions of the estrogen that women produce naturally.

It is well-known that estrogen can fuel so-called hormone-dependent cancers of the breast and uterus. Dr. Burke says it may be that soy phytoestrogens compete with natural estrogen for molecules on the surfaces of cells that recognize and bind to estrogen. If soy phytoestrogens fill these receptors, the more potent natural estrogen can't, thereby helping to prevent cancer.

High cholesterol. Soy may lower both "bad" low-density lipoprotein (LDL) and total cholesterol levels without reducing "good" high-density lipoprotein (HDL) cholesterol. In one large study conducted at the University of Kentucky, the LDL cholesterol of people who consumed about 2 ounces of soy protein a day plunged 12.9 percent, and their total cholesterol dropped 9.3 percent. Their levels of "good" HDL cholesterol stayed steady.

No one knows exactly how soy might lower cholesterol. But one theory is that soy phytoestrogens help transport LDL cholesterol from the bloodstream to the liver, where it's broken down and excreted. Phytoestrogens may also keep LDL from turning rancid (a process known as oxidation), making it less likely to clog the walls of your arteries.

Osteoporosis. Soy phytoestrogens appear not only to repair bone but actually to build it. In one study, women who consumed 40 grams of soy protein (containing high concentrations of isoflavones) a day for 6 months significantly increased the thickness of the bone in their lower spines. And there's another reason to bone up on soy: Animal protein seems to speed up the body's excretion of calcium. Apparently, soy protein doesn't, says Dr. Burke.

Menopausal symptoms. Sometimes isoflavones block a woman's natural supply of estrogen, and sometimes, they actually supplement it. This is a boon for women in menopause, when declining levels of estrogen and progesterone can trigger hot flashes and night sweats. In one study, women who consumed 60 grams of soy protein a day for 12 weeks cut their rate of hot flashes by nearly half.

Supermarket Soy

By now, the soy revolution has probably reached your supermarket. With tofu in the produce section, soy milk in the dairy case, and soy-based frozen yogurts next to the Häagen-Dazs, it has never been easier to add soy to your diet. But if you haven't yet joined the revolution, read on to get acquainted with these commonly available soy foods.

Tofu. The mother of all soy foods comes in three varieties, one as versatile as the next. Firm tofu is solid, so it's often stir-fried, grilled, or added to soups and stews. Soft tofu, which has a creamy consistency, and silken tofu, which has a custardlike texture, can be mashed or pureed and added to blender drinks, dips, dressings, and puddings. Don't be put off by its taste. Standing alone, tofu is bland, but it takes on the flavors of other foods that it's mixed with.

Tempeh. Pronounced "TEM-pay," this traditional Indonesian food is made of cooked, fermented whole soybeans. The result is a chunky, tender cake with a smoky or nutty flavor. Tempeh is a tasty, low-fat alternative to meat—in fact, many women marinate it and grill it, just like a steak. Tempeh can also be added to soups, casseroles, or chili.

SEARCH OUT SOY "EXOTICS"

When it comes to soy, tofu isn't the only game in town. Explore your local natural foods store or Asian market for the more exotic fare below.

Edamamé. These are large soybeans, harvested when they're still green and sweet. Boil them for 15 to 20 minutes, and you have a high-fiber, high-protein, cholesterol-free, soy-rich snack or main vegetable dish.

Okara. Okara is the pulpy fiber by-product of soy milk. It tastes similar to coconut, so try adding it to baked goods, such as cookies or muffins, or sprinkling it over your breakfast cereal.

Soybeans (whole). As soybeans mature in the pod, they ripen into a hard, dry bean—yellow, black, or brown. Whole soybeans are an excellent source of protein and dietary fiber; add the cooked beans to sauces, stews, and soups.

Soy nuts. This nutty-tasting snack food is actually whole soybeans that have been soaked in water, then roasted. High in protein and a concentrated source of isoflavones, soy nuts are similar in texture and flavor to peanuts. Soy nuts can be found in a variety of flavors, including chocolate-covered.

Soy nut butter. If you're a peanut butter junkie, give this nutty-tasting spread a try. Made from whole, roasted soy nuts, soy nut butter contains significantly less fat than peanut butter.

Soy milk. This creamy liquid comes from soybeans that are soaked, finely ground, and strained. It's a good source of protein and B vitamins, and many brands are fortified with calcium. Lots of folks pour it over their breakfast cereal or use it in cooking. And since soy milk comes in a variety of flavors, including vanilla and chocolate, some folks drink it straight. Because it isn't dairy milk, look for "soy beverage" or "soy drink" on the labels when you are purchasing soy milk.

Sneaking Soy into Your Diet

Many women have come to enjoy soy foods. Others . . . well, it might take a little longer. If you fall into the latter category, take the stealth approach to soy, in which you sneak the stuff into already familiar dishes. These ideas will get you started.

Cook up some pudding. You could get 30 to 50 milligrams of isoflavones by consuming 1 cup of soy milk or ½ cup of tofu or tempeh. Or you could savor some creamy pudding. Pudding mixes are made to be blended with firm tofu. One brand, Mori-Nu, contains 30 milligrams of isoflavones per ½ cup. Or simply add 2 cups of soy milk to your favorite fat-free pudding mix.

Savor a smoothie. For another quick dessert, blend ½ cup silken tofu with ½ cup each fresh berries, nonfat yogurt, and skim milk. Add a dash of vanilla or honey if you like.

Dig into pizza. "Soy can transform pizza from everyone's favorite 'fun' food into serious nutrition," writes Patricia Greenberg in her book *The Whole Soy Cookbook*. Start with a homemade crust that contains soy flour, add tomato sauce and shredded soy mozzarella cheese, then top it with crumbled soy sausage or soy pepperoni. Delicious.

Kick back with a latte. Microwave 1 cup of vanilla soy milk for 60 seconds, then add 1 teaspoon of instant coffee. No need for sugar— vanilla soy milk is sweet. This elegant beverage packs 30 milligrams of isoflavones.

Go nuts. If you're hooked on roasted peanuts, try soy nuts. They are a concentrated source of isoflavones and a tasty, high-protein alternative to other roasted nuts, says Patricia Murphy, Ph.D., professor in the food science and human nutrition department at Iowa State University in Ames. "They taste somewhat like peanuts and make a great snack."

Slip soy into sweets. Bake with soy flour, suggests Dr. Murphy. Just ½ cup contains 30 to 50 milligrams of isoflavones. When baking quick breads and muffins, replace one-quarter to one-third of the total flour with soy flour. In yeast-raised recipes, use only 15 percent soy flour, or just a little more than ⅛ cup. (Soy flour is gluten-free, so expect yeast-raised breads to be denser in texture.)

You can find soy flour in natural food stores. Keep it in the fridge or freezer; soy flour goes bad more quickly than processed white flour.

Play hide-the-tofu. If you're exploring the countless delicious ways to prepare tofu, take a bow. But if you just want to hide the stuff, add cubed tofu to soups, stews, chili, and spaghetti sauce.

Take a powder. Add 2 to 3 tablespoons of powdered isolated soy protein (ISP) to milk, juice, or health shakes, suggests Dr. Burke. Available at health food stores, ISP is a simple way to get soy protein *and* isoflavones. Pass up ready-made soy shakes, however. "They tend to contain a lot of sugar and fat and may not be as healthy as you think," he says.

Get out the ketchup. Try the new breed of soy hot dogs, burgers, and sausage (as well as the many soy cheeses and yogurts), suggests Dr. Burke. While these products contain few or no isoflavones, they are still lower in total and saturated fat and cholesterol than their full-fat counterparts. "And that's still to your benefit," he says.

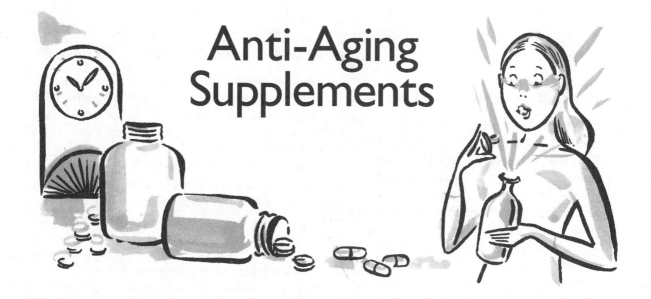

Anti-Aging Supplements

Phosphatidylserine. It doesn't exactly spell P-R-O-M-I-S-I-N-G, does it?

It looks more like one of those unpronounceable ingredients listed on the label of a hair shampoo. But actually, it's brimming with promise. This natural supplement is on the cutting edge of anti-aging medicine. It has been shown to renew brain cells and sharpen mental performance.

Where can you find this exotic stuff? (It's pronounced "foss-fuh-TID-ill-SEER-een," by the way.)

It's sitting on a shelf at your local health food store or just a click away on the Internet, along with other exciting, cutting-edge anti-aging substances that you may not know much about yet. Among them are alpha-lipoic acid, coenzyme Q_{10}, and melatonin, to name just a few.

"I'm sure these supplements seem somewhat mysterious," says Ronald Klatz, M.D., D.O., author of *Brain Fitness* and president of the American Academy of Anti-Aging Medicine, a Chicago-based society of physicians and scientists who believe aging is not inevitable. "After all, we've known about the role of vi-

tamin C in good health for the past 30 years, and vitamin E for longer than that. These are quite new."

What makes these substances so special?

For one thing, many of them are potent antioxidants, says Dr. Klatz. Only antioxidants can neutralize free radicals, the unstable oxygen molecules that punch holes in cell membranes, destroy vital enzymes, damage cellular DNA—and, ultimately, lead to the diseases of aging.

For another, their antioxidant power is, in some cases, many times more powerful than that of better-known antioxidants such as vitamins C and E. Some actually recycle vitamins C and E, giving them new life in the endless war against free radicals. Still others dissolve in both fat and water, enabling them to neutralize free radicals wherever they occur, from our watery blood to our fatty brains.

These new substances have the potential to extend life span and stave off age-related degenerative diseases, says Dr. Klatz. Future youth is out there!

To decide whether these supplements might be of any benefit to you, here's a primer on some that have longevity experts and medical researchers buzzing.

Alpha-Lipoic Acid (ALA)

What it is: An antioxidant made by the body, ALA also helps break down food into the energy needed by your cells. It helps the body recycle and renew vitamins C and E, making them serviceable again. And unlike many antioxidants, which dissolve only in fat or only in water, ALA fights free radicals in both the fatty and watery parts of cells, protecting both from free-radical damage. "Lipoic acid can zip in and out of any cell in the body, even those in the brain," says Lester Packer, Ph.D., professor of molecular and cell biology at the University of California, Berkeley.

How it delays aging: Clinical studies suggest that ALA may help prevent the nerve damage, caused by free-radical attacks, that frequently accompanies diabetes. In one German study, intravenous ALA significantly reduced pain, tingling, and numbness in the feet of people with diabetes.

What you'll find: ALA comes in capsules and tablets, in dosages from 50 to 300 milligrams.

How much to take: The general recommended dose is 50 to 100 milligrams a day. In the treatment of diabetes, the recommended dosage is 300 to 600 milligrams a day, says Dr. Packer.

Be aware: If you have diabetes and are being treated for symptoms of nerve damage, Dr. Packer suggests that you talk to your doctor before taking ALA supplements.

DON'T FORGET YOUR MULTI

"A multivitamin/mineral supplement is the cornerstone of any smart supplement regimen," says Jeffrey Blumberg, Ph.D., chief of the antioxidants research laboratory at the U.S.D.A. Human Nutrition Research Center on Aging at Tufts University in Boston.

But how can you know if the multi you are taking is a good one? Read the label. Look for a multi supplement that contains 100 percent of the Daily Value (DV) for most essential vitamins and minerals. None contains them all. The label should also have the letters USP on it. This stands for United States Pharmacopeia. Also, check the expiration date and don't buy more than you can use before then.

Your multi should contain these essential nutrients.

VITAMINS

Nutrient: Vitamin A or preformed Vitamin A (beta-carotene)
Daily Value: 5,000 international units (IU)
What it does: Helps your eyes adjust to dim light; maintains immunity; and forms and maintains normal structure and function of the epithelial cells (cells that act as a barrier between your body and the environment) in your mouth, eyes, skin, hair, gums, and various glands
Nutrient: Vitamin B_6
Daily Value: 2 milligrams
What it does: Helps your body make red blood cells; helps maintain your immune system; and helps produce insulin (the hormone that aids in converting food to energy)
Nutrient: Vitamin D
Daily Value: 400 IU
What it does: Helps bones mineralize properly by transporting bone-building calcium and phosphorus to the blood and, eventually, to the bones
Nutrient: Folic acid (folate)
Daily Value: 400 micrograms
What it does: Helps you produce DNA and RNA, the genetic code for cell reproduction. It is needed to form hemoglobin, which carries oxygen in red blood cells.

MINERALS

Nutrient: Chromium

Daily Value: 120 micrograms

What it does: Helps your body convert carbohydrates and fats into energy; works with insulin to help your body use glucose (blood sugar)

Nutrient: Copper

Daily Value: 2 milligrams

What it does: Helps your body make hemoglobin, which carries oxygen in red blood cells; and helps your body absorb iron

Nutrient: Iron

Daily Value: 18 milligrams

What it does: Carries oxygen in your blood and removes carbon dioxide, which is formed as your body produces energy; helps protect against infection. Multis come in regular or low- or no-iron formulas. If you have heavy periods, aim for the DV; otherwise, you should look for a multi that contains low or no iron.

Nutrient: Magnesium

Daily Value: 400 milligrams (The most you'll find in a regular multi is 100 milligrams; adding more would make the multi too big to swallow.)

What it does: Helps your body make proteins; helps maintain the cells in your nerves and muscles; plays a role in the mineralization of bones and immune-system function

Nutrient: Selenium

Daily Value: 70 micrograms (Most multis contain less; look for a minimum of 10 micrograms.)

What it does: Works with vitamin E to protect cells from damage by free radicals, unstable oxygen molecules thought to speed up the aging process by damaging our cells and tissues

Nutrient: Zinc

Daily Value: 15 milligrams

What it does: Helps keep your immune system strong; promotes cell reproduction; and helps heal wounds. It is crucial for sperm production and fetal development.

Bioflavonoids

What they are: Bioflavonoids are a group of plant pigments that give fruits and flowers some of their color. Some bioflavonoids act as powerful antioxidants, "many of which are more potent than better-known antioxidants such as vitamins C and E," explains Shari Lieberman, Ph.D., a nutrition scientist and exercise physiologist in New York City.

How they delay aging: Bioflavonoids may help lower the risk of heart disease. In 1996, a Finnish study found that women who ate the most flavonoids had a 46 percent lower risk for heart disease than those who ate the least.

Bioflavonoids keep the tiny disks in our blood (called platelets), which help blood clot, from clumping together and forming clots that can block the arteries. They also keep harmful low-density lipoprotein (LDL) cholesterol from oxidizing and sticking to artery walls.

Some bioflavonoids can stop cancer before it starts. To give just a few examples, quercetin, found in apples, yellow and red onions, and tea, has been shown in test-tube studies to discourage the growth of tumors and prevent malignant cells from spreading. And rutin, found in buckwheat, helps reduce cancer risk through its action as an antioxidant.

What you'll find: You can get bioflavonoids by eating fruits and vegetables or by taking them in supplement form. Supplements may contain either a single bioflavonoid or several in combination, says Michael Janson, M.D., president of the American College for Advancement in Medicine and author of three books including *Dr. Janson's Vitamin Revolution*. These usually contain extracts of quercetin, hesperidin, rutin, and citrus bioflavonoids and come in 500- or 1,000-milligram doses.

How much to take: Dr. Janson recommends taking 1,000 milligrams once or twice a day. As powerful antioxidants themselves, bioflavonoids increase the absorption of vitamin C.

Be aware: They are generally regarded as safe.

Coenzyme Q$_{10}$

What it is: An antioxidant made by our bodies, coenzyme Q$_{10}$ helps make ATP (adenosine triphosphate), the fuel that allows our cells to do their jobs. Every cell in our bodies contains this antioxidant, but it's most concentrated in heart muscle cells, which require the most fuel. We have plenty of coenzyme Q$_{10}$ until we hit age 40. After that, our levels take a nosedive.

How it delays aging: Coenzyme Q$_{10}$ may help prevent or treat many common forms of heart disease, says Peter Langsjoen, M.D., a staff cardiologist at Mother Francis Hospital and the East Texas Medical Center in Tyler. "It provides such dramatic improvement, it's unthinkable for me to practice medicine without it."

Research shows that people with various types of heart disease are deficient in coenzyme Q$_{10}$, and that the more severe the heart disease, the lower these levels drop. This substance appears

REAL-LIFE SCENARIO
She's Messing with Disaster

After years of working overtime and weekends in her career as a computer programmer, Terri, age 39, has finally snagged that project manager's position. To celebrate, she's treating herself to a week in the Bahamas, and she's determined to transform herself from an ivory-skinned redhead to a bronzed beachcomber. Of course, she knows the dangers of sun exposure, but she has a plan. First, she'll load up on antioxidants, like Pycnogenol, that promise to keep her skin supple and youthful. Then she'll apply some artificial tanning oil to herself. She figures that if she's brown to start with, she'll enjoy natural protection against the sun's harmful rays, and she won't even have to use any of those slimy sunblocks that make her feel as if she's just showered in grease. Besides, it's only a week. How much damage could the sun do?

Considerable damage. In fact, Terri's "plan" leaves her skin vulnerable not only to lines and wrinkles but also to skin cancer.

Some animal and test-tube studies have found that antioxidants such as vitamins C and E and Pycnogenol may help prevent sun damage. While in humans there's not much conclusive evidence of this, long-term use of topical vitamin C has been shown to provide a little protection.

Even if they do work, there's no way to know the dosages that would be needed to prevent sun damage, or how long they'd need to be taken prior to sun exposure. Sunless tanners, if they don't contain a sunscreen, don't protect skin either, regardless of how "brown" they make skin appear.

The best thing Terri could do to protect her skin is to avoid the sun between 10:00 A.M. and 4:00 P.M., when its rays are strongest. If she won't do that, she can wear protective

to improve the heart's ability to contract. And because it's a powerful antioxidant, coenzyme Q$_{10}$ also helps prevent "bad" LDL cholesterol from sticking to the walls of the arteries and clogging blood vessels.

Coenzyme Q$_{10}$ is used to treat a variety of

clothing and a broad-brimmed hat, slather herself with a sunscreen, spend as much time as possible under an umbrella, and get out of the sun completely for 15 to 20 minutes every hour.

Whatever sunscreen Terri uses should be applied ½ hour before exposure. She could opt for a product that contains a physical sunblock, such as zinc oxide or titanium dioxide. These substances prevent two types of the sun's ultraviolet (UV) rays—UVA and UVB—from being absorbed by the skin.

Or Terri could use what's called a broad-spectrum sunscreen. An active ingredient in these products, avobenzone, also known as Parsol 1789, blocks both UVA and UVB rays.

Whatever product Terri uses, it should have a sun protection factor (SPF) of at least 15. Because her skin is so fair, she should reapply it every few hours, whether she thinks she needs it or not. And she needs to remember that as protective as sunscreen is, it still allows some UV rays to penetrate skin. During her "sun breaks," Terri should also check to see if her skin is turning pink, a sign that she's on her way to a skin-damaging sunburn. If her skin is turning pink, she should get out of the sun for the rest of the day.

As for becoming a "bronzed beachcomber," the brown of a real tan means that the skin has already been damaged and at some point may shown signs of premature aging and skin cancer. If sun-kissed is the look Terri really wants, the artificial tanning oil will give it to her without any sun exposure at all.

Expert consulted
Karen Keller, M.D.
Dermatologist
Burlingame, California

heart conditions, from heart pain (angina) to cardiomyopathy (any noninflammatory disease of the heart muscles). Some studies suggest that this antioxidant helps treat angina by allowing heart muscle cells to use oxygen more efficiently. In a small study of 19 people with cardiomyopathy conducted by Dr. Langsjoen, those who took 100 milligrams of coenzyme Q_{10} a day along with their conventional therapy did far better than those who got conventional therapy and a placebo.

Coenzyme Q_{10} also helps treat congestive heart failure, which occurs when the heart is too weak to pump blood through the body. In a large study conducted by Dr. Langsjoen, 58 percent of people taking coenzyme Q_{10} improved by one New York Heart Association classification (the standard doctors use to assess heart patients' condition), 28 percent improved by two classes, and 43 percent stopped using one or more drugs.

What you'll find: Coenzyme Q_{10} can be found in 10- to 200-milligram capsules. Dr. Langsjoen prefers the soft-gel supplements prepared with oil because they're better absorbed by the body.

How much to take: As a preventive measure, take from 30 to 60 milligrams per day, says Dr. Langsjoen. He prescribes higher doses—120 to 360 milligrams—for people with heart problems.

This nutrient dissolves only in the presence of fat, so if you're using coenzyme Q_{10} supplements that aren't in gel form, take them with a meal or snack that contains a small amount of fat, says Dr. Langsjoen.

Be aware: Some medications deplete the body's supply of coenzyme Q_{10}. These include cholesterol-lowering drugs such as lovastatin (Mevacor). In rare occurrences, a slight decrease in the effectiveness of the blood thinner warfarin (Coumadin) has been observed. Also, if you have heart disease, consult your doctor before taking coenzyme Q₁₀, says Dr. Langsjoen.

Flaxseed Oil

What it is: A polyunsaturated vegetable oil that's a rich source of omega-3 fatty acids. Studies have repeatedly suggested that omega-3's lower blood levels of cholesterol and triglycerides and reduce the stickiness of platelets, thus reducing the risk of heart attack or stroke. Other studies have found that omega-3's raise high-density lipoproteins (HDLs), the "good" cholesterol that helps whisk artery-clogging LDL out of the blood. While fish oils are the best-known sources of omega-3's, flaxseed oil contains twice the amount of omega-3's that fish oils do.

How it delays aging: Researchers have conducted numerous studies on flaxseed to study its potential in preventing and treating cancer, particularly breast and colon cancer. In animal studies, flaxseed helps keep breast cancer from starting and slows the growth of breast tumors already in place.

Research suggests that the cancer-fighting substances in flaxseed are lignan precursors, compounds that the body converts into lignans. These are estrogen-like compounds that may prevent breast cancer by taking up estrogen receptors on breast cells, thereby blocking stronger, cancer-causing estrogen.

Lignans also act as antioxidants and contain other beneficial plant chemicals. An accumulating body of research suggests that they may help protect against age-related chronic conditions such as heart disease.

What you'll find: There are a wide variety of flaxseed oils on the market, but not all are equally beneficial, notes Michael T. Murray, N.D., a faculty member at Bastyr University in Kenmore, Washington, in his book *Understanding Fats and Oils.*

He recommends choosing a brand that has been processed using a technique called modified atmospheric packing (MAP). This method squeezes the oil from the seed at low temperatures while also protecting it from the damaging effects of light and oxygen. Some trade names for MAP processing include Bio-Electron Process, used by Barlean's Organic Oils; SpectraVac Cold-Pressed, used by Spectrum Naturals; and the Omegaflo process, used by Omega Nutrition.

Because lignan precursors are found only in the hull of flaxseeds, many brands of flaxseed oil don't contain these beneficial compounds. Some brands that do are Barlean's Organic High-Lignan Flaxseed Oil, Spectrum Naturals' High-Lig Flax Oil, and Hi-Lignan Flax Seed Oil from Omega Nutrition. They are available in some health food stores or by mail order.

One more thing: Buy only those brands that come in light-resistant plastic containers. Light causes any oil, including flaxseed oil, to break down and turn rancid.

How much to take: Take 1 tablespoon per 100 pounds of body weight a day, suggests Dr. Murray.

Keep flaxseed oil in the freezer until you open it. This will keep its beneficial substances intact. After you open it, keep it in the refrigerator. Also, take flaxseed oil with food (perhaps mix it into yogurt). Your body will absorb and use its essential fatty acids more efficiently. Flaxseed is easily damaged by heat, so don't use it in cooking.

Be aware: Due to its high calorie content, you could gain weight if you don't figure flaxseed oil into your total calorie intake.

Ginkgo

What it is: Ginkgo is an herb extracted from the fan-shaped, leathery leaves of the ginkgo tree.

How it delays aging: This herb helps the brain function more efficiently. Already used in Germany to treat dementia, ginkgo enhances blood circulation, so more nutrients reach brain cells, enabling them to work more efficiently. In European studies, ginkgo has also been found to improve mental performance and short-term memory.

While there's no proof that taking ginkgo now will prevent Alzheimer's disease later, a growing body of research suggests that a concentrated extract of this herb improves the mental functioning of people who already have the disease.

In one of the biggest studies, researchers found that among people with Alzheimer-type dementia and those with dementia caused by blood vessel disease of the brain, those taking ginkgo were better able to think and interact with others than were those taking a placebo.

What you'll find: Ginkgo usually comes in 40-, 60-, or 120-milligram capsules.

How much to take: Take from 120 to 240 milligrams a day in two or three separate doses, says Varro E. Tyler, Ph.D., Sc.D., dean emeritus of the Purdue University School of Pharmacy and Pharmacal Sciences and author of *The Honest Herbal*. The supplement you buy should contain 24 percent flavone glycosides and 6 percent terpenes, says Dr. Tyler. (You might see "24/6" on the label.)

Be aware: According to Dr. Tyler, you should be cautious about using ginkgo if you are taking

ARE HORMONE SUPPLEMENTS SAFE?

Some of the anti-aging hormones normally made by your body are now available in bottles at your local health food store. And while the government classifies these "bottled hormones" as dietary supplements, some experts say that they shouldn't be.

"These products are powerful substances and should be viewed as drugs," says Alan R. Gaby, M.D., professor of nutrition at Bastyr University in Kenmore, Washington. "They have potential for great benefit, but they can also cause significant harm."

One example is DHEA (dehydroepiandrosterone). In animal studies, this male hormone (which a woman's body makes, too) appears to boost immunity and help protect against diabetes, heart disease, and even cancer.

Here's the problem. Our bodies convert DHEA into estrogen and testosterone. So if even a small amount is converted to estrogen in a woman with a family history of breast cancer, she may be increasing her risk of developing the disease, says Dr. Gaby.

Pregnenolone, the precursor to DHEA, is another bottled hormone that's flying off the shelves. But clinical research on this hormone is sparse. "There's an animal study that suggests that it improves memory, and that's about it," says Dr. Gaby.

In the body, pregnenolone may be converted into DHEA, increasing our bodies' amounts of estrogen and testosterone. There are potential risks in using pregnenolone, says Dr. Gaby. It hasn't been used long enough to determine if it is safe.

The bottom line: Don't self-prescribe hormone supplements, says Dr. Gaby. Consult a doctor, who will advise you if hormone supplements are appropriate, prescribe them at the appropriate dosage (if necessary), and monitor your progress.

herbs that help prevent blood clotting such as garlic, ginger, and feverfew. Also, don't take it if you are currently using aspirin, warfarin (Coumadin), or an MAO inhibitor drug.

Melatonin

What it is: Melatonin is a hormone secreted by a pea-size gland, called the pineal gland. The hormone helps regulate our sleep patterns. Our levels of melatonin peak by the time we are 3 years old and remain at high levels until after middle age.

How it delays aging: Melatonin is a powerful antioxidant, says Russel J. Reiter, Ph.D., a cellular biologist at the University of Texas Health Science Center at San Antonio, author of *Your Body's Natural Wonder Drug: Melatonin*, and editor of the *Journal of Pineal Research*.

"Melatonin is one of the most powerful antioxidants there is," says Dr. Reiter. As such, it protects against age-related diseases such as cardiovascular disease and cancer, which may be linked to free-radical damage.

But there's more. Unlike many other antioxidants, melatonin is able to cross what's called the blood-brain barrier, which means that it penetrates the brain more easily than some other antioxidants, says Dr. Reiter. So it's better able to fight the free-radical damage in the brain.

Recent evidence suggests that melatonin may also slow the progression of Alzheimer's disease. "Much of the dementia associated with aging, including Alzheimer's disease, is due to loss of neurons as a result of free-radical damage," says Dr. Reiter. "While very high doses of vitamin E, a well-known antioxidant, given for long periods of time can slightly delay Alzheimer's, a recent study on a pair of identical twins found that as little as 6 milligrams of melatonin taken every day for 3 years substantially reduced the progression of Alzheimer's disease."

In some laboratory studies, melatonin has also been found to prevent the growth of cancer cells and to slow the growth of some tumors.

What you'll find: Melatonin usually comes in 3-milligram capsules and tablets. While less common, you can find it in 1-milligram and 0.5-milligram (or 500-microgram) doses as well. Avoid so-called natural melatonin supplements, which probably don't contain enough to be effective, says Dr. Reiter. The synthetic variety, which is probably what you will find, is fine.

How much to take: You take less than you'd think. Although the generally recommended dose is 1 milligram, Dr. Reiter takes 0.5 milligram per day. "And I have the melatonin levels of a young person," he says.

Also, always take melatonin before bed, says Dr. Reiter. And keep your room dark: Darkness stimulates the production of melatonin.

Be aware: Since melatonin makes you drowsy, don't drive or engage in any activity that requires you to be alert after taking it, says Dr. Reiter. Before you start using melatonin, talk with your doctor. Though rare, interactions with prescription medications can occur.

Phosphatidylserine

What it is: This substance is a phospholipid, a kind of a fat concentrated in the nerve cells of the brain. In elderly people, low levels of phosphatidylserine have been linked with impaired mental functioning and depression.

How it delays aging: Phosphatidylserine improves memory and age-related brain changes, says Timothy Smith, M.D., an expert in anti-aging medicine in Sebastopol, California, and author of *Renewal*. It also helps regenerate damaged nerve cells, so they can send and receive their "messages" more effectively.

Researchers at Stanford University and at Vanderbilt University in Nashville studied the effects of phosphatidylserine in 149 people between the ages of 50 and 75 with "normal" age-related memory loss. The most memory-impaired people reversed an estimated 12-year decline in memory. In other words, the average scores attained by 64-year-olds rose to match the average scores of 52-year-olds.

What you'll find: Phosphatidylserine supplements are made from lecithin, a derivative of soy. In this country, it's available in 20- to 100-milligram capsules and tablets.

How much to take: Dr. Smith recommends taking 100 milligrams of phosphatidylserine two or three times a day. After a month, he says, switch to a maintenance dose of 100 to 200 milligrams a day.

Be aware: Phosphatidylserine appears to be safe with no serious side effects, notes Dr. Smith.

Pycnogenol

What it is: A trademarked supplement derived from the bark of the French maritime pine tree, Pycnogenol (pronounced "pik-NA-je-nal") contains about 40 bioflavonoids with antioxidant powers. Its active ingredients—a class of flavonoids called proanthocyanidins, also found in grape seeds—make it a potent antioxidant. Pycnogenol also recycles vitamin C and, indirectly, vitamin E, making them effective again, says Dr. Packer.

How it delays aging: Pycnogenol reduces the risk of heart disease by keeping platelets unstuck so that they can't adhere to artery walls and by keeping LDL cholesterol from oxidizing, says Dr. Packer.

Pycnogenol also strengthens the body's smallest blood vessels, called capillaries, and prevents free-radical damage to blood vessels. Pycnogenol also suppresses the overproduction of nitric oxide (NO) by immune system cells, which has been linked to rheumatoid arthritis and Alzheimer's disease, says Dr. Packer.

LIFE EXTENDER
Evade Cancer the One-a-Day Way

Colon cancer is the third most common cancer in women, killing 24,900 of us every year. But taking a daily multivitamin/mineral supplement or a vitamin E supplement may reduce your risk of developing the condition, suggests a study conducted at the Fred Hutchinson Cancer Research Center in Seattle.

Researchers analyzed vitamin use in 444 men and women with colon cancer, focusing on the 10-year period ending 2 years before diagnosis. Then, they compared vitamin use in this group to vitamin use in 426 people without cancer. Researchers found that people who had regularly taken multivitamins for 10 years reduced their risk of colon cancer by 51 percent, and those who took vitamin E may have lowered their risk by 57 percent.

This does not necessarily mean that vitamin supplements are your best protection against cancer. Eating plenty of fruits and vegetables is still the best advice, according to the researchers, because they contain just the right balance of vitamins.

What you'll find: Pycnogenol comes in tablets or capsules, in dosages from 20 milligrams to 100 milligrams.

How much to take: The generally recommended dose is from 50 to 100 milligrams per day, says Dr. Packer.

Vitamin C

What it is: An antioxidant nutrient, vitamin C is found in citrus fruits, strawberries, broccoli, kiwifruit, and other fruits and vegetables.

How it delays aging: Studies suggest that people who consume a high-C diet have lower rates of cancer, heart disease, and high blood pressure. There's also evidence that vitamin C supplements may help stave off cataracts and may help thicken bones during the early postmenopausal years and in women who never used estrogen-replacement therapy. Clinical studies suggest that it can fight high blood pressure.

What you'll find: Vitamin C supplements come in 250-, 500-, 1,000-milligram and even higher dosage tablets and capsules as well as powder that you can mix into water or juice.

Whatever form you buy, don't waste your money on natural vitamin C supplements. "There's no difference between synthetic and natural vitamin C—it's exactly the same molecule," says Jeffrey Blumberg, Ph.D., chief of the antioxidants research laboratory at the U.S.D.A. Human Nutrition Research Center on Aging at Tufts University in Boston.

How much to take: The Daily Value is 60 milligrams, an amount researchers now concede is too low to prevent disease. Aim for 200 to 500 milligrams a day, says Dr. Blumberg.

Be aware: Taking more than 1,000 milligrams of vitamin C a day can cause diarrhea in some people. If this happens to you, immediately stop taking vitamin C. If you want to take more than 1,000 milligrams, start with 250 milligrams and increase the dose every few days as your tolerance increases, says Dr. Blumberg.

Vitamin E

What it is: An antioxidant nutrient, vitamin E is found in nuts, seeds, and vegetable oils.

How it delays aging: Research suggests that vitamin E's antioxidant power may help prevent heart disease and cancer, boosts the immune system, and possibly helps normalize blood sugar levels in people with diabetes.

Vitamin E also seems to slow the progression of Alzheimer's disease. Researchers at Columbia University and other centers gave 341 people with moderately severe Alzheimer's disease 2,000 international units (IU) of vitamin E a day for 2 years. At the end of the study, researchers concluded that E had slowed the mental deterioration of those people by about 25 percent, mainly in their ability to perform everyday tasks such as dressing, using the toilet, and eating.

What you'll find: Vitamin E comes in 100-, 200-, or 400-IU capsules. It's also available in liquid.

Recent studies have found that our bodies absorb the natural form of vitamin E (d-alpha tocopherol) more effectively than the synthetic kind (dl-alpha tocopherol). You'll pay more for the natural kind, however.

How much to take: The Daily Value is 30 IU—not enough, suggests some research, to head off heart disease or other illnesses. Aim for 100 to 400 IU, recommends Dr. Blumberg. Take vitamin E with a meal that contains a small amount of fat. You'll absorb it better.

Be aware: If you are taking anticoagulant drugs, use vitamin E only with medical supervision, says Dr. Blumberg.

Water: The Ultimate Anti-Aging Tonic

The Spanish explorer Juan Ponce de León sailed halfway across the world looking for the fountain of youth. He never found it. You or I, on the other hand, can make it appear instantly by turning on the kitchen tap.

Sound like magic? Not really. Today we know something that Ponce de León didn't: The power of that fountain lies in simple, fresh, clean water.

Your body needs water for all the basic processes of life, which include everything from transporting nutrients to regulating internal temperature. But drinking plenty of water—at least eight 8-ounce glasses a day—can give you benefits above and beyond the basics. It can also help you maintain healthy, younger-looking skin and prevent certain diseases and conditions that can make you feel far older than your years.

Water Down Wrinkles

Nature makes the lesson obvious: Dry out a grape, you get a raisin. Dry out a plum, you get a prune. Wrinkles, wrinkles, wrinkles.

On the other hand, if you're ironing out the wrinkles from a cotton shirt, you moisten it with steam. And if you want to keep roses from wilting, you put them in a vase with water.

So it is with skin. If you want to keep it smooth, supple, and radiant, water is one of the secrets you're looking for. "Healthy skin is about 10 to 20 percent water," says Diana Bihova, M.D., a dermatologist in New York City and coauthor of *Beauty from the Inside Out*. If your skin loses more than half its moisture, it becomes dry and flaky. Even fine lines become more pronounced. Over time, dry skin can age more quickly.

One way to fight back is by using moisturizers. When you moisturize your skin, it plumps up and looks smoother, and fine lines seem to disappear.

The problem is that time makes the going tougher. Our skin gets drier as we get older. Around age 30, oil and sweat glands slow their production and skin is less able to retain moisture, says Dr. Bihova. And as we get closer to menopause and our estrogen levels drop, our skin may dry out even more.

pruny by the last plate, bathing or showering in steamy-hot water may send you hankering for hand-and-body lotion hours later. That's because hot water can dry out your skin. To save face, try soaking or showering in lukewarm water instead of hot.

Switch your soap. Washing with harsh soaps can leave your skin feeling like sandpaper—so stick to gentle cleansers like Cetaphil. They cleanse your skin without irritation and leave behind a moisturizing film. Buy cleansers with ingredients such as water, glycerin, sodium lauryl sulfate, cetyl alcohol, and stearyl alcohol.

Time it right. The best time to moisturize is right after a shower or bath, when your skin is still wet and the moisture can be sealed in.

Water the air. Dry winter air wicks moisture away from your skin, leaving it dull and dry. But running a humidifier adds moisture to the air and prevents water loss through your pores.

Drink to Your Health

That's where water comes in. Drinking plenty of water is important. Whether you sip it or soak in it, water moisturizes your skin. But that's not all you need to do. "Drinking an ocean of water is not, by itself, going to repair your dry skin," says Dr. Bihova. And simply slathering on lotion won't end your dry skin dilemma either. Here, Dr. Bihova shares some secrets to getting the most from moisture.

Keep your cool. Just as washing a sinkful of dishes in hot water leaves your hands dry and

Water not only lubricates your skin, it keeps everything inside your body flowing smoothly as well. "Most people are minimally dehydrated, and that can impact practically everything a person does," says Felicia Busch, R.D., a nutritionist in St. Paul, Minnesota, and a spokesperson for the American Dietetic Association. You can lose 1 to 2 percent of your body weight in water without ever feeling thirsty. And once you have lost that much water, your body can't function at its best. You start to feel tired, unfocused, weaker, and slower. You may even get a headache—all things that make you feel sluggish and older than you really are.

A well-watered body has what it needs to stay young and healthy. Here are some ways you can use water to help you feel your best.

Keep your colon healthy. Drinking the standard eight glasses a day may lower your risk for colon cancer. Researchers have found that women who drink more than five glasses of water a day have about half the risk of colon cancer of those who drink two or fewer glasses.

Stay regular. Older people are five times more likely to be constipated than younger folks. And chronic constipation can lead to uncomfortable and painful conditions like hemorrhoids or diverticulitis.

To keep your bottom end feeling as young as a baby's bum, drink up. Having enough water in your pipes can help prevent and relieve constipation, especially if you eat a high-fiber diet. That's because water softens your stools so that they can move more easily through your system.

Slim down. Drinking lots of water keeps you trim—first, by helping you burn fat more efficiently. And second, if you drink it right before meals, it fills you up, so you eat less.

Beat bladder infections. Almost half of the 16,000 women surveyed by *Prevention* magazine and the American Medical Women's Association a few years ago had experienced a bladder infection and had tried drinking plenty of water

---

LIFE EXTENDER
Green Tea: The Longer-Life Elixir

Trading in your coffeepot for a tea kettle could add years to your life. Research shows that drinking green tea may offer you a slew of benefits, from helping to lower your cholesterol and blood pressure to reducing your risk of heart attack and stroke. This Chinese pot of gold also helps protect the immune system, aids digestion, and prevents cavities and gingivitis. But someday we may find that green tea's most impressive life-extending benefit comes from cancer-fighting antioxidants called polyphenols.

Animal studies show that substances in green tea may protect against several types of cancer, including tumors of the skin, breast, stomach, colon, liver, lung, and pancreas. Studies on humans are less clear but suggest that drinking green tea may lower the risk of getting certain cancers such as stomach, colorectal, and pancreatic. A study of more than 35,000 middle-aged women in Iowa found that those who drank at least 2 cups of black, green, or oolong tea a day significantly reduced their risks of getting digestive tract and urinary tract cancers.

What's more, a study found that women with early-stage breast cancer who were regular green tea drinkers had a better prognosis than those who weren't. Green tea drinkers also develop cancers much later in life. In one study done in Japan, women cancer patients who had consumed more than 10 cups of green tea a day developed the disease an average of 8.7 years later than those who drank fewer than 3 cups a day.

---

to treat it. Eight out of 10 said it worked for them. Doctors say that all those fluids may help by flushing infection-causing bacteria out of your system.

Stave off kidney stones. When you don't drink enough water, wastes that are normally dissolved and removed in your urine may become concentrated in crystals, which could lump together to form a kidney stone.

scopic muscle damage, which shows up as soreness the next day, says Scott Hasson, Ed.D., chairperson of the department of physical therapy at the University of Connecticut in Storrs.

A good rule of thumb is to drink a glass of water before and after physical activity as well as a half-cup every 15 to 20 minutes during the activity, he says.

A Female Disadvantage

Your body's about 50 percent water, so think of yourself as a glass that's half full. To keep that level from dropping, you have to drink at least eight 8-ounce glasses of water a day. Staying hydrated is especially important for women because their bodies store less water than men's, says Busch. That's because women have less muscle, which holds a lot of water, and more fat, which doesn't. As a result, a woman's well runs dry more quickly than a man's, so you have to be more faithful about replenishing what you lose each day. Women who are pregnant or nursing need to drink even more water, Busch adds—at least 10 to 12 glasses a day.

Still others need extra water to keep their skin supple and their bodies working at their best. Here's how to know if you are getting your fill.

Check the conditions. You need to drink more than the average eight glasses a day if you're sick, if you live in a hot climate, if you spend a lot of time inside heated or air-conditioned buildings, if you do a lot of public

Prevent muscle soreness. When you're physically active—whether you're doing work around the house, gardening, or playing tennis—water can ward off the day-after aches that make you feel all washed up. If you're slightly dehydrated, your body taps the water that's stored in your muscles. That can decrease your strength and increase your risk of micro-

speaking (like a teacher), or if you're larger than average, Busch says.

Drink before you're thirsty. You can't use thirst to determine when you need to fill up, because you can lose as much as 5 percent of your body's water supply before feeling thirsty, Busch says. To prevent this, try water breaks: when you first wake up, when you get to the office, at break times, before meals, and before bed. One glass of water at each of these times will keep you well-hydrated on regular days.

As you get older, your sensitivity to thirst decreases, so it becomes even more important to drink throughout the day, whether you're thirsty or not, adds Joanne Curran-Celentano, Ph.D., associate professor of nutritional sciences at the University of New Hampshire in Durham.

Clear things up. Check the color of your urine. "It should be almost clear, a pale yellow," says Lucia Kaiser, R.D., Ph.D., a nutrition specialist at the University of California, Davis. If it's not, you need to drink more fluids.

Ways to Fill Your Tank

If downing 2 quarts of water a day sounds like more than you can stomach, don't dry-dock just yet. These tips from our experts will help you get a handle on staying hydrated.

Call in a substitute. All eight glasses don't have to be water. Other beverages like milk, juice, seltzer, and sparkling water can also count toward your daily intake. So can foods that contain lots of water such as soups and juicy fruits such as watermelon, cantaloupe, grapes, and oranges. But don't count beverages that contain alcohol or caffeine; they actually cause you to lose more water than you take in.

Punch up the flavor. If water's too plain for you, try flavored water or squeeze in fresh fruit like lemon, lime, orange, or pineapple. Or toss frozen-juice ice cubes into your water—they add flavor as they melt. For soft-drink fans who miss the carbonation, try adding sparkling water to $1/4$ cup of juice.

Sip before you snack. People often think that they're hungry when they're actually thirsty. So have a drink first; it may take care of your hunger pang.

Measure it out. Fill a 64-ounce pitcher and try to empty it by the end of the day.

Keep it close. Have a glass or bottle of water with you when you're at your desk, outdoors, in your car, or at the gym.

Take it slow. Sipping rather than gulping will prevent you from feeling bloated.

Make a pit stop. Every time you pass a water fountain, take a drink.

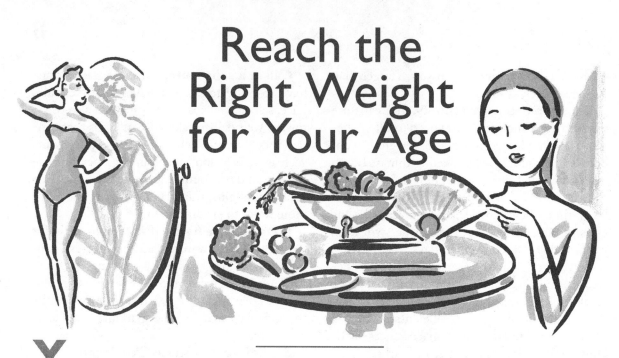

Reach the Right Weight for Your Age

You gain a lot as you reach your middle years: understanding, control, self-confidence, wisdom, stature, freedom—and, unfortunately, weight. Whether it's a joke of Mother Nature's or an accident of evolution, a woman's scale and her age creep up together as she reaches her thirties, forties, and beyond.

All sorts of factors fight against you in your battle with extra pounds during this time of your life. "It's not hard to gain weight. There are all kinds of metabolic changes that promote weight gain as you get older," says Susan Roberts, Ph.D., professor of nutrition and psychiatry and chief of the energy metabolism laboratory at Tufts University in Boston.

First off, your body's metabolism slows down. In other words, you burn fewer calories during an activity now than you would have 20 years ago. "Even athletes have decreased energy expenditure with aging," Dr. Roberts says.

You also tend to be less physically active at this stage of your life than when you were younger, which slows the calorie burn even more. And to top it all off, muscle mass naturally decreases with age. Since muscle uses up more

energy fuel than any other kind of tissue, including fat, having less muscle diminishes your calorie burn still further.

It sounds as if we're doomed, but there's reason to take heart. We aren't supposed to look like we did when we were 25, and a little extra weight may not hurt us, especially if we are physically active. On average, women gain 10 to 15 pounds by age 60, says Michael Hamilton, M.D., program and medical director of the Diet Fitness Center at Duke University in Durham, North Carolina.

The key during these years is to find a *healthy* weight. Here's how to find what's the right weight for you and what you need to do to keep it there.

Weighing In

Ahh, the dreaded scale. Women have learned to treat its revolving numbers as the measure of truth when it comes to their worth and health. They look for that one magic number that will tell them everything is all right. But science has moved beyond the actual digits that show up on the scale and has found that factors other than weight alone have much more significant influence on your health.

Many weight experts now rely on the body mass index, better known as the BMI, to gauge your well-being. The BMI compares your height to your weight. A healthy BMI usually falls into the 20 to 25 range, says Susan Fried, Ph.D., associate professor of nutritional sciences at Rutgers University in New Brunswick, New Jersey. So if you had a BMI of 21 when you were in your twenties but now have a BMI of 23, you are still considered to be at a normal, healthy weight.

If you're in the over-25 range, it may be time to make some changes. A BMI of 25 to 30 is considered overweight; and a BMI over 30 is in the obese category. If you find yourself in either of those ranges, you'd do your health a favor by losing some weight. Why? Because numbers above 25 have been linked to increased rates of heart disease, diabetes, and breast cancer. Numbers above 30 have been even more closely linked with these problems.

Here's how to determine your BMI: Multiply your weight in pounds by 705. Divide the result by your height in inches, then divide that result by your height in inches again. So if you are 145 pounds and 66 inches tall, your BMI would be 23.4, well within the healthy range.

But BMI isn't the whole story. Where you add on weight may be as important as how much, says Dr. Fried. Women who carry extra fat in their abdomens are at greater risk for weight-related diseases than are those who gain in their thighs, hips, or butts. So researchers

---

THE PRICE OF PREGNANCY

After gaining anywhere from 20 to 50 pounds per child, you'd think that pregnancy would contribute to the weight problem of many women. Not so, at least for a majority of moms. Two studies have discovered that most women go back to either their pre-pregnancy weight or just a few pounds above it.

A study at the Karolinska Hospital in Stockholm, Sweden, followed 1,423 pregnant women until a year after their deliveries. On average, the women were about a pound heavier than they were before their pregnancies. Thirty percent actually dropped below their pre-pregnancy weight, while 56 percent gained anywhere between zero and 11 pounds. Only 14 percent kept more than 11 pounds. Another study at the University of Iceland looked at 200 women 2 years after giving birth. About 89 percent of the women got back to their pre-pregnancy weight.

Studies haven't shown any metabolic process that would keep weight on after a pregnancy, says Jill Kanaley, Ph.D., assistant professor of exercise science and director of the human performance laboratory at Syracuse University in New York. Whether a woman gains or loses weight after a pregnancy depends on how much she eats and exercises.

---

have devised another guideline to assess weight and health risk: your waist circumference. If your waist is larger than 35 inches, says Dr. Fried, you may be at higher risk for heart disease, stroke, diabetes, high blood pressure, and certain cancers.

The BMI and waist circumference act as good general guidelines, but it is possible to be perfectly fit with a BMI over 25. And you can be out of shape and live a nonhealthy lifestyle and have a BMI under 25. Here are some other criteria to help you decide where your weight should be.

Fitness level. If you carry an extra 10 to 15 pounds but are physically active and can do daily tasks—walk up and down hills, climb steps, run to catch a bus—without a problem, then you are probably fine, says Jill Kanaley, Ph.D., assistant professor of exercise science and director of the human performance laboratory at Syracuse University in New York. If you aren't fit and you have a problem getting around, then your weight may pose a health risk.

Family history. If your parents are overweight and have problems such as high blood pressure, high cholesterol, or diabetes, chances are the extra weight may cause the same problems for you, says Dr. Kanaley. But if Mom and Dad were overweight all their lives, yet were fit and lived into their eighties or nineties, you have less to worry about.

Other risk factors. Women who are carrying a few extra pounds but are otherwise healthy shouldn't worry too much. "They shouldn't beat themselves up over their weight," Dr. Kanaley says. But if you have high cholesterol, high blood pressure, or diabetes, losing the extra weight could lessen your risk of developing serious health problems in the future.

If you do need to lose weight, you don't necessarily have to go from a BMI of 30 to the low 20s to get health benefits. Expert panels and government guidelines have determined that a 5- to 10-percent drop in body weight—maintained for one year—should be considered a success, says Gary Foster, Ph.D., clinical director of the weight and eating disorders program at the University of Pennsylvania School of Medicine in Philadelphia. In other words, if you weigh 200 pounds and are considered overweight, a loss of 20 pounds would be a reasonable and

---

REAL-LIFE SCENARIO
Why Is She So Thin and Old-Looking?

Marie is 39 years old, although from the look of her, you'd guess she was closer to 59, which someone recently did say. She was crushed. She had thought she looked great because she had never allowed herself to put on an ounce since she'd gotten out of college, as so many other women her age had. Then, after the birth of her last daughter, she'd gotten back down to within 7 pounds of her normal weight, when she plateaued. She was horrified. To her, fat meant unattractive. She immediately cut her food intake down to 1,000 calories a day. She's never been so thin—right down to the hollows in her cheeks, her sunken eyes, and her frail-looking shoulders. And lately her back and knees have been hurting, and more often than not, she has a cold. She thought she'd chosen a healthy way to live. What's gone wrong?

Marie has two serious misconceptions about her weight. Her first is equating low weight—even lower-than-normal weight—with attractiveness and good health. Her second is allowing her weight to control her self-esteem. Both beliefs are making her look and feel old before her time.

The key to reaching and maintaining a healthy weight is to do the all right things *within reason*. If Marie ate a balanced diet and exercised regularly, her weight would fall to where

---

healthy goal. Why 10 percent? It is a realistic goal, it is easier to maintain, and various studies have shown that just a 10-percent loss improves many of the medical conditions associated with excess weight such as diabetes and high blood pressure, Dr. Foster says.

Say Goodbye to Dieting

There's a reason trendy diets go out of style as fast as go-go boots and beehive hairdos: They don't work. As you talk to weight-loss experts, you'll hear over and over again that there is no

her body needed it to be. When Marie was 7 pounds over her pre-pregnancy weight, she was at no higher risk for health problems than she had been before getting pregnant. But now that she has reached what she considers a "healthy" weight, she's experiencing all kinds of symptoms, and she looks unhealthy.

Why? Her body is telling her that it doesn't want to be that thin. If she insists on remaining at that weight, she'll have to live like a Spartan for the rest of her life. No person could keep up such a lifestyle.

Marie must also begin to recognize that a number on a scale does not define her worth as a person. Right now, her identification with what she weighs has turned into an unhealthy obsession. There's a very good chance that, no matter how many pounds she loses, she'll never be satisfied. And as long as she links her body weight with her self-esteem, she'll never feel good about herself.

If Marie wants to move beyond the scale and live life completely, she'll have to start defining herself in different ways—by her value as a mother, a friend, a wife, a worker.

Expert consulted
Gary Foster, Ph.D.
Clinical director of the weight and eating disorders program
University of Pennsylvania School of Medicine
Philadelphia

magic weight-loss diet. If you drastically cut back on calories to lose weight, the pounds will come flocking back once you start to eat normally again.

The not-so-secret secret to weight loss and control is not an eating plan with a sexy name and lots of hype, but a healthy, low-fat diet that emphasizes fruits, grains, and vegetables. If you make it part of your lifestyle, you won't have to worry about gaining pounds back. "Fad diets come and go. Over and over we see that the only thing that really works is a balanced, healthy diet with moderation," says Lorna Pascal, R.D., nu-

trition coordinator at the Dave Winfield Nutrition Center at the Hackensack University Medical Center in Hackensack, New Jersey.

When it comes to planning and eating meals, remember these tips to help keep the pounds off.

Fill up with fiber. Not only is fiber good for you, but it fills you up more quickly and with fewer calories, which prevents you from eating more. A study at the Brooke Army Medical Center at Fort Sam Houston, Texas, found that pectin, a soluble fiber found in the skins of fruits and vegetables, made people feel fuller longer. To get more fiber, base your meals on fruits, vegetables, legumes, and whole grains, such as whole-wheat bread, brown rice, and whole-grain breakfast cereals, says Melanie Polk, R.D., director of nutrition education at the American Institute for Cancer Research in Washington, D.C.

Get low-fat and lean. Each gram of fat contains more calories than a gram of protein or carbohydrate. Eating a high-fiber diet full of fruits, vegetables, and whole grains naturally helps you cut down on fat, Polk says. Also, limit your use of oils and butter and switch to dairy products like fat-free milk, low-fat cheese, and low-fat yogurt. If you eat meat, choose moderate portions of skinless chicken and turkey and lean cuts of red meat, such as top round, bottom round, and top sirloin.

Be moderate. No food is bad if you don't eat too much of it. "We live in a super-sized world," Pascal says. Even people who choose low-fat fare will gain weight if they eat too much. You can enjoy just about any food as long as you enjoy it in moderation.

Eat with all your senses. It's easy to gulp down a meal without enjoying it, then end up still feeling unsatisfied. If you focus more on your food, a little will go a long way, Polk says. Look at the plate and study the colors and textures. "Get the visual enjoyment," she adds. Then close your eyes and smell the aroma of the meal. As you put a small bite into your mouth, pay attention to the texture and taste of each and every morsel. Slowly chew and savor the food before swallowing, she says. "You'll satisfy all your senses and realize that you don't need to eat as much food to get the enjoyment out of it."

Size up serving sizes. When is a bagel not a bagel? When it's really four bagels. Just because you eat one of something doesn't mean it's a single serving. Many foods—such as a big bagel—are actually four servings of bread. When you're eating foods that come in bulk, such as rice or pastas, read their labels and figure out exactly what a serving size is, Pascal says. Measure out how much food you eat and compare it to the label to see how many calories and grams of fat you are actually getting. Once you learn servings, you'll be able to judge with your eye how much you should eat.

Ask for a doggie bag first. Because they're so busy, many women find themselves eating out a lot these days. Restaurant serving sizes can be up to four times what a regular serving size should be. To make sure that you don't overdo it, ask for the doggie bag first, Polk says. Put half of the meal away before you even start to eat.

Make veggies the centerpiece. In a typical American meal, meat is often the star. Vegetables and whole grains just garnish the main

event. Break out of that mindset, Polk says. Make vegetables and whole grains the centerpiece. If you do have meat, make it a small side dish.

Utilize spices and flavors. Fat isn't the only way to flavor food. Polk suggests using nonfat sauces such as teriyaki, flavored vinegars, or no-fat salad dressing. Season vegetables and meats with herbs and spices to add flavor without fat.

Be prepared. If you don't have any healthy low-fat food around, it's easy to fall into a fat-eating trap. Stock up your pantry with a few items to make sure that you can always fix a

really attracted to women who have low self-esteem. So when an attractive man did approach, I was skeptical of his motives.

On top of all that, I was terribly frustrated that I couldn't get the scale to move. In fact, I got to a point where I felt so frustrated that I went to my doctor and told him, "Here is what I have eaten for the last 7 days." I tracked every morsel I put into my mouth, and it was my typical diet. What was wrong with me? And he said that I was basically starving myself and had been for years—that I actually wasn't eating enough. He told me my blood pressure was low, my cholesterol was low, and that I was extremely fit. He said, "Maybe you weren't meant to be a thin person."

After that, I decided that I was going to have to be satisfied with myself or I was going to waste all this energy on excessive dieting and exercise. Life is too short for that. I still lead a very active and healthy lifestyle: I swim three or four nights a week, I weight train and I eat right, but I don't worry about the number on the scale.

I am happier and I feel younger now than I did 5 years ago because I am not obsessed about my weight. I wish I had had this kind of self-confidence 5, 10, 15 years ago. It feels great walking down the beach in my bathing suit. I am who I am, and I am proud of it.

Putting Exercise into Everyday Events

Exercise is important at every stage of life. It makes you stronger and helps battle high blood pressure, heart disease, and osteoporosis. But as you get older, exercise takes on a much more important role in your weight-loss/weight-control regimen.

Exercise not only helps you lose weight but also helps you keep it off. Studies have shown that women who continue to exercise regularly are more successful at maintaining weight loss than those who do not, Dr. Foster says.

Aerobic exercise also gets rid of abdominal fat, which causes more health problems than extra pounds on any other part of the body, Dr. Fried says.

Experts now say that making movement part of your everyday life is just as effective as going to a gym a couple of times a week, Dr. Fried says.

"A lot of people think, 'If I am not out there running 5 miles a day, I am not exercising.' Now we are recommending 15 to 20 minutes of some activity—no matter how simple—every day," Dr. Kanaley adds. A study at the Cooper Institute for Aerobics Research in Dallas revealed that lifestyle physical activity—like taking a brisk walk or raking leaves—was as effective as a structured exercise program in improving physical activity, heart and respiratory fitness, blood pressure, and body fat on healthy but sedentary adults.

Whether you already have an exercise program or you're just starting out, read the following to learn how easy it is to mix physical activity into everyday tasks.

quick-and-easy, tasty meal: brown rice, whole-grain spaghetti, beans, salsa, frozen vegetables, canned fruit, low-fat pasta sauce, and low-fat chicken broth. Polk points out that many combinations of these items can make a quick, tasty meal.

Snack on fruits and vegetables. Snacking isn't evil when you're trying to lose or maintain weight—as long as you pick healthy, low-fat snacks, Polk says. When you feel the hunger set in before meals, try fresh or canned fruit, whole-wheat crackers, vegetables such as baby carrots, or a glass of low-fat or fat-free milk.

AGE ERASER

Making Weight Disappear

How can you make a few pounds disappear? By opening your closet. Here are some slimming fashion secrets that will make you appear thinner without all that hard work.

Go vertical. Vertical lines and stripes make the eye go top to bottom, giving you the appearance of being taller and slimmer.

Avoid the horizontal. Horizontal stripes draw attention to width, making you look heavier than you are.

Become a princess. Princess lines—a cut-in at the torso of your dress—create the appearance of a smaller waist.

Walk this way. Exercise trends may come and go (remember Jazzercise?), but walking is still the cheapest and easiest exercise you can do. A ½-hour walk a day is a good way to start. If you can't do it in one chunk, take several shorter walks throughout the day. If you can, make walking your primary mode of transportation, Dr. Fried says. If you can walk to the store instead of driving, do so.

Count your steps. According to Dr. Hamilton, you should take at least 10,000 steps a day. Instead of boggling your mind counting each step in your head, you can track your daily physical activity with a pedometer. Dr. Hamilton wears his, which cost him about $24, on his belt or underwear. It measures every step you take so that you can make sure you reach your 10,000 steps a day, he says. If Dr. Hamilton comes up short some days, he knows he needs to take a walk or make it up the next day. "I had to drive someplace one day, so I only made 6,000 steps. But the next day, I took a 2-mile walk and registered 13,000," he says.

Get down in the dirt. Whether you get dirty in your garden or clean your house, both activities burn off calories. "Spending a day in your garden is a great workout," Dr. Kanaley says. And although cleaning may not sound like fun, think of it as a weight-loss exercise instead of housework.

Become a fidget. Don't think that finger tapping and stretching at your desk help you lose weight? Guess again. Researchers at the Mayo Clinic in Rochester, Minnesota, fed an extra 1,000 calories a day to 16 volunteers for 8 weeks. The volunteers also wore instruments that measured their energy output. The study found that those who fidgeted stayed slim. Small movements such as finger and toe tapping, maintaining good posture, stretching, and standing up often burned calories that would have been stored as fat. You too can become a fidget. Get up and walk around every 15 minutes or so, stretch, and just keep moving during the day.

Count the little things. By taking an extra few steps, you burn off a few more calories and get a little more exercise into your day. "Be as inefficient as possible," Dr. Hamilton says. He suggests some simple yet worthwhile things to do.

- Park your car a few blocks away and walk.
- Avoid revolving doors. Open the door yourself.
- Carry your own bags. Never use the wheels on luggage.
- Use the stairs whenever possible.
- Make several trips when taking out the trash, carrying in the dishes, doing the laundry.
- Make the most of litter. When you see it, squat down, pick it up, and throw it away.

Lifting the Pounds

Getting rid of the pounds isn't always the best way to fit into a smaller dress size. In many cases, adding weight—as in free weights—is the perfect way to slim down. "Resistance training deserves its place in the components of fitness for women," says Harvey Newton, a certified strength and conditioning specialist and executive director of the National Strength and Conditioning Association (NSCA) in Colorado Springs, Colorado.

Even if you don't lose a single pound on the scale, weight training tones and firms up the body you have, making it appear sleeker and slimmer. After all, a toned 145-pound body looks much better than a nontoned 145-pound body, Newton says. And it can add a little lean body mass as well. Even this small amount will help increase your metabolism so that your body will burn more fat even at rest.

You can learn the basics of weight lifting easily from a good book or an exercise video. If you want personal guidance, check with your local health club to see if it has trainers. Be sure to ask about academic qualifications, certification from organizations such as NSCA, and references from satisfied customers.

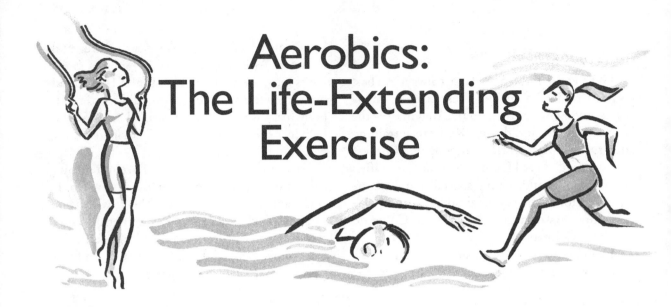

Aerobics: The Life-Extending Exercise

Air. We can't see it, and we don't think about it. But each of us breathes about 5,000 gallons of the stuff every day, and without it, we'd survive only 8 short minutes.

It's also one of the keys to staying young and healthy.

All day long our muscles and organs get a minimal amount of oxygen as we breathe normally, but if we want to take advantage of oxygen's anti-aging effects, we need to get a little extra. It turns out that the best way to do that is with aerobic exercise. That means huff-and-puff movement, like brisk walking, swimming, biking, and hiking.

When we exercise aerobically, our muscles demand more oxygen and blood than when we're just sitting on the sofa watching television. To fill the demand, our hearts beat faster and stronger, and we start to breathe more heavily.

Cash In on the Benefits

All that huffing and puffing—along with everything else that happens when we exercise—does us a great deal of good. It's like a low-risk investment that yields tremendous short- *and* long-term profits. Here are some of the immediate youth-enhancing benefits exercisers can cash in on.

Boosts metabolism. All that heart-pounding, lung-filling exercise burns a lot of calories and elevates our metabolism, says Miriam E. Nelson, Ph.D., director of the Center for Physical Fitness at Tufts University School of Nutrition Science and Policy in Boston and author of *Strong Women Stay Young*.

As women, we can use all the help we can get. When we hit our thirties, our metabolisms begin to slow by 2 to 5 percent per decade.

Our metabolic rates are already 10 to 12 percent lower than men's. That's partly because pound for pound women have more fat and less muscle than men—and fat burns virtually no calories. Muscles, on the other hand, burn lots of calories as they contract and stretch, making them our metabolism's best buddy.

Why is our metabolism so important? Because it's what helps us control our weight. As it slows, so does our body's ability to use up the calories we eat before they're converted to fat,

Dr. Nelson says. Exercise for at least 30 minutes every day, and you'll maintain or even *lose* weight by giving your metabolism a daily boost.

Boosts energy. Try this the next time you're falling asleep at your desk: Go take a brisk 10- to 15-minute walk. Chances are that you'll feel refreshed and energized when you return. "After it's over, you feel like your energy level is really surging," says John Duncan, Ph.D., an exercise physiologist at Texas Woman's University Center for Research on Women's Health in Denton. A number of things probably go on in your body to create that energy boost, he says. One is that your brain releases feel-good chemicals called endorphins—the same ones that, in excess, create the "runner's high" that marathoners often experience.

Reduces stress. Studies show that exercise is a great stress buster. And the best part is that you don't have to run a 3-minute mile to take that load off your shoulders. Researchers at the University of Georgia in Athens found that anxious college women cut their anxiety in half just by leisurely riding an exercise bike for 20 minutes.

Makes falling asleep E-Zzz. If you've been counting more sheep than a shepherd lately, you're not alone. Women age 40 and older are especially prone to insomnia as they begin to experience the hormonal changes that usher in menopause. Aerobic exercise can improve your sleep by reducing stress, tiring you out, and regulating your body temperature.

The best time to exercise for improved sleep is in the late afternoon, according to Peter Hauri, Ph.D., co-director of the Sleep Disorders Center at the Mayo Clinic in Rochester, Minnesota. The body goes through a cycle of rising and falling temperatures throughout the day. When your temperature is at its lowest point, it's easiest for you to fall asleep. Vigorous exercise in the afternoon can boost your body temperature for up to 5 hours, so your temperature will drop just in time for bed.

The worst time to work out is less than 1½ hours before you normally hit the sack, when your body temperature will still be elevated. But everyone is different, adds Dr. Nelson. As long as you cool down adequately before tucking yourself in and you don't have problems sleeping, exercising at night is fine.

Revs up your sex drive. If your libido is in low gear, exercise may give it a turbo-boost. Experts say that aerobic exercise can put the sizzle back in your sex life in a number of ways. First, it reduces stress.

When we're more relaxed, we're often more interested in having sex, says David Case, Ph.D., a research specialist in the department of psychology at the University of California, San Diego.

Exercise can also make you feel better about your body as you find yourself becoming more fit. The more attractive we feel, the friskier we usually are, he says. And finally, exercise has been found to boost the levels of the hormone responsible for sex drive in men, according to a study done by Dr. Case and colleagues at the University of California, San Diego. And that effect may be similar in women, Dr. Case says.

Eases menstrual cramps. When cramps hit, you're probably not in much of a mood for a jog. But women who exercise regularly experience fewer and less painful menstrual cramps. "We're not sure exactly how exercise helps, but it may be that fit women have tighter abdominal muscles, and that may be beneficial somehow," says Mary Lang Carney, M.D., medical director of the Center for Women's Health at St. Francis Hospital in Evanston, Illinois. Exercise also relaxes us and produces those "happy hormones" called endorphins, which may help relieve the discomfort as well.

Treats you to a natural facial. Ever hear the term *pregnant glow*? Well, exercise can give your face that same rosy radiance. The glow probably occurs after exercise because of the extra blood your heart pumps throughout your body, explains Priscilla Clarkson, Ph.D., professor of exercise science and associate dean of the University of Massachusetts School of Public Health in Amherst. What's more, women who exercise regularly may feel better about themselves. And when you're happier, your face tends to exude that charisma, she says.

Disease-Proof Your Body

While the immediate benefits of aerobic exercise may be remarkable, its long-term benefits are even more impressive. Regular exercise increases your vitality, endurance, flexibility, and balance—all things that tend to decline as we age. Fit women not only live longer, they also function as well as unfit people 20 years their junior. But the most significant benefit of exercise is undoubtedly its role in disease prevention. "If you look at a list of all the health problems that occur as you age, exercise has been shown to reduce almost all of them," Dr. Clarkson says. "There's no pill, no medicine that can do that, but exercise can." Here are just some of the conditions exercise can counteract.

Heart disease. Regular aerobic exercise helps prevent heart disease by improving several risk factors: It lowers blood pressure and cholesterol, controls weight, reduces stress, and improves cardiovascular fitness, says Elizabeth Ross, M.D., a cardiologist at Washington Hospital Center in Washington, D.C. The link between exercise and heart health is so strong that even people who already have heart disease can lower their risk of having a heart attack by exercising.

CELLULITE: IS IT INEVITABLE?

Dimples on our cheeks are cute. Dimples on our thighs and butts are not. In fact, cellulite ranks with wrinkles and gray hair as one of the most unwelcome signs of aging.

To get rid of the ripples, women have tried everything from exotic creams to deep massage. But as you might expect, a low-fat diet and regular aerobic exercise turn out to be the most effective therapies. That's because the primary cause of cellulite is weight gain.

When you put on weight, your fat layers expand, but not in a smooth, uniform way, explains Grant J. Anhalt, M.D., acting chief of dermatology at Johns Hopkins University School of Medicine in Baltimore. There are areas where the skin is anchored down by fibrous bands that tunnel through the fat and attach to the muscle. It's those anchors that cause dimpling.

"It's more pronounced in women who are overweight," says Toby Shawe, M.D., assistant professor of dermatology at the Medical College of Pennsylvania–Hahnemann University Hospitals in Philadelphia. "But practically every woman—overweight or not—will get some degree of cellulite," she says.

We can thank our hormones for that. Part of the female hormone estrogen promotes weight gain on the thighs and butt, says Dr. Shawe.

When fat cells take residence on the lower half of the body, they are more likely to get crowded and push against the skin, which creates the bulged and puckered look of cellulite.

Cancer. Exercisers have a lower risk of developing breast and colon cancer. An 11-year study of more than 1,800 women (average age 75) conducted by James R. Cerhan, M.D., Ph.D., and researchers at the Mayo Clinic in Rochester, Minnesota, found that those who walked, gardened, or did housework several times a week cut their breast cancer risk to half that of inactive women, while those who did more vigorous activity—such as swimming or running—at least once a week were 80 percent less likely to develop

As we age, our skin also tends to lose its tautness, especially if we don't exercise. Exercise tones the muscles underneath the skin, which keeps skin taut and eliminates surface lines that can show up on skin stretched by fat. And that can add to the rippling effect.

Genetics play a role as well. "Cellulite is often more noticeable in some people because of heredity," Dr. Anhalt says.

But the years don't have to deposit dimples where they aren't wanted. "The best way to get rid of cellulite is to prevent it," says Jessica Fewkes, M.D., assistant professor of dermatology at Harvard Medical School. "That means starting early with good habits like exercise and a healthy diet."

If the dimples have already developed, you have a few choices. First, you can simply learn to live with them—and still be a very attractive woman. "It's not going to detract from you as a woman unless you let it," Dr. Fewkes says.

Or you can lose those extra pounds and tone your hips, thighs, and buttocks with exercise. Two other options are liposuction, which removes the excess fat, or a mechanical massage called Endermologie, which smooths out the dimples. But either of those will cost you a bundle—from several hundred to several thousand dollars, depending on the procedure. Endermologie averages $1,400 for a series of treatments.

As for massage and those creams that claim to reduce cellulite: "They don't work," Dr. Anhalt says.

Stroke. Regular exercise can cut your stroke risk in half, according to a recent study conducted by researchers at the Harvard School of Public Health. Swimming 5 hours a week, gardening 6 hours a week, or walking an hour a day for 5 days a week are all ways of dramatically reducing your chances of having a stroke.

Depression. Exercise can help relieve mild depression by raising levels of feel-good substances in the brain and by reducing stress, according to June Primm, Ph.D., a clinical psychologist and associate professor of pediatrics and psychology at the University of Miami School of Medicine. In fact, several studies have shown that aerobic exercise is just as effective as psychotherapy at treating mild depression.

Osteoporosis. Regular exercise can help prevent osteoporosis, the disease that causes women's bones to become so weak that they easily break. A study of nearly 240 postmenopausal women between the ages of 43 and 72 found that those who walked about a mile a day (7.5 miles a week) had denser bones than women who walked less than a mile a week.

Arthritis. At one time doctors told patients with arthritis *not* to exercise. But now we know that exercise—especially walking—can actually ease arthritis pain. A study at Wake Forest University in Winston-Salem, North Carolina, assigned elderly people with arthritis of the knee to do aerobic exercise, strength training, or no exercise. After a year, those who did best were in the aerobic exercise group. They reported less pain and disability than the nonexercise group and were able to walk, climb stairs, and get in and out of the car more easily.

breast cancer. And when it comes to colon cancer, in 1996 the Surgeon General's report concluded that physical activity protects against it.

Diabetes. People who exercise regularly have a significantly lower risk of developing type 2 diabetes. A 6-year study of more than 8,600 subjects, conducted by researchers at the Cooper Institute for Aerobics Research in Dallas, found that those who were least fit had a four times greater risk of developing diabetes than those who were most fit.

WOMAN TO WOMAN

She Walked Off the Weight and Feels Years Younger

As she approached the big 4-0, Terri Politi was 25 pounds over-weight—and painfully aware of every extra pound. Her clothes didn't fit right, she felt flabby, and, perhaps worst of all, increasingly sluggish. In other words: old. Then, 5 months before her birthday, the Sedalia, Missouri, resident, now 41, found the secret to weight loss and peeled off 20 pounds in 4 months. Here's how she turned back the clock.

There I was, hitting one of those big milestones in life, and I was feeling heavier than ever—even heavier than when I was pregnant. I thought, "It's going to be hard enough just to turn 40. I want to do this gracefully." I knew that I could feel better and look better if I just set my mind to it. So in September, I started my quest and gave myself only a few months—by my birthday in January—to reach my goal.

Weight Watchers helped me get a handle on my eating, and that was important, but I wanted to do more. So I began working out with free weights early in the morning, at least three times a week for about 20 minutes each session.

I did start to feel better, yet even that wasn't enough. I decided to start walking on our treadmill for 30 to 35 minutes after every weight workout. I had just enough time to do that, see the kids off to school, jump in the shower, and be at work by 8:00 A.M.

Then, one of my girlfriends at the office and I decided to start a walking program. We have a big church here in town, which had put in a gymnasium, so during lunch break, we went over to check it out. When we found out that 14 times around the gym was a mile, we made it our goal to walk a mile or more three times a week.

Sure enough, by the time January rolled around, I had lost 20 pounds—so I bought myself a little brown dress with a border print along the bottom. I had never owned a simple straight-cut dress before because I always felt my hips were too big to wear something like that. But I like how I look and feel in it.

I have so much energy now and feel so much better about myself that I don't feel like I'm over 40 anymore. I feel as if I'm in my midthirties again.

Liven Up Your Lifestyle

Escalators. Leaf blowers. Riding lawn mowers and self-propelled vacuum cleaners. Remote controls. Power windows.

Little by little we have managed to engineer physical activity out of our lives, says Russell Pate, Ph.D., professor and chairperson of the department of exercise science at the University of South Carolina in Columbia. In fact, a Scottish researcher estimates that people in the United Kingdom burn 800 fewer calories a day compared to 25 years ago.

In the United States, 60 percent of the population incorporates little or no physical activity into their lives. If you're among America's legion of couch potatoes, here's some good news: You don't have to take up tennis or become a marathon runner to enjoy the benefits of exercise. Research shows simply increasing your physical activity provides the same health benefits as a structured exercise program—which is why most experts now recommend trying to work 30 minutes of accumulated moderate activity into your day.

The key word here is *accumulated*. Ten minutes here and there of raking, vacuuming, walking, and playing catch with the kids all adds up. "To make your lifestyle more active, think about what you need to do each day and how you can make those tasks more physical," Dr. Clarkson suggests. That may mean selling the leaf blower and canning your cleaning lady. Or you can try some of the following lifestyle-makeover tips from our experts.

Turn off the TV. "The first step toward improving your fitness is limiting your sedentary activity," Dr. Nelson says. And one of the most common inactive pastimes is watching TV. Even if you're not a channel-surfing TV junkie, you probably turn on the set at least a few times a week. Try to cut back by 1 hour every week until you've managed to trim an hour of sitcoms, soaps, or game shows from each day. You'll be surprised at how much time you'll have on your hands.

If you can't bear to miss an episode of *NYPD Blue*, then put a piece of exercise equipment—like a treadmill or stationary bike—in front of the tube and turn your TV time into a workout, suggests Dr. Ross.

Walk and talk. If you have a cordless telephone, take advantage of your wireless freedom. Walk around the house or up and down the stairs while chatting on the phone. You'll catch up with your friends while you catch a short workout.

Dodge the drive-through. More and more service businesses are installing drive-up windows for our convenience: banks, fast-food restaurants, even drugstores and photo developers. "As we take on these conveniences, we don't realize how much they decrease the amount of physical activity in our daily lives," Dr. Clarkson says. So resist the quick convenience of the drive-up window and walk into the bank to make your transaction.

Pick the farthest spot. When it comes to your health, the best parking spot is not the one that's closest. Park a few blocks away, and you can work in a quick walk, Dr. Pate says.

Take the stairs. Make a conscious effort to use the stairs instead of an elevator or escalator,

Dr. Pate says. It may not seem that significant, but think about how often you'd opt for stairs. Every day? Once a week? A few times a month? No matter what, it can really add up.

Eliminate e-mail. If you send e-mail to coworkers who are in the next office or just down the hall, consider taking an e-mail vacation. Deliver the message in person, and you'll save yourself from gaining 11 pounds over a decade. That's how much weight a Stanford University researcher calculated you would gain if you spent 2 minutes an hour sending e-mails to coworkers instead of walking down the hall to speak to them.

Pay the pound a visit. Getting a dog may help get you off your duff. Pups make great walking partners—and they don't let you off the hook easily when a walk may not be what you had in mind.

Plant a garden. Playing in the dirt was fun when we were kids. And now that we're grown-ups, we can make more than mud pies. Whether you grow flowers, herbs, or vegetables, you'll burn almost as many calories as taking a moderate aerobics class—plus you'll connect with the earth, says Dr. Nelson.

12 Tips for a Better Workout

Fitness is a step-by-step progression, Dr. Nelson says. If you're already fairly active—or you've recently succeeded in adding more physical activity to your lifestyle—the next step to getting fit is simple: Whatever you're doing now, do *more*.

This is where aerobic exercise comes in. But don't worry. You still don't have to join a health club or take an aerobics class (unless you want to). The great thing about aerobic exercise is that there are so many different activities to choose from—dancing, biking, swimming, playing tennis. The list goes on and on.

No matter which activities you choose, you'll get the most out of your workout if you follow these practical pointers.

Put on your dancing shoes. If you're dancing, that is. And running shoes if you're running. Walking shoes if you're walking. You get the idea. "As we get older, our feet, ankles, shins, and knees are more vulnerable," says Joan Price, certified fitness instructor, speaker, and writer from Sebastopol, California, and author of *Joan Price Says, Yes, You Can Get in Shape!* "Wearing the right shoes for your activity can protect you by cushioning and stabilizing your feet and basically serving as mini-shock-absorbers."

Seek out support. When you work out, make sure that you wear an appropriate sports bra that holds your breasts close to your body, Dr. Nelson suggests. Otherwise, all the movement that's involved in aerobic exercise can start your breasts sagging southward. "It amazes me that a lot of women don't wear a sports bra when they exercise," she says. "When you don't, the repeated movement will actually stretch the breast tissue and make it less elastic."

Warm up. Your car isn't the only thing that needs to be warmed up before all its parts are lubricated and ready to roll—you have your own engine and parts that need to run a few minutes before shifting into high gear. "A warmup provides a gradual transition from rest to the physiologic demands of exercise," Dr. Pate says. Basically, a good warmup gets your blood pumping, limbers up your ligaments and tendons, and loosens your muscles so that you reduce your risk of injury.

Light stretching and a slow version of the activity you're about to do work best, Dr. Pate says. Walk more slowly before you pick up the pace, for example, or swing the racket and hit a few balls before playing a round of tennis. You could even march or jog in place—anything that gets your arms and legs moving for 5 minutes.

Cool down and stretch. Your body needs to downshift its gears slowly, rather than going from brisk walking to a sudden halt. The cooldown is similar to the warmup, only instead of gradually picking up the pace, you gradually slow it down. This lowers your heart rate gradually so that you don't feel dizzy or faint, Dr. Nelson explains.

After your workout is also the best time to stretch because your muscles are still warm. A good 20- to 30-second stretch of each of the major muscle groups—that's your arms, legs, abdomen, back, and rear end—helps to build flexibility and prevent injury.

Beat blisters. Whether you walk, jog, hike, or hit the tennis courts, a bad case of blisters can put the brakes on your physical activity fast. To prevent blisters before they start, cover your clean, dry feet with your regular antiperspirant, suggests lead researcher Joseph Knapick, Sc.D., at the U.S. Army Center for Health Promotion and Preventative Medicine in Aberdeen Proving Ground, Maryland.

You can use any kind—spray, stick, or roll-on. Just make sure to hit every nook and cranny of your feet. Try it every day for 5 days before your run or hike, or use it once or twice a week indefinitely. It works by reducing sweat, which creates the friction that causes blisters. And it helped 80 percent of U.S. Army cadets stay blister-free after a 13-mile hike.

One note of caution: If you develop a rash or experience any skin irritation, try using the antiperspirant every other day or switch brands. If the irritation continues, stop using it.

Drink up. When you exercise, you sweat out more fluids than you would just sitting on the couch. And since your muscles are about 70 percent water, you need to replenish those fluids so that you don't start to feel weak before your workout's over. A good rule of thumb is to drink an 8-ounce glass of water before and after you exercise and to have half a cup every 15 to 20 minutes during your workout, says Felicia Busch, R.D., a nutritionist in St. Paul, Minnesota, and a spokesperson for the American Dietetic Association.

Leave your worries behind. To get the relaxation benefit of exercise, you have to wind down while you're working out. We already mentioned a study conducted at the University of Georgia in Athens where stressed-out college students cut their anxiety in half by riding exercise bikes for 20 minutes. Simply taking time out from daily worries may have been responsible for the drop in anxiety, the study authors say, because another group of women who studied while riding still had high anxiety levels afterward.

Add weights to firm flab. Many experts recommend combining your aerobic exercise with strength training. Why? Because together they give your flab a one-two punch. "Aerobic exercise burns fat while strength training tones muscle," Dr. Nelson says. And the result is a firmer, shapelier body.

What's more, strength training gives your metabolism an extra boost by building muscle, which burns more calories.

And the stronger your muscles are, the more you'll get out of your aerobic workout. "You'll be able to exercise longer, and you won't feel as tired afterward," Dr. Nelson says.

Slow down the music. The aim isn't to add romance to your workout, but to keep the music at a comfortable pace, especially if you're participating in an aerobics class that requires fancy footwork or using a step. "The music should be slow enough for you to put your foot all the way down," Price says. "Staying on your toes because the music is too fast puts you at risk to injure your foot or leg." If you feel uncomfortable asking the instructor to use slower music, or if you're using a workout video and can't change

the music's speed, then do the move at half-speed, she suggests.

Make it fun. When we were kids, exercise was a ball. We sprinted up the stairs, we ran home for dinner, we jumped when we heard something exciting, and we looked forward to recess. "Exercise should still be playtime," Dr. Ross says. "Most women have so many responsibilities in addition to their jobs that if exercise becomes just one more thing on our 'must do' list, we won't stick with it. That's why I encourage women to find something that's fun. Put the kids in a stroller and the dog on a leash and go for a walk. Dance with your husband for 15 minutes before you sit down to eat. Take the kids roller-skating or ice-skating. Or go for a bike ride."

Grab a partner. Even if you're not square dancing, a partner can help you out in several ways. First, she can motivate you when you're feeling tired or discouraged, Dr. Nelson says. Second, exercising with a friend can turn your workout into a social activity—so it's more fun. And most important, a friend can help you stay committed. If you don't feel like exercising but your friend is counting on you, you're more likely to put on those sneakers and hit the road.

Stick with it. Cardiovascular fitness requires maintenance. If you work out 5 days a week for several weeks, for example, and then cut back to exercising just 1 day a week, you'll lose 90 percent of your gains in 12 weeks, Dr. Duncan says. So do yourself—and your heart—a favor and make exercise a permanent part of your routine.

Weather Your Workout

Many women use their workouts as a way to take in some scenery. But exercising outdoors brings with it comfort and safety issues. These simple tips will help you weather your workout so that you can enjoy your time in the great outdoors.

WOMEN ASK WHY

Both of my knees are the same age, so why is one causing me all kinds of trouble when I exercise?

While both of your knees are the same age, they aren't always subject to the same punishment. Do you favor one hand over another when you write, drive, or toss a ball? Chances are good that you've battered one of your knees more often when walking, jumping—or even falling—over the years.

That cumulative punishment is called microdamage. But as we get older, it can cause big problems. Like a dried-out rubber band, our connective tissues simply become less flexible, making them more prone to tearing.

So how can you avoid knee pain while—or after—you exercise? For one thing, you need to start slowly. Our bodies do change and adapt to our workouts, but not if we try too much all at once. The key is to increase your activity and intensity gradually over time.

If you do begin to experience some pain—whether it's in a knee, ankle, or some other joint—that's your body's way of telling you that you need to slow down. If your pain is minor and goes away in a day or so, you probably won't have to stop exercising, but proceed with caution.

If your pain persists or is severe, you'll need some rest and treatment. One of the most common therapies for knee or ankle pain is called RICE—an acronym that stands for rest, ice, compression (wrapping with a bandage), and elevation. When using ice in a pack or bag, make sure to cover it with a thin towel to protect the skin. If you don't feel better after 2 or 3 days' rest, you may need to see a doctor.

Expert consulted
Russell Pate, Ph.D.
Professor and chairperson of the department
of exercise science
University of South Carolina
Columbia

Save your skin. Always apply sunscreen to any part of your body that's exposed. This simple habit will help prevent wrinkling and skin cancer, says Grant Anhalt, M.D., acting chief of dermatology at Johns Hopkins University School of Medicine in Baltimore. Wear a sunscreen with a sun protection factor (SPF) of 15 if you're out in the morning or late afternoon. But switch to an SPF of 30 to 45 if you're out between 10:00 A.M. and 2:00 P.M. for substantial periods of time—like if you're shooting 18 holes, fishing, or boating, he says.

Shade your eyes. Eye doctors at Johns Hopkins University School of Medicine polled more than 2,500 people on their history of sun exposure. Those who had been in the sun the most had a 57 percent greater likelihood of having a cataract. The best way to protect your peepers is to wear sunglasses or clear prescription glasses and a wide-brimmed hat whenever you exercise outdoors—even in the winter when snow causes sun glare, says Dr. Pate.

Follow the dress code. If you bike, walk, or jog during the day, wear bright colors so that drivers can easily spot you. If you work out at night, dawn, or dusk, outfit yourself with some type of reflective gear so that you can be seen from the front and rear. And make sure to sport bright or reflective clothes on rainy and foggy days, too.

Layer it on. If you weather winter workouts, make sure to put on several layers of clothing. That way you can shed layers as needed so that you don't overheat. It may feel frigid outside, but your body temperature will rise as you exercise, and you may get hot, Dr. Duncan explains.

If it's really cold, experts suggest wearing three layers. Use fabrics such as Coolmax, polypropylene, or ThermaStat blends as an inner layer to wick moisture away from the skin. As a middle layer, insulate by trapping a layer of warm air next to your body with fleece, wool, or Bipolar fabric. The outer layer should shield you from weather extremes. Gore-Tex, fleece, and wind jackets and pants are all good outer protectors.

Outsmart hay fever. If you find yourself sneezing and rubbing your eyes during allergy season, avoid exercising in the morning or move your workout indoors, suggests Carol Wiggins, M.D., clinical instructor of allergy and immunology at Emory University in Atlanta. During fall and spring hay-fever seasons, the pollen count is highest between the hours of 5:00 and 8:00 A.M. and lowest at night.

Slather after laps. Whether you swim indoors or out, slather on a moisturizer after finishing those laps. Swimming washes away the natural lipids in your skin, making it dry and itchy, says Dr. Anhalt. The best time to moisturize is right after getting out of the pool when your skin is still wet. Doing so helps seal in the moisture that's still on your skin. Moisturizing immediately after getting out of the shower will help to further prevent dry skin.

Toning: The Full-Body Face-Lift

The average newborn in the United States weighs 7 pounds. The average grocery bag weighs even more. And the average piece of furniture . . . well, women know a lot about heavy lifting.

And since we're doing so much of it anyway, we may as well turn all that lifting to our advantage. After all, if we do it in a regular, organized way, it can make us look younger, feel stronger, and live longer. We don't necessarily want to use the baby, a sack of cantaloupes, or the sofa, of course. Dumbbells are more like what the doctor ordered—and not the kind of dumbbell that gets all your toppings wrong when you order pizza over the telephone, but rather the kind that bodybuilders use.

Pump Iron to Stop the Clock

Did the word *bodybuilder* make you cringe? Don't worry. You won't bulk up like a female Arnold Schwarzenegger. Instead, you'll slow the sagging and bulging that begins as gravity starts to get the better of us in our midthirties. That's when many of us start to lose one-fourth to one-third of a pound of muscle every year and replace it with fat because of slowing metabolism and a less active lifestyle.

The problem is that fat takes up more space than muscle, so even if you don't gain a pound, your clothes will gradually feel tighter as you grow older. It doesn't look good, and it doesn't feel good.

So if the problem is to keep fat off, why don't we just diet?

It's true that as we get older, we can ward off wiggly arms and thighs by controlling our weight. But eventually, even thin women will see signs of sagging. That's where strength training comes in. "I think if there's one thing that really is the elixir of youth for women as they age, it's strength training," says Joan Price, a certified fitness instructor, speaker, and writer from Sebastopol, California, and author of *Joan Price Says, Yes, You Can Get in Shape!*

Shed Excuses, Shed Years

But I'm too old to start lifting weights. Is that what you're thinking? Think again.

"We have women in their nineties who are strength-training and doing really well," says Miriam E. Nelson, Ph.D., director of the Center for Physical Fitness at Tufts University School of Nutrition Science and Policy in Boston and author of *Strong Women Stay Slim* and *Strong Women Stay Young*. "Certainly, we love for women to start at a younger age, but if you're already 75 or 92, then that's the right age to start."

Okay, maybe I'm not too old, but I'm barely able to take the time to eat, let alone spend a few hours in a leotard lifting weights at a gym. This is an excellent excuse. You're to be commended. Unfortunately, it won't work. Just ditch the leotard and plan to stay home.

All it takes to tone your trouble zones are two or three at-home sessions a week. You can even break up the sessions into smaller workouts. Best of all, you will see dramatic changes in your body in about a month, and most women get a big energy boost right away, says Dr. Nelson.

More Than Skin Deep

The benefits to resistance training go way beyond reshaping your body.

A study done by Dr. Nelson and her colleagues at the Jean Mayer USDA Human Nutrition Research Center on Aging at Tufts University found that 20 women who began a strength-training program sometime after menopause com-

WOMAN TO WOMAN

She Looks and Feels Far Younger Than Her Years

Filomena Warihay, president of an international consulting firm in Downingtown, Pennsylvania, still slips into her size 4 bikini at age 61. But she hasn't always been so fit and trim. Her body was slowly giving in to time and gravity, when a chance invitation from her daughter introduced her to a whole new way of life. From that day on, her body seemed to grow younger. Here's her story.

I haven't always had the body I have today. I really struggled to fit in workouts when I had four small children to take care of. I would sit them in a wagon and pull them up and down the street to get in a walk. I parked my car a mile from work and walked the rest of the way.

Then, when I was 40, one of my daughters was awarded a full athletic scholarship to college. When she received her summer training schedule, she realized that she'd have to go to the gym 3 days a week. She begged me to go with her. I did, but my primary motivation was to help her get her college education paid for.

After we'd gone to the gym for a while, my daughter said, "Mom, I bet you could run a mile." Well, I tried, and I couldn't. We went over to the track, and it was pitiful. But we stayed with it, and by the middle of the summer, I ran in a local 5-K race. To my surprise, I came in second or third in my age category. I've won a medal in that race every year since.

Now I'm even more disciplined about exercising. I work out 6 days a week, either running 6 miles outdoors, chugging away on my stairclimber, or going to the gym. I lift weights and do 400 crunches every other day and stretch daily for about 15 minutes. I actually feel better now than when I was 30. And I'm within 5 pounds of what I weighed when I graduated from high school.

Most people think I'm in my forties, and I'm not ashamed to tell them the truth. Nor am I embarrassed to wear any of my six or so bikinis. Still, every year I say to my husband, "Maybe this is the last year I'll be able to wear a bikini." And he always says, "I'll tell you when."

pletely transformed their bodies—inside and out. After a year of doing a five-exercise workout twice a week, the women were in the same physical condition as women 15 to 20 years younger, says Dr. Nelson. Here are some of the anti-aging benefits these women gained from strength training.

Thinner physique. The women in the study were told to stick with their normal diet so that they wouldn't gain or lose weight during the 1-year period. The women doing the strength training may not have dropped pounds, but they lost fat and gained muscle. They looked much leaner, and some even dropped as many as two dress sizes.

Higher metabolism. Although your metabolism tends to slow down as you get older, making it more difficult to maintain your weight, there are ways to speed it up again. Increasing the amount of muscle you have is one. That's because muscle tissue burns more calories than fat. One woman in the study gave her metabolism a major boost: She lost 29 pounds of fat and, as a result, now burns 160 extra calories a day.

Increased strength. Dr. Nelson's study showed that within 2 months, women typically double the amount of weight they can lift. That's good news for a lot of people. According to one study of 10,000 women ages 40 to 55, more than one-fourth struggle with everyday tasks such as carrying groceries or walking up a flight of stairs.

More energy. As the women in Dr. Nelson's study became stronger, they felt more energized

REAL-LIFE SCENARIO
Is She Destined to Look Like Her Mom?

Every time Nancy, 44, looks at her mom, she gets a sinking feeling in the pit of her stomach. What she sees is a woman, only in her sixties, who is hunched over, shuffling in her step, overweight, and covered with age spots. Her mother's face seems leathery and more wrinkled than it ought to be, covered with fine lines, especially around the lips. What unsettles Nancy most is looking through old family albums. Her mother had been such a beauty. There's one picture, in particular, of her lounging on a veranda in a hotel in sunny Puerto Rico, a martini in one hand and a cigarette in the other, and the most dazzling smile on her face. She was breathtaking, sophisticated. But that person seemed to have disappeared entirely over the years, and in her place is a woman whom Nancy still very much loves . . . but doesn't want to become. She's desperate to find some way to avoid her mother's fate.

Nancy is not on a predestined path to premature aging. Although genetics *does* play a role in how we look as we age, the health and lifestyle habits we follow when we're younger can determine much of how we look when we're older.

The photo of Nancy's mother reveals several habits that may have added years to her appearance.

For starters, smoking can cause premature and pronounced wrinkling—especially around the lips—because it robs the skin of two things it needs to be healthy: oxygen and vitamin C. Not to mention that smoking increases your risk for more serious conditions, such as heart disease and cancer. Her mother's smoking habit also may have contributed to her hunched-over posture, which is a sign of os-

and began doing things that they hadn't done in years—or had never done at all. They went canoeing, river rafting, dancing, bicycle riding, and skating. By the end of the study, the women in the strength-training group were 27 percent

teoporosis. That's a condition that turns your bones so brittle that they easily break. Smoking weakens your skeleton in two ways: It interferes with bone formation and promotes bone loss. Because osteoporosis is often genetic, Nancy may be at increased risk. But she can reduce her risk by not smoking and by getting 1,000 milligrams of calcium a day through diet and supplements.

The martini in her mother's hand may seem innocent enough, but regular alcohol intake can weaken bones and contribute to wrinkling as well. And alcoholic beverages are loaded with "empty" calories, meaning they provide no nutrition, which may have led to another one of her mother's problems—weight gain. To protect her bones and maintain her weight, Nancy should stick to drinking no more than one alcoholic drink a day.

From the photo, it appears her mother was also a sun worshiper. Sun damage is the number one cause of wrinkles and leathery skin—as well as those age spots. Unprotected exposure to the sun can also lead to skin cancer. For the health of her skin, Nancy should avoid sunbathing and should wear sunscreen with a sun protection factor (SPF) of at least 15 whenever she goes outdoors.

Another important stay-young strategy is regular exercise. Aerobic exercise combined with strength training can help Nancy maintain her weight, prevent osteoporosis, and improve her posture and balance—so instead of shuffling, she'll be *springing* in her step when she hits 60.

Expert consulted
Clarita E. Herrera, M.D.
Clinical instructor of primary care
New York Medical College
Valhalla

same USDA laboratory, strength training was found to be comparable to antidepressant drugs at fighting depression, which affects far more women than men.

Added bone. After menopause, women typically lose 1 percent of their bone mass each year. Over time, eight million women develop osteoporosis, a condition in which bones become so brittle that they easily break. The strength-training group in Dr. Nelson's study *gained* 1 percent of bone density, while those who didn't strength-train *lost* about 2 percent.

Better balance. Our balance deteriorates as we age, making us more likely to suffer a bad fall. The women in the study who didn't do strength training experienced an $8\frac{1}{2}$ percent decline in balance, while those who lifted weights improved their balance by 14 percent.

Gearing Up: What You Need to Get Started

For hundreds of dollars less than a one-year gym membership, you can buy everything you need to start our body-shaping program now. And just imagine what you'll save on leotards. Here's how to equip yourself.

Pick up some dumbbells. Also called free weights, they are available in 1-pound increments from 1 to 20 pounds. Beginners may want to start out with lighter weights. Pairs of 3-, 5-, 8-, and 10-pound dumbbells should do the job and will run anywhere from around $25 to $55 for all four pairs.

more active than a year before, while the group that hadn't done strength training had become 25 percent *less* active in that year.

Improved mood. Lifting weights can lift your spirits. In another study conducted at the

They even come in pretty pastel colors.

Purchase some padding. A foam mat can turn any floor into a home gym. Mats are great for floor stretches, pushups, and crunches, and they cost around $10.

Have a seat. You will need a sturdy chair without arms for at least one exercise we describe later. A few others—such as the biceps curl and the overhead press—can be done either standing or seated. A chair from your dining room set may fill the bill.

Dress the part. As promised, no leotard. But you will need a pair of athletic shoes. "A good pair of athletic shoes offers both stability when you're doing the exercises and some protection, just in case you drop a free weight," says Price. You should also wear comfortable clothes made of a breathable fabric like a cotton/synthetic blend.

"Avoid wearing anything that could impair your range of motion or anything so baggy that a weight could become lodged in your clothing," says John Duncan, Ph.D., an exercise physiologist at Texas Woman's University Center for Research on Women's Health in Denton.

Strength Training 101

Like any sport or activity, strength training has tricks to learn and techniques to master. Strength training can involve using weights or your own body weight to challenge and build muscle. Here's a quick lesson to help you get the most from your workout.

Know the lingo. The words *rep* and *set* are the jargon of gym junkies. We will decode

> ### SHAPE UP WITH THE STARS
>
> How do Hollywood celebs keep their sleek physiques? With a hot strengthening and stretching program called the Pilates Method of Body Conditioning.
>
> This method, developed over 70 years ago by German gymnast, boxer, and circus performer Joseph Pilates, caught on in the 1950s among top dancers who wanted to stay in shape and prevent injury. Unlike most exercise programs, Pilates simultaneously works on strength, flexibility, and balance. Now it's toning up stunning stars like Madonna, Sharon Stone, Jane Seymour, Vanessa Williams, Uma Thurman, Julia Roberts, and Jodie Foster. What's more, because of its effect on conditioning, suppleness, and balance, it may be one secret to staying young.
>
> The Pilates Method (pronounced "puh-LAH-teez") promises to make you look taller and leaner and to build strength and flexibility—without developing bodybuilder-size muscles. It will leave you with a slimmer shape, improve your posture and balance, and give better overall function to your body. And best of all, you'll start to see results in a matter of weeks. The method's inventor offers this guarantee: "You will feel better in 10 sessions, look better in 20 sessions, and have a completely new body in 30 sessions."
>
> Here's how it works. Each session lasts 45 minutes to an hour and takes you through a series of precise, controlled movements that require concentration and controlled breathing. The main focus of the Pilates Method is to

them for you. One rep, or repetition, describes one complete exercise. So one pushup, for example, would be one rep. A set is just that—a set of repetitions. Dr. Nelson recommends doing two sets of 8 to 12 repetitions for each exercise. Start with 8 repetitions in each set. When you can easily do 12, you can add a little more weight.

Work out between meals. Right after eating a Thanksgiving feast is not the best time to pick up a pair of dumbbells. "If your stomach

strengthen the "powerhouse" of your anatomy—the abdomen, lower back, and buttocks—to enable the rest of your body to move more freely. You use continuous, flowing movements and low repetitions to tone without bulking. There are 19 apparatuses with unusual names like Pedipull, Reformer, and Cadillac, which help strengthen your muscles through a full range of motion. Or you can do your entire workout on a mat. Ideally, you should do two to three sessions per week.

The method incorporates 500 exercises, but you'll probably do only 30 to 40 per session and may learn only a total of 50 to 60. That's because certified Pilates trainers design a workout to meet your personal fitness goals.

"This is probably the most widely adaptable exercise system that's available today," says Sean P. Gallagher, a physical therapist and national director of the Pilates Studio in New York City. "You can use this system whether you're completely out of shape or you're a superstar athlete. I've worked with amputees, people with head injuries, young people, and even people in their eighties."

Women who've tried Pilates rave about the results. After just 40 sessions, 49-year-old Patricia Scanlon of Philadelphia feels more than a decade younger. "My waist is smaller, my stomach is tighter, my posture is better, and I'm stronger and more energetic," she says. "The strengthening you do with Pilates is so deep. I'm getting down into muscles I never felt before. It's sort of like a massage from the inside out."

is really full, you're going to feel uncomfortable," Dr. Nelson says. It is also unwise to work out when you haven't eaten for several hours. "If you're starving, you may get light-headed," she says. To be at your best, try to work out midway between meals or have a light meal or snack an hour or so beforehand.

Warm up. We're not talking about drinking hot cocoa by a toasty fire. We mean warming up your muscles for 5 to 10 minutes so that you don't go directly from sitting in front of the TV to lifting 12-pound weights over your head. Muscles much prefer being eased into exercise. To warm up, you can take a brisk walk, do jumping jacks, march or jog in place, or do toning exercises for 5 to 10 reps without weights. If you do an aerobic workout in addition to resistance training, says Dr. Nelson, you can do the aerobics first, in place of a warmup.

Pick the right weight. If you lift weights that are too heavy, you could hurt yourself. On the other hand, lifting weights that are too light won't do much to firm your flab. Here's a good rule of thumb: If you can't lift the weight in good form 8 times, then it's too heavy, Dr. Nelson says. But if you can easily lift the weight more than 12 times, it's too light.

Lift with a friend. Beginners may want to find a weight buddy. That person serves three purposes. First, she can lend a hand if you tire and struggle through that last repetition, Dr. Duncan says. Second, she can watch to make sure that you are using good form. And third, she can offer the encouragement that first-time lifters often need.

Don't wait to exhale. Strange as it may sound, many weight lifters literally hold their breath, which can cause their blood pressures to spike. The proper way to breathe, says Dr. Nelson, is to exhale on the exertion—when you lift the weight or do the crunch—and inhale as you lower the weight or return to the starting position.

Tame the tension. "When we contract one muscle, we have a tendency to tense the others as well. But during strength training, only the muscles you're working should contract," writes Dr. Nelson in her book *Strong Women Stay Young*. Some common trouble spots to check: Make sure that you're not clenching your teeth, furrowing your brow, or tensing your shoulders up around your ears.

Take it slow. Fast, herky-jerky movements can cause injury. They can also cause you to use momentum, rather than muscle, to lift weight. Slow, controlled movements, on the other hand, are safer and take more effort—so you get more benefit, Price says. Each repetition should take about 6 seconds: 2 seconds to lift the weight, a 2-second pause, and then another 2 seconds to lower the weight.

Perfect your form. Good form—doing an exercise in exactly the right way—helps you get the most benefit from lifting and prevents injury, says Price. An easy way to watch your lifting form is to position yourself in front of a full-length mirror. Make sure that your wrists are straight, not bent backward or forward. And be sure that you are doing the exercise precisely as it is shown.

Pay attention to posture. Whether you're sitting or standing when you lift dumbbells, keep your back, neck, and head straight to prevent muscle strain and injury. And good posture doesn't mean standing stiff. Stand tall but relaxed. If you're seated to do the exercise, sit up straight with your feet flat on the floor, recommends Dr. Nelson.

PERK UP YOUR POSTURE

Let's play detective. We walk along a dimly lit street and see two feminine figures looming in the shadows. Without seeing their faces, it's clear that one woman is far older than the other. What gives away her age? Posture. One woman stands straight as a pencil and the other bends over like a banana.

The good news is that even banana-shaped women can take steps to straighten up—and there are plenty of reasons to undo the hunch. For starters, correct posture prevents muscle and bone pain and allows us to breathe properly. Standing up straight can make us look taller, thinner, younger, and more confident. And good posture helps our clothing to fit its best. That's because clothes are cut for people with "normal" posture, says Margit L. Bleecker, M.D., Ph.D., director of the Center for Occupational and Environmental Neurology in Baltimore.

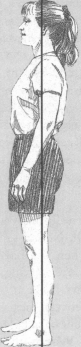

But we don't have to have the posture of a ballerina to reap the benefits. "There is no such thing as perfect posture," Dr. Bleecker says. "There's a spectrum of what is acceptable posture." A good rule is to keep your ears, shoulders, hips, knees, and ankles in a straight line as much as possible. Doing so can actually *prevent* the unsightly slump. That's because women who have good posture before they hit menopause—when their bones start to demineralize—are less likely to end up hunched over, she says.

But if your posture needs perking up, one easy way to do that is to adjust your work habits. If you do a lot of computer work, for example, take short breaks. "Working at a keyboard promotes poor posture, so it's important to stand up whenever possible and move around," Dr. Bleecker says.

If you have a job that requires you to stand most of the day, such as working a cash register, try putting one foot up on a box or telephone book. "When standing for a long time, the lower back tends to arch and the hips lean forward," Dr. Bleecker explains. "Elevating one foot can prevent this."

Correcting poor posture may also mean doing a balancing act. "Most posture problems are caused by an imbalance of muscles," Dr. Bleecker says. Women who tend to bend slightly forward as they stand usually have tight, shortened muscles in the front of their bodies and weak, elongated muscles in the back. Stretching the tight muscles and strengthening the weak ones with the proper exercises can help stop the slump.

Perhaps most important, we should pay attention to how we're sitting, standing, and walking and make any necessary adjustments to correct our posture. After a while, it will become automatic. When sitting at your computer, keep your back in contact with the chair and your feet flat on the floor. Your thighs should be parallel with the floor, and your shoulders should stay relaxed, with your elbows at a right angle to your body.

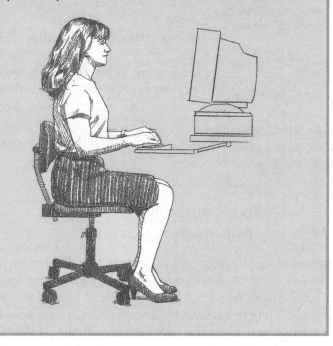

Be kind to your joints. Avoid locking your elbows or knees when lifting weights. "Anytime you lock a joint, the joint bears the stress of the weight, not the muscle," Price says. "To prevent joint pain, end the move just short of locking your knees or elbows."

Break between sets. Take a 1- to 2-minute break after completing each set to give your muscles a chance to recuperate and prepare for the next set. To save time, Dr. Nelson points out, you can do an exercise that works another muscle group. Try alternating between leg and arm exercises, for example.

Finish with flexibility. The ideal time to stretch is after you finish your workout, when your muscles are warmed up. Lifting weights actually contracts and shortens your muscles, which makes them less flexible. But stretching after lifting restores their length and keeps them supple, which helps to prevent injury in the long run.

"When you're inflexible, you're much more prone to injury," Dr. Nelson says, "because instead of your muscles being elastic and allowing some give, they're quite tight."

Take a day off. Your muscles need at least a day to rest in between resistance-training sessions. It's actually during that time that your muscles get stronger, Dr. Nelson says. That's because lifting weights causes tiny tears in the muscle tissue. As your muscles repair that damage, they become stronger, she explains.

Everything that is tight and firm in our youth starts to sag as we edge over 40. Our bellies. Our butts. Our breasts. Even our skin. Exercise can no doubt help tighten our tummies, derrieres, and chests. But is there a way to tone up sagging skin?

In a word—yes.

Our skin sags as we age for two reasons, says Toby Shawe, M.D., assistant professor of dermatology at the Medical College of Pennsylvania–Hahnemann University Hospitals in Philadelphia. First, the skin's elasticity naturally declines over the years. Second, we tend to gain weight around midlife, which stretches out the skin. If you lose those extra pounds, the decreased elasticity doesn't allow the skin to bounce back as well as it once did. As a result, it will look as though it's sagging—especially in the areas around the belly and butt and under the chin and arms.

To stop the sag before it starts, your best bet is to lose weight very slowly. "Try losing only a pound or two a month," Dr. Shawe says. And while you're losing weight, you can further prevent the sag by toning the underlying muscles with light weight lifting.

Toning those muscles also helps reduce any sagging you may already have. "When the muscle becomes larger, it takes up more space, so the skin won't appear to sag as much," Dr. Shawe explains.

And of course, cosmetic surgery to remove the extra skin can help, too. "A combination of surgery and weight lifting often brings women the best results," Dr. Shawe adds.

decrease the weight, says Dr. Nelson.

Mix up your routine. After lifting weights consistently for a few weeks or months, you may hit a plateau. That's when you find that you can't seem to progress to the next level with heavier weights. This is a sign that your muscles have become used to your workout and need a new challenge to grow further. "When you hit a plateau, try changing something in your routine," Price suggests.

Alter the exercise slightly, try a completely different exercise to work the same muscle, or lift and lower the weight even more slowly. For example, take 4 seconds to lift the weight, a 2-second pause, and then 4 seconds to lower it.

Pay attention to pain. Pain may be a sign that a muscle, tendon, or joint has been overworked or strained. "If something doesn't feel right, don't keep training it," Dr. Nelson says. Rest a few days before trying your routine again.

Work through soreness. You're probably going to feel a little sore for the first few weeks after starting a new body-toning program. Only when the soreness subsides should you increase the amount of weight you're lifting, and then add no more than a pound per session. If the soreness is significant, so that even everyday movement is painful, you may need to

Give Yourself a Full-Body Face-Lift

With the help of Price and Dr. Nelson, we've put together a total-body workout to firm up all the female trouble spots—the legs, rear end, chest, back, abdomen, shoulders, and arms—so you'll get the best results without putting in hours of effort.

Squat

BODY ZONES TONED: buttocks (gluteus maximus) and thighs (quadriceps and hamstrings)

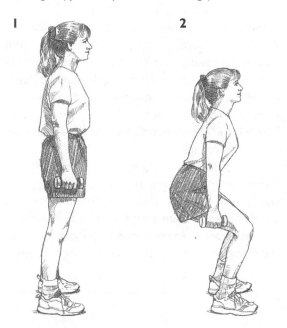

MASTER THE MOVE: (1) Stand with your feet slightly more than shoulder-width apart. Your toes should point forward or slightly out. Holding the dumbbells, keep your arms straight down at your sides. (2) Keep your back straight, your heels on the floor, and your eyes focused straight ahead. In a slow, controlled movement, lower your body as if you were sitting down in a chair. Sit back over your heels rather than squatting straight down. Your knees should be directly above (never beyond) your toes. Hold for a second and return to the starting position by pushing up from your heels and straightening out your legs. Squeeze your buttock muscles, then repeat.

PLAY IT SAFE: If this is your first time doing resistance training, do this movement without weights for a few sessions. If you feel any stress to the knees, make sure you're sitting back over your heels and not allowing your knees to go beyond your toes. Women who have knee problems should check with their doctors before doing this exercise.

Lunge

BODY ZONES TONED: buttocks (gluteus maximus), thighs (quadriceps and hamstrings), front of hips (hip flexors), and calves (gastrocnemius)

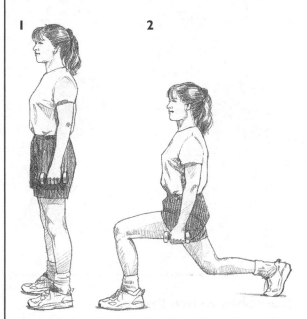

MASTER THE MOVE: (1) Stand with your feet hip-width apart and your arms straight down, holding the dumbbells at your sides. (2) Take a large step forward with your left foot, keeping your back and torso upright and bending both knees. Your left knee should be bent at a 90-degree angle and should not be beyond your toes. Your right knee should be bent a little wider than 90 degrees, and your heel should lift off the floor. Hold for a second and return to the starting position by bringing your back leg forward. Repeat on the opposite side.

PLAY IT SAFE: If you're a beginner, use weights only after you have mastered the move without them. If you have knee problems, check with your doctor before doing this exercise.

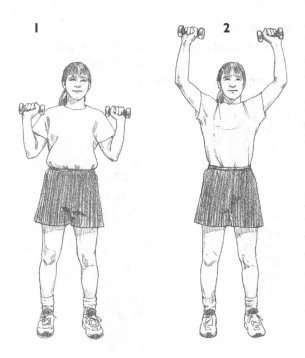

Overhead Press

BODY ZONES TONED: shoulders (deltoids), back of upper arms (triceps), and lower neck and upper middle back (trapezius)

MASTER THE MOVE: (1) Start with your feet shoulder-width apart. Hold the dumbbells with your elbows bent and your palms facing front. The inner ends of the dumbbells should touch your shoulders. (2) Push the dumbbells straight up and extend your arms overhead just short of locking your elbows. Slowly lower the dumbbells back to the starting position and repeat.

MIX IT UP: Try changing the move slightly by starting with your palms and forearms facing in toward your chest rather than facing front. As you raise the dumbbells, rotate your forearms and palms so they face front when your arms are extended. Rotate and lower your arms back to the starting position.

Dumbbell Bench Press

BODY ZONES TONED: chest (pectoralis major), front of shoulders (anterior deltoids), and back of upper arms (triceps)

MASTER THE MOVE: (1) Lie back on a bench with your feet flat on the floor. If you find yourself arching your back to reach the floor, put your feet flat on the end of the bench with your knees bent. Keep your buttocks, upper and lower back, and head in line and in contact with the bench during the exercise. Extend your arms above your head with the weights directly above your shoulders and your elbows just short of locking. The inner ends of the dumbbells should touch each other. (2) Slowly lower the dumbbells by bending your elbows and bringing your arms down to your sides. At the end of the move, the weights should be about chest-high and close to your body. Return to the starting position by pushing the dumbbells upward and together. Repeat.

MIX IT UP: If you don't have a workout bench, try lying on a step bench designed for step aerobics.

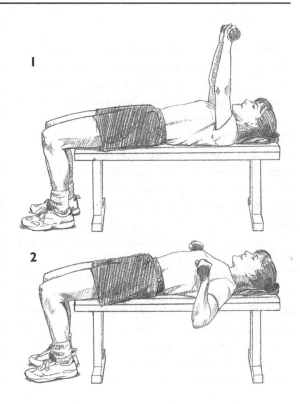

Pushup

BODY ZONES TONED: chest (pectoralis major), arms (biceps and triceps), and shoulders (deltoids)

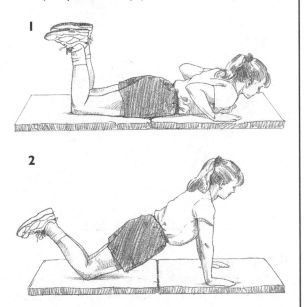

MASTER THE MOVE: (1) Lie facedown on an exercise mat with your palms flat on the floor just outside your shoulders. Your fingers should point forward and your elbows should point upward. Bend your legs at the knees so that your feet and lower legs are raised in the air to form a 90-degree angle with your upper legs. (2) Push your torso up. Rest your body weight on the padded part of your lower thigh, slightly above the kneecap. Your thighs, buttocks, back, neck, and head should be in a straight line, and your abdominal muscles should be tight. Make sure that your shoulders are directly above your hands and that your elbows aren't locked. Hold for a second, then lower your torso back to the floor. Repeat.

MIX IT UP: To make this move more difficult, do a full pushup with your legs straight. Only your toes and hands should remain on the floor. Your legs, back, neck, and head should form a straight line.

PLAY IT SAFE: Do not do this exercise if you have carpal tunnel syndrome or if you feel any wrist pain in the pushup position.

Abdominal Crunch

BODY ZONE TONED: abdominals (rectus abdominis)

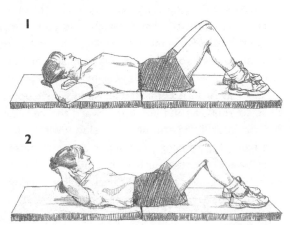

MASTER THE MOVE: (1) Lie on your back on the exercise mat with your legs bent, keeping your feet flat and your lower back relaxed against the floor. Place your fingers behind your head for support with your elbows pointing out to the sides. Be careful not to pull your head forward with your hands. (2) Use your abdominal muscles to slowly lift your chest and shoulders, making sure not to arch your lower back. Hold for a count of five and slowly return to the starting position. Don't rest between repetitions.

MIX IT UP: For a more advanced workout, lift your lower body toward your chest as you do the crunch. Your legs should be bent slightly at the knees, and your feet should be crossed at the ankles. Raise your torso and lower body at the same time as if you were trying to touch your knees to your shoulders.

PLAY IT SAFE: If you have lower-back pain, try the crunch with your feet and lower legs resting on a chair. Bend your legs at a 90-degree angle, and keep your lower back against the floor when you do the move.

Triceps Extension

BODY ZONES TONED: back of upper arms (triceps)

MASTER THE MOVE: (1) Sit toward the front of a sturdy chair with your back straight and your feet flat on the floor. Bring the arm holding the dumbbell straight up over your head. Bend your arm at the elbow and slowly lower the weight back to your shoulder as far as is comfortable. Keep your elbow close to your ear and pointed toward the ceiling. Support your lifting arm near the elbow with your free hand. (2) Keeping your upper arm still, raise your lower arm over your head just short of locking your elbow. Lower the weight back to the starting position and repeat. Switch arms for the next set.

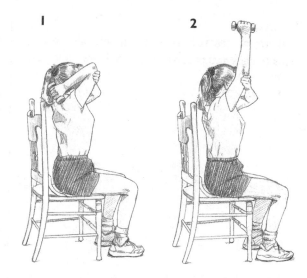

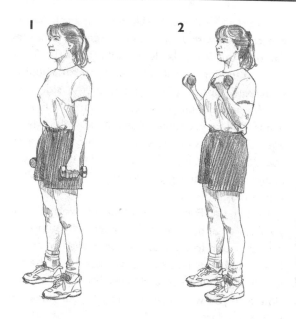

Biceps Curl

BODY ZONES TONED: front of upper arms (biceps)

MASTER THE MOVE: (1) Stand with your feet about shoulder-width apart and with your arms straight down at your sides, holding the dumbbells so that your palms are facing your thighs. (2) Lift the weights in one smooth motion by bending your elbows, rotating your forearms so that your palms face up, and raising the dumbbells to shoulder height. Keep your wrists and back straight. Slowly lower the weights back to the starting position and repeat.

MIX IT UP: To make this move more difficult, try what is called a concentration curl. Sit on the end of a bench or chair with your feet flat on the ground and your legs bent at a 90-degree angle. Your feet should be slightly more than shoulder-width apart. Hold a dumbbell in one hand. Lean your torso forward a bit and rest the elbow and upper arm you are working against your inner thigh. Keep your free hand on your other knee for support. Slowly lift the dumbbell to your shoulder, keeping your elbow and upper arm firm against your thigh.

Stretch Your Limits

Follow your workout with these stretches to increase your flexibility and lower your risk of injury, says Dr. Nelson.

Lying Quadriceps Stretch

BODY ZONES STRETCHED: front of thighs (quadriceps) and front of hips (hip flexors)

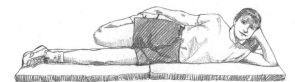

MASTER THE MOVE: Lie on your side with your legs straight and together, one on top of the other. Support your head with the hand closest to the floor by resting your upper arm on the floor and bending it at the elbow. Bend your lower leg slightly if you need to for balance.

Bend the knee of the top leg so that your foot comes back toward your buttocks. Grasp your foot with your free hand and pull the heel in toward your buttocks until you feel a comfortable stretch in the front of your thigh. Hold it there for 20 to 30 seconds, then slowly release. Roll onto your other side and stretch the opposite leg.

Standing Hamstring Stretch

BODY ZONES STRETCHED: back of thighs (hamstrings), inner thighs (adductors), and buttocks (gluteus maximus)

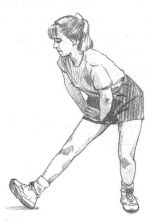

MASTER THE MOVE: Stand with your feet together and take a very large step forward with your right leg. Keep your right foot pointing straight ahead and turn your back leg slightly so that your left foot points a bit to the left.

Bend the knee of your back leg, place your hands on the upper thigh of your front leg, and slowly lean forward with your torso as far as you comfortably can. Keep your back, neck, and head in a straight line. Bend your back leg further while pushing your hips and buttocks down and back. Lift the front of your right foot off the floor, while maintaining pressure on your front heel. You should feel a comfortable stretch in your back and in the inner thigh of your outstretched leg. Hold for 20 to 30 seconds, then stretch the other thigh.

Shoulder Stretch

BODY ZONES STRETCHED: shoulders (deltoids) and arms (biceps and triceps)

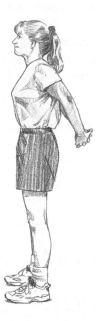

MASTER THE MOVE: Stand with your feet shoulder-width apart and your arms down at your sides. Extend your arms straight behind your body, stretching them back and upward as far as you comfortably can. If your hands reach far enough, clasp them together. Hold for 20 to 30 seconds.

Side Bend

BODY ZONES STRETCHED: mid- and lower back (latissimus dorsi) and side abdominals (obliques)

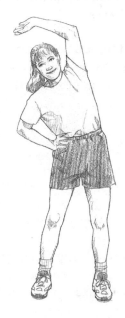

Without leaning forward, bend at the waist toward the hand on your hip while slowly reaching over your head with the other hand as far as you comfortably can. Hold for 20 to 30 seconds and then stretch the other side.

Bowing Shoulder Stretch

BODY ZONES STRETCHED: mid- and lower back (latissimus dorsi), shoulders (deltoids), and arms (biceps and triceps)

MASTER THE MOVE: Get down on all fours on an exercise mat with your hands and knees about shoulder-width apart. Keep your back flat, your neck straight, and your eyes looking down at the floor. Sit back on your heels, extending your arms out in front of you. Push down slightly with your palms and hold for 20 to 30 seconds.

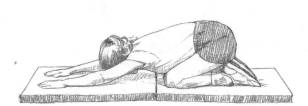

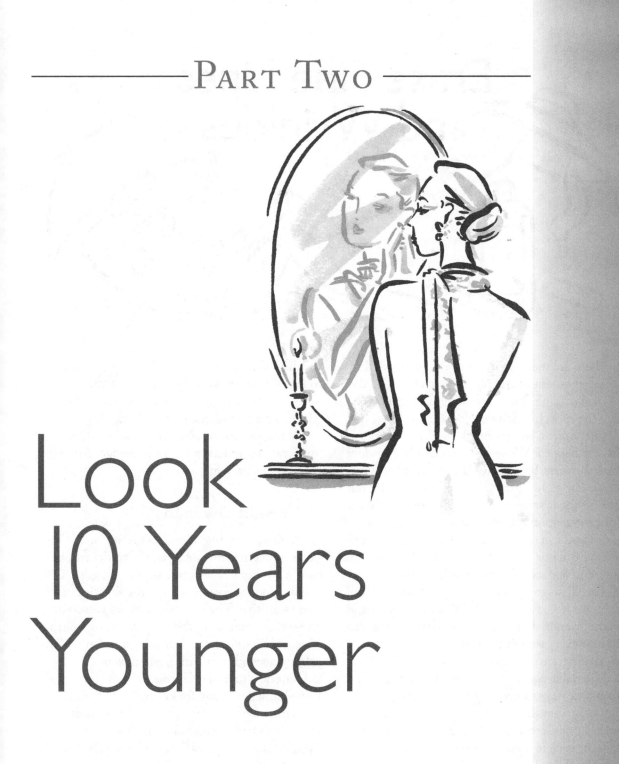

PART TWO

Look 10 Years Younger

Erase Fine Lines and Wrinkles

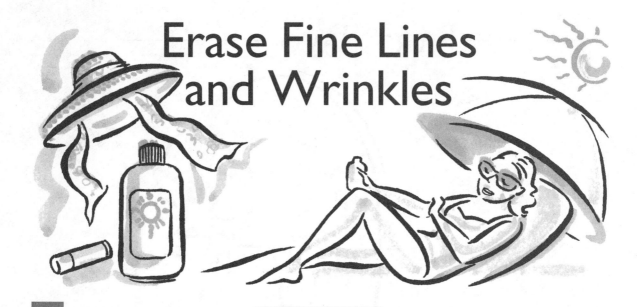

There are many milestones in a woman's life: The beginning of her monthly cycles. The day of her wedding. The birth of her first child. The day she spots her first wrinkle . . .

Oh, mirror, mirror on the wall, why does it have to happen? We know we accumulate wisdom with the years, but must we also accumulate wrinkles? The sight of those tiny crinkles under our eyes or the first faint creases along our foreheads (not to mention the appearance of broken capillaries and age spots), can make us want to turn away from our own reflections (or, like the evil queen in *Snow White*, just smash the mirror).

Faced, so to speak, with less-than-youthful skin, we have two choices. We can accept it and make friends with our frown lines. Or we can fight it every step of the way.

Want to arm yourself for battle? We have considerable control over how our skin ages and plenty of ways to keep it glowing and youthfully smooth, ways that don't include weird facial exercises, skin creams with hundred-dollar price tags, or trips to a plastic surgeon's office.

Even if you haven't yet spied that first wrinkle, you still have good reason to lavish your still-youthful skin with TLC. "The earlier you start to care for your skin, the bigger the difference you'll see as you age," says Francesca J. Fusco, M.D., a dermatologist in New York City.

To achieve more youthful-looking skin, it's important to understand how it changes through the years—and why.

Why Skin Gives In

Obviously, aging alone takes its toll. Our skin's protective outside layer, the epidermis, becomes thinner and increasingly fragile. Oil glands produce less oil, leaving the skin drier and more sensitive. The number of blood vessels decreases, so you lose the rosy glow of youth. Moreover, aging slows down the speed at which you replace old cells with fresh, new ones.

Genetics, too, plays a role in how skin ages. Fair-skinned women, for example, show signs of premature aging faster than women with darker skin. That's because fair skin contains less melanin, the substance that gives skin its pigment and helps protect it from the sun, explains Linda K. Franks, M.D., a dermatologist in New York City.

DON'T NEGLECT YOUR NECK

No matter how young you may look from the chin up, if you don't lavish some care on your neck, your age will be an easy read. Like the skin around our eyes, neck skin is a prime age-revealer. "It's thinner than facial skin, with practically no oil glands, so it's extremely vulnerable to dryness and sun damage," says Jennifer Ridge, M.D., a dermatologist in Middletown, Ohio.

To prevent further damage, start using these save-your-neck strategies now.

Pamper your throat. It's not necessary to use special neck creams, says Dr. Ridge. Simply lavish your neck with the same gentle cleanser and rich moisturizer you use on your face. Apply the moisturizer with firm upward strokes.

Take the Teflon approach. Coat your neck daily with a sunscreen, moisturizer, or makeup foundation that has a sun protection factor (SPF) of at least 15. If you are using sunscreen alone, use a chickpea-size dollop.

Apply sunscreen to your chest, too. "Open collars and scoop-neck dresses expose your chest to the sun," says Dr. Ridge.

To further protect your neck, keep a small tube of sunscreen in your handbag and apply it several times a day—every 2 hours if you're out in intense sun. Why? Because a single application in the morning won't protect your neck all day. "Sunscreen sweats off, it rubs off—in a few hours, it's gone," says Dr. Ridge.

Protect while you sleep. When we sleep on a pillow, we tend to squash our chins against our necks, says Dr. Ridge. Over the years, as our skin loses its ability to snap back into place, these "sleep wrinkles" on our necks will become permanent.

To keep your neck smoother, trade in your regular pillow for a neck roll, suggests Dr. Ridge. These small, log-shaped pillows, available in medical supply stores and catalogs, are designed to keep your chin and neck in alignment. They also keep your neck skin taut. Be warned, however: Neck rolls can have an unfortunate side effect. "You may snore more," says Dr. Ridge, "but your neck will look better."

Defy nature. To reduce the wrinkles on your neck, use lotions or creams containing glycolic acid, one member of a group of substances known as alpha hydroxy acids (AHAs), says Dr. Ridge. These natural fruit and milk acids chemically slough off, or exfoliate, the buildup of dead cells on the surface of your skin, exposing the newer, fresher skin underneath.

You'll find products containing AHAs, most of which use glycolic acid, in the skin-care aisle of any drugstore. Look for brands that contain 10 percent glycolic acid. To get the most dramatic results, however, you may need a stronger concentration—up to 25 percent—for which you'll have to see a dermatologist.

A dermatologist may also suggest tretinoin (Retin-A or Renova). Like glycolic acid, these products chemically exfoliate the skin's top layer. They also penetrate its second layer, the dermis, where they help form collagen, the fibrous material that gives skin its youthful plumpness. Although they both work well, says Dr. Ridge, Retin-A and Renova are both prescription drugs, so you can get them only under a doctor's supervision.

But that's only part of it. No matter how many candles may decorate your birthday cake or how fair your complexion is, to a large extent, your skin's "age" depends on how well you take care of it.

The cardinal skin sins are basking in the sun and smoking cigarettes. Both speed the breakdown of collagen and elastin, the structural proteins that give skin its youthful plumpness and

OUT, DAMNED SPOTS

Freckles on kids' faces? Cute. Freckles on *our* faces? Unless we were blessed with them at birth, not cute at all.

"If you're 35 or 40 and have 'freckles' in areas that you never did as a kid, your skin has sustained sun damage," says Jennifer Ridge, M.D., a dermatologist in Middletown, Ohio.

What we commonly call freckles actually fall into two categories, she explains. True freckles, or ephelides, are the little brown spots we're born with. They're simply spots of melanin, the substance that gives skin its pigment. We inherit them from our parents; those of us with light skin and hair are more likely to have them. While true freckles come out in the sun, they also tend to disappear as we age.

Like true freckles, false freckles, or solar lentigines, are made of melanin. But unlike inherited freckles, lentigines sprout for a specific reason: They are the skin's attempt to defend itself from the sun. And they don't fade with the years. They get worse.

While lentigines aren't dangerous, they do mean we've sustained sun damage, which makes skin more vulnerable to sun-induced skin cancers, says Dr. Ridge. The antidote to future sun damage? Sunscreen. Coat your face and neck with a product that has a sun protection factor (SPF) of at least 15. Or use moisturizers and makeup with SPF 15 sunscreen.

---

ability to snap back. The result is premature sagging, wrinkles, roughness, age spots, and blotches.

Other skin agers include chronic emotional stress, poor nutrition, excessive dieting, and drinking alcohol, says Debra Jaliman, M.D., a dermatologist in New York City.

Skin Enemy Number One: The Sun

Ask dermatologists to name the most treacherous skin villain of all, and the sun wins hands down. Sun damage, or photoaging, gives skin the texture of leather and can leave a formerly peaches-and-cream complexion riddled with wrinkles, spots, blotches, and broken blood vessels.

How can something that feels so good on our bare skin wreak so much destruction? In a word: radiation.

The sun gives off two types of ultraviolet (UV) radiation: both UVA, sometimes called tanning rays, and UVB, the so-called burning rays. Until recently, UVA rays were thought to be harmless. In fact, UVA light is still used in tanning beds. But dermatologists now know that both UVA and UVB rays are equally destructive to the skin. Over the years, these rays slowly but steadily break down collagen and elastin, until one fine day—presto! You've entered the Face-Lift Zone.

The damage starts earlier than you may think. "Eighty percent of the sun damage takes place before the age of 20," says Rhoda S. Narins, M.D., clinical associate professor of dermatology at New York University Medical Center and a dermatologist in New York City and White Plains, New York.

Most vulnerable to photoaging are women with fair skin and light hair and eyes, and women who have grown up in high altitudes, where UV rays are at their most intense, says Dr. Franks. "I see women in their twenties who have grown up in Colorado or skiers who have spent years in high-intensity sun, and they already have fine lines and wrinkles under their eyes."

Think your darker skin is immune to solar assault? Think again, says Dr. Franks. Even African-Americans and olive-skinned people of Mediterranean ancestry, whose skin contains more melanin than that of lighter-skinned people, can sustain sun damage. "I've seen many olive-skinned women who have extremely sun-damaged skin," she says. "They seem to develop sunspots, or so-called liver spots, earlier."

Sunscreen to the Rescue

Wouldn't it be great if there was a miracle product that could protect skin from the sun's assault? That could actually *prevent* sun-induced wrinkles?

There is. It's called sunscreen.

Think of sunscreen as Armor All for your skin. No matter what your age, slathering on sunscreen *right now* can help prevent future sun damage, say dermatologists.

It may also fend off the formation of wrinkles. "It takes years of sun exposure to make wrinkles, but the skin is damaged before wrinkles actually appear," says Dr. Franks. "By using sunscreen now and turning off the ongoing assault, you can delay or even prevent wrinkles."

There are two types of sunscreens. Physical blocks, the first type, contain zinc oxide or titanium dioxide and act as a force field, literally blocking UVA and UVB rays from reaching the skin. Zinc oxide—that pasty white stuff lifeguards used to slather on their lips and noses—is the more powerful of the two.

Thankfully, it's now possible to reap the benefits of zinc oxide without looking as though you just came from a Halloween party. Nowadays, most nonprescription physical blocks, which are

WOMEN ASK WHY

Why does my skin look so awful when I don't get enough sleep?

The baggy eyes, dark circles, puffiness, and sallowness your skin manifests after a bout of insomnia or an all-nighter happen for the same reason people with jet lag look lousy: Your body clock—and your hormones—are out of whack.

Most people's body clocks are set to let them sleep at night and wake them up in the morning. These internal clocks are also programmed to release certain hormones at certain times of the day.

You may have noticed that at night, before you go to bed, your eyes are swollen and you look tired and puffy. Why don't you look that way in the morning? Assuming that you have had adequate sleep the night before, your hormones rebound for the morning ahead and "prepare" your skin to wake up.

One hormone that peaks primarily in the morning is cortisol, which is secreted by the adrenal glands. Cortisol has a dramatic impact on skin: It aids in regulating swelling. With changes in the levels of cortisol, swelling can go up or go down.

When you get enough sleep, cortisol peaks on schedule—in the morning. It helps reduce morning puffiness and contributes to your skin's looking rested and refreshed. On the other hand, a late night or a bout of insomnia throws off your body clock, so cortisol doesn't peak when it is supposed to. You arise with a pale, puffy face.

Expert consulted
Andrew Pollack, M.D.
Chief of dermatology
Chestnut Hill Hospital
Philadelphia

available at a dermatologist's office, contain zinc oxide that has been micronized (that is, crushed into virtually invisible particles). You can also check on the Internet for these products, since they aren't commonly available in stores.

Chemical sunscreens, the second type, contain specific chemicals that absorb both UVA and UVB rays. Avobenzone, also known as Parsol 1789, is one of the most widely used and most effective chemical sunscreens, notes Dr. Franks.

But using sunscreen alone can't keep the sun from aging your skin if you insist on starting—and finishing—the latest 300-page bestseller while you bake on the beach. "Even the best sunscreens allow some UV rays to penetrate the skin," says Dr. Fusco.

A Sunscreen Primer

So now you're convinced that the sun turns skin to toast? You've sworn to use sunscreen every day? Great. Now all you have to do is choose the right product and use it correctly. Here's how.

Follow the numbers. For everyday protection, use a sunscreen that contains a sun protection factor (SPF) of at least 15, says Dr. Franks, and apply it 30 minutes before going out into the sun. Every day. Even when you don't see a hint of sun. (Clouds can block brightness, but they may allow as much as 80 percent of UV light to reach your skin.)

If you plan to spend time on the golf course, tennis court, or ski slope, use a sunscreen with an SPF of 30, says Dr. Fusco. Ditto, if you spend a lot of time on a boat or at the beach. Sun reflects off water and bounces onto your skin, which intensifies its damage. And since perspiration, excessive toweling, and water can wash sunscreen away, reapply it occasionally. You may want to try one of the many waterproof sunscreens avail-

---

GLOW FOR IT—WITHOUT THE SUN

To get a sun-kissed glow minus the wrinkles, try a self-tanning lotion, says Mary Ronnow, a paramedical aesthetician (skin-care specialist working in a doctor's office) at Northern Nevada Plastic Surgery in Reno. Unlike the "bottled tans" of the past, the new generation of sunless tanners is less likely to streak—and, better yet, won't turn you the color of a carrot.

The active ingredient in self-tanners, dihydroxyacetone (DHA), interacts with the amino acids in your skin's top layer, turning skin darker in the process. This "tan" fades within a few days, as your skin sheds dead cells.

To get the best bottled tan possible, follow this step-by-step plan from Ronnow.

Shower, then rinse well. Self-tanners "take" better when they are applied to skin free of body oils, perspiration, and cleanser residue.

Slough off roughness. While you're in the shower, exfoliate with a loofah, body mitt, or exfoliating cleanser to remove dry skin and rough patches. Smooth skin absorbs DHA more evenly, so your tan won't look splotchy.

Moisturize. To smooth skin even more, slather on your favorite body lotion. Let it penetrate until you can no longer see or feel it on your skin.

Take it from the top. Apply a self-tanner thinly and evenly, from face to feet. Use a dime-size amount on your

---

able, but remember that it also has to be reapplied.

Broaden your protection. A sunscreen's SPF factor measures only its UVB coverage, says Dr. Franks. So make sure that the sunscreen you buy is labeled "broad-spectrum," meaning that it absorbs both UVB and UVA rays. Most broad-spectrum sunscreens contain Parsol 1789 or titanium dioxide.

Don't be stingy. Use a marble-size amount of sunscreen to cover your face, two "marbles" to cover your neck and chest, says Dr. Fusco. If you

face, another to cover your neck, but don't apply tanner on the eyelids or into the eyebrow. Blend down your chin and into your neckline. To tan the backs of your hands, put a dollop of self-tanner on a cotton ball, then wipe across the backs of your hands and fingers. Don't use too much tanner around your hairline or on knees, elbows, and ankles; these areas seem to "grab" more DHA and can become especially dark.

If you're using a spray-on tanner, spray the product lightly and evenly on one body part at a time. Then blend quickly, following the guidelines above. To apply to your face, spray the product on your hand and blend evenly and well.

Whatever product you choose, don't use it in a hot, steamy bathroom. The heat will turn it runny, making it difficult to apply.

Tan-proof your palms. When you're finished, immediately scrub your hands with a loofah or a product with scrubbing grains. Get between your fingers, too.

Keep glowing. Reapply a sunless tanner a second time the same day until you're as dark as you want to be. To maintain your tan, reapply it every few days.

One caution: Self-tanners won't protect your skin from the sun. So choose a brand that contains a sunscreen with a sun protection factor (SPF) of 15 or above. Two that do are Bain de Soleil and Physician's Formula. You can also apply sunscreen over your new "tan" to get the same protection.

use makeup or moisturizer and a sunscreen, apply the sunscreen first. You want it as close to your skin as possible.

Use "built-in" sunscreens. To save time, money, and medicine-cabinet space, use a moisturizer or foundation with an SPF of at least 15. "For everyday use, these products are as effective as sunscreen alone, when used properly," says Dr. Fusco. "But you must remember to apply the equivalent of 1 teaspoon of foundation to assure the sun protection factor promised."

Wrinkle-proof your kisser. Sun damage can eventually crinkle lips, too. So wear a lipstick or lip balm with added sunscreen to help keep lips soft and youthful looking, says Dr. Fusco.

Skin Tips for Sun Junkies

Ask any dermatologist, and she'll tell you to stay out of the sun between 10:00 A.M. and 4:00 P.M., when the sun's rays are strongest. While that's sound advice, we're women, not vampires. Some of us live in sunny climates, some of us spend weekends in our gardens, and others love to golf or play tennis. If you must bask, follow the tips below. They will help to "super-boost" your sun protection.

Use your head to save your skin. While in intense sun, wear a hat with a brim that's at least 4 inches wide (think: a Mae West–size chapeau). Forget the sailor hats and baseball caps; neither offers much protection from full-bore sun, says Dr. Jaliman.

Take a cue from Foster Grant. Wear wraparound sunglasses designed to block 95 to 100 percent of UVA and UVB rays, says Dr. Jaliman. Why wraparounds? They will protect your eyes from harmful UV rays while completely blocking the crow's-foot zone.

Be slightly shady. While out in intense sun, periodically retreat to a shady spot, says Dr. Jaliman. At the beach, park yourself under a big umbrella. Also, while on hikes or on the water, if it's not too hot out, wear tightly woven clothing. It will help keep UV rays from penetrating your skin. But if you'll fry, wear at least a hat, sunglasses, and plenty of sunscreen.

Clean Up Your Act

When dentists say that good oral hygiene protects your teeth and gums, you know exactly what they mean. Extending the metaphor, practicing good *skin* hygiene can help protect skin from premature wrinkling. The tips below can help you clean up youth-stealing skin habits.

Don't be a smoke face. Here's another good reason to quit. Current smokers are two to three times more likely to develop premature wrinkling than nonsmokers, according to research conducted at the University of California, San Francisco. That's because smoking causes the fibers of the skin to lose their elasticity sooner and become more susceptible to wrinkling. It also literally strangles skin. The nicotine in cigarettes narrows blood vessels, preventing oxygen-rich blood from reaching the tiny capillaries in the top layers of the skin. This oxygen deprivation makes skin dull, gray, and leathery—a condition so well-known that it has a name: smoker's face.

The good news is that smokers will see an improvement in the appearance of their skin in just 60 smoke-free days, says Dr. Franks, the time it takes for skin to replace itself twice.

Get enough Zzzs. As obvious as it sounds, try to sleep at least 8 hours a night. "Like any other organ, your skin needs time to repair itself, and sleeping is excellent downtime," says Dr. Franks.

Sleep on your back. If you can't, learn. Scrunching your face into your pillow for 30 to 40 years will eventually press wrinkles into your skin, says Dr. Jaliman.

The Perfect Cleanser

The skin-care industry spends millions trying to convince us that their products hold the secret to smooth, line-free skin. Dermatologists say, "Bah!"

"I'm a big fan of simple, basic skin care," says Dr. Franks. "All you need is a gentle cleanser and a moisturizer." The mini-guide below can steer you toward cleansers that work best for *your* skin.

As mentioned earlier, the skin's oil glands produce less oil as we age. The right cleanser washes away dirt and makeup but leaves oil where it belongs—on your face.

If you're dry, go creamy. "The drier your skin, the more gentle your cleanser should be," says Dr. Fusco. She suggests Oil of Olay Foaming Face Wash or Cetaphil. Cetaphil is a soap-free cleanser that's free of skin-irritating fragrances, additives, and preservatives.

Dissolve away oil. Oily skin tends to be thick, so it can tolerate a stronger cleanser. Try an oil-binding liquid cleanser formulated for oily skin, such as Neutrogena Oil-Free Acne Wash, a cleanser with salicylic acid. If you prefer a bar cleanser, try Neutrogena Oily Skin Formula Facial Cleansing Bar, suggests Dr. Fusco. Or try a gel cleanser formulated for oily skin.

If you're sensitive, pick a kinder, gentler cleanser. Try Cetaphil, says Dr. Fusco. Dermatologists often recommend this product for people with sensitive skin. If not, pick a cleanser such as Almay that's labeled hypoallergenic, meaning that it contains fewer ingredients than regular products and few or none of the ingredients known to cause allergic reactions.

Cleanse correctly. The way you cleanse your skin is just as important as the product you use, says Dr. Fusco. Here's the correct way to wash your face. If you're using a liquid, lotion, or gel cleanser, place about a teaspoon of cleanser in the palm of your hand. Massage it gently into your skin using the balls of your fingers. Rinse your face with warm water until all the cleanser is removed (about five or six times) or wipe off the cleanser with a soft, damp washcloth. If you're using a bar cleanser, hold it under water to wet it, then work up a lather in the palm of your hand. Using the balls of your fingers, massage your face in a circular motion for 30 seconds, then rinse, as above. Pat skin dry—never rub it.

Avoid scrubbing grains or pads. "Prolonged exfoliation can actually make the skin become drier and accent fine lines," says Dr. Fusco. Enough said.

How to Navigate the Moisturizer Maze

Moisturizers are like diet books—there's a new one on the market every day. But don't be seduced by high-priced, high-tech products: All a moisturizer can do, says Dr. Fusco, is soften skin and moisturize. It cannot erase lines.

If you're dry, oil up. The drier your skin, the more hydrating elements your moisturizer should contain, says Dr. Fusco. So pick a product formulated with ingredients such as glycerin, hyaluronic acid, or dimethicone. Eucerin and Moisturel are two of many good choices, she says. They slow down natural moisture loss throughout the day and prevent further skin dehydration.

Or go the natural route. "Olive oil is a great moisturizer," says Dr. Jaliman. Of course, it's not for someone who is acne-prone, and it's best used as a before-bed treatment because olive oil can't protect your skin from the sun. (Plus, you'll smell like a Greek salad while you're at work.)

If you're oily, go light. Oily skin may feel dry, the result of harsh cleansing products formulated with ingredients such as alcohol that strip away the skin's natural oils, says Dr. Fusco. Try a moisturizer that contains humectants (ingredients that attract and hold water), such as glycerin and sodium PCA, she says. These ingredients trap water in your skin with no greasy shine. Also, choose a lotion. Lotions are lighter than creams and tend to contain less oil, so they won't clog pores.

If you're sensitive, think basic. Use a hypoallergenic moisturizer, says Dr. Fusco. Apply it to a test area first to see if you tolerate it well. Pure glycerin (available at drugstores) or petroleum jelly can be effective, she adds, but you should avoid them if you're acne-prone.

Consider eye creams. It's fine to use your regular moisturizer around your eyes. But if you have sensitive skin or your eyes are easily irritated, consider buying moisturizing eye cream, says Dr. Fusco. Creams made to be used specifically around the eyes are less likely to aggravate delicate undereye skin—or your peepers themselves.

The Care and Feeding of Youthful Skin

Years ago, we thought that chocolate and french fries could cause zits. Much too late, we found that it wasn't true. What *is* true: Consuming a *healthy* diet shows on the face. To feed your skin young, read on.

Quench your skin. The Great Water/Skin Debate has raged since your own mother was a girl. But according to Dr. Franks, "Drink, drink, drink—eight glasses a day, at least." Drink more during the winter, when the indoor air is dry. Skin continually loses moisture to the air, so it draws on the reserve of water that's in the skin's deeper layers.

Back off the booze. Alcohol dilates blood vessels. In some women, consuming more than moderate amounts of alcohol will cause their vessels to continually dilate and constrict, stretching them like rubber bands until they have no more snap, says Dr. Franks. Eventually, vessels just stay dilated, she says, leading to spider veins and broken capillaries.

Alcohol also causes the skin to lose water, "and dehydrated skin is more sensitive to sun damage," says Dr. Franks.

Eat your skin vitamins. Consume a mother lode of fruits and vegetables rich in the antioxidant nutrients vitamin C, vitamin E, and beta-carotene, says Dr. Fusco. Antioxidants help protect skin from the damaging effects of free radicals, unstable oxygen molecules that are generated after exposure to the sun.

Strawberries, papayas, kiwifruit, navel oranges, and sweet red peppers are especially rich sources of vitamin C. Vitamin E can be found in cooking oil, wheat germ, nuts, and seeds. Spinach and other dark green leafy vegetables, along with deep orange fruits and vegetables such as carrots, sweet potatoes, cantaloupe, and pumpkin, are bursting with beta-carotene.

Take extra C. Consider taking extra vitamin C, which the skin needs to build collagen, says Dr. Jaliman. She suggests 1,000 milligrams of vitamin C a day. You can choose a multivitamin that contains this amount or consume a separate vitamin C supplement.

Say no-no to yo-yo dieting. Avoid gaining and losing weight over and over. "It leads to wear and tear on collagen and elastin," says Dr. Jaliman. Steer clear of starvation diets, too. Very low calorie diets deprive your skin of the nutrients it needs to thrive, she says.

Special Problems of Aging Skin

As if coping with laugh lines and crow's-feet wasn't enough, we also have to deal with other

> ### OUR EYES AT 30, 40, 50
>
> According to Jennifer Ridge, M.D., a dermatologist in Middletown, Ohio, here is a general idea of what your face can expect as time marches on.
>
> *In our thirties:* We may get dark circles under our eyes, as the skin under our eyes thins and exposes the pigment beneath. We may also notice our first lines or wrinkles. They may be barely noticeable or quite prominent, depending on whether we have dark or light skin and how much sunlight we were exposed to in our teens and twenties. In some of us, the fat pad under our cheeks (the malar fat pad) begins to droop, pulling the skin under our eyes with them.
>
>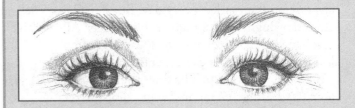
>
> *In our forties:* Our skin begins to lose its youthful plumpness and elasticity, and we may see our first lines and wrin-

age-related skin problems, from puffy eyes to large pores. But take heart. Here's what experts suggest you can do on your own to brighten, tighten, or just plain hide these bothersome flaws.

To shrink puffy eyes: Believe it or not, some women use the hemorrhoid product Preparation H. This product contains hydrocortisone, a topical steroid that reduces inflammation, says Dr. Jaliman. Does it really send eye bags packing? "My clients say it does," she says, "but the tightening effect is temporary." Be warned that long-term use can thin the skin and lead to acne, premature wrinkling, and broken blood vessels. Consult your physician before using this product around your eyes.

kles. We also develop deeper lines at the corners of our eyes. These crow's-feet, as they're called, are especially prominent if we have fair skin, if we've smoked, or if we were sun junkies in our youth.

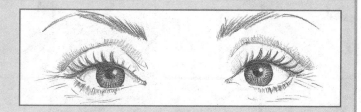

In our fifties: Wrinkles become deeper, especially in the crow's-foot zone. Sagging becomes more prominent, causing our upper lids to droop toward our lash line.

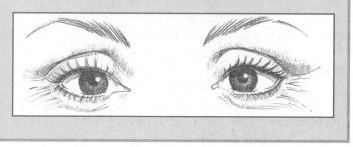

If daubing hemorrhoid cream under your eyes sounds less than appealing, reduce eye baggage with more conventional tactics, says Dr. Jaliman. Sleep with your head elevated so that fluid doesn't pool under your eyes. Reduce your intake of salt, which encourages fluid retention. Or keep a stash of teaspoons in the freezer and place them over your eyes when you wake up with puffs. The cold metal will reduce the swelling.

To brighten sallow skin: Ask a dermatologist about glycolic acid, suggests Sheryl Clark, M.D., a dermatologist in New York City. This alpha hydroxy acid (AHA), derived from sugarcane, removes dead, complexion-dulling cells from the skin's top layer, revealing the new, fresh skin beneath. And you can see results in as little as 2 weeks. You can obtain glycolic acid through your dermatologist. Over-the-counter formulations often are too low in concentration to be effective.

To hide spider veins or broken capillaries: These fine red lines that squiggle across the cheeks or nose can be removed with either a laser or an electric needle, says Dr. Jaliman. It's easier just to conceal them with makeup.

To minimize large pores: Use pore-cleansing strips, like Bioré or Pond's, on your nose, forehead, chin, or cheeks, suggests Dr. Fusco. "Dirt dilates pores," she says. "If they're not all plugged up with gunk, they'll look smaller." While these products are safe and effective, don't use them more than once every 2 weeks.

Astringents and clay masks can also temporarily minimize pores, says Dr. Fusco. The skin temporarily plumps up, which makes pores appear smaller. Use this trick only on special occasions, however. "Overuse of these products can leave skin tight, dry, and flaky," she says.

To discourage frown lines: Place a piece of waterproof cloth tape across your forehead before bed, suggests Dr. Jaliman. "The tape will keep you from frowning in your sleep, which will prevent some wrinkling." Tape won't prevent crow's-feet, however. "You don't scrunch your eyes when you sleep," she says.

Cosmetics That Nourish Your Skin

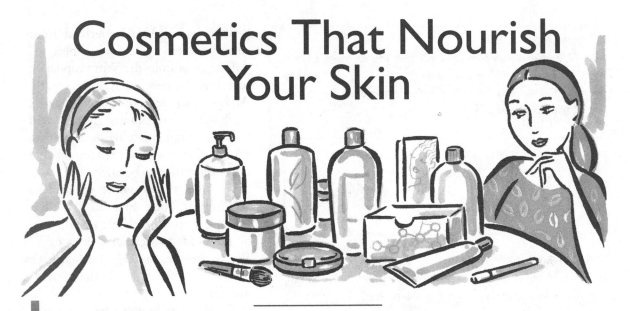

Let's face it: We're bedazzled by so-called anti-aging products that promise smoother, more youthful skin. But do these lotions and potions, so temptingly packaged (and often, so astronomically priced), actually work?

That depends on how you define *work*.

Some over-the-counter anti-aging products contain specific ingredients that can help skin look better temporarily, says Debra Price, M.D., clinical assistant professor in the department of dermatology at the University of Miami. The first ingredient is glycolic acid, a member of a group of fruit acids called alpha hydroxy acids (AHAs). The second is topical vitamin C— more specifically, L-ascorbic acid, a particular form of vitamin C.

If your skin appears dull and has lost its glow, an over-the-counter glycolic acid product may make it appear smoother and fresher, says Dr. Price. And when teamed with sunscreen, vitamin C gives skin extra protection against sun damage, the primary cause of wrinkles, roughness, age spots, and discoloration.

But the weak concentrations in over-the-counter products cannot—repeat, *cannot*—permanently alter the skin. So while they may exfoliate and smooth your skin, they won't erase wrinkles. "If they could, they would be classified as drugs, and they wouldn't be available at the cosmetics counter," says Dr. Price.

There is one substance that research shows *can* permanently alter the structure of skin: tretinoin, a derivative of vitamin A and the active ingredient in Retin-A and Renova. These products are drugs, so they're available only with a doctor's prescription. But they are the way to go if you want to reduce fine wrinkles and crinkles, roughness, or pigment changes such as age spots, says Nia Terezakis, M.D., clinical professor of dermatology at Tulane University School of Medicine in New Orleans.

Still, we know how irresistible those tiny jars, bottles, and perky cosmetics-counter salespeople can be. This guide to the hottest anti-aging skin products will tell you how they work, how to use them, what they can (and can't) do, and whether to buy them over-the-counter or from a dermatologist or skin-care salon.

Get Glowing with Glycolic Acid

Derived from sugarcane, glycolic acid is the most common AHA in over-the-counter anti-aging products. It's also the most effective, says Sheryl Clark, M.D., a dermatologist in New York City.

Research has shown that the chemicals in glycolic acid slough off, or exfoliate, the buildup of dead cells on the skin's top layer. "Removing these dead cells makes skin look smoother and gives it a glow," says Francesca J. Fusco, M.D., a dermatologist in New York City.

The average drugstore glycolic acid product costs around $10. But expect to pay $20 or more—sometimes much more—for the ritzier glycolic acid products offered by major cosmetics companies.

At the cosmetics counter. Most over-the-counter glycolic acid products contain less than 10 percent glycolic acid. These low concentrations won't do a thing for lines and wrinkles, say experts. But some women who use these products like the way they make their skin look smoother and fresher.

Research suggests that at concentrations of 10 percent or higher, glycolic acid may stimulate the formation of collagen, the connective tissue in the skin's second layer (the dermis) that gives skin its youthful plumpness and strength. A few over-the-counter products, such as the Alpha-Hydrox and Aqua Glycolic lines, do contain 10 percent glycolic acid.

Glycolic acid products are easy to use. Once a day, you simply apply two to three pea-size

"BETA" THAN ALPHA HYDROXYS?

If your skin stings and burns when you use products containing glycolic acid, which is an alpha hydroxy acid (AHA), try a kinder, gentler wrinkle fighter: salicylic acid, also known as beta hydroxy acid (BHA).

Found naturally in the bark of willow and sweet birch trees, salicylic acid works at much lower concentrations than glycolic acid, says Albert M. Kligman, M.D., emeritus professor of dermatology at the University of Pennsylvania School of Medicine in Philadelphia. That means that it causes less redness, stinging, and burning.

In one study involving hundreds of women, those who used salicylic acid on their faces reported much less irritation than the group who used glycolic acid.

Apparently, their skin looked better, too. A panel of 30 judges who looked at before-and-after photos concluded that the salicylic acid group showed more improvement in their skin than the glycolic acid group. The judges specifically looked at fine lines, blotches, and abnormal pigmentation of the skin.

Those of us who battle breakouts along with wrinkles may also want to use salicylic acid, says Dr. Kligman. Like glycolic acid, salicylic acid sloughs off, or exfoliates, the top layer of skin. It also penetrates into our pores, liberating the trapped dirt and oil that lead to acne. That's why it's the active ingredient in many over-the-counter acne medications.

Anti-aging products formulated with BHA can be found in your local drugstore. Three examples are Oil of Olay's Daily Renewal Cream with Beta Hydroxy Complex, Almay's Time-Off Revitalizer Daily Solution, and Aveda's Exfoliant.

amounts to the clean, dry skin of your face and neck, says Dr. Clark.

At the dermatologist's office. If you are sporting a few faint lines, consider seeing a dermatologist, who can offer a variety of products that can contain up to 25 percent glycolic acid. "It's clear that higher concentrations of glycolic acid—12 percent and above—are more likely to benefit aging skin," says Dr. Price. Expect to pay from $10 to $60, depending on the product line and how much glycolic acid it contains.

The advantage of going to a dermatologist is that she can examine your skin and recommend the concentration of glycolic acid that's right for you. If you have dry or sensitive skin, she may recommend using a product formulated with 8 percent glycolic acid, says Dr. Clark. Then in a month or so, after your skin adjusts, she may jump you to a higher percentage.

Oily skin can tolerate higher concentrations of glycolic acid, she says. So a dermatologist may recommend, right off the bat, a gel or oil-free cream that contains 10 to 20 percent glycolic acid.

You use doctor's-office glycolic acid products the same way as the over-the-counter variety, says Dr. Clark. You're likely to see a noticeable difference in your skin tone within 2 weeks of the first application.

If these products are going to minimize fine lines, expect to wait at least 3 months, says Nicholas V. Perricone, M.D., associate clinical professor of dermatology at the Yale University School of Medicine.

Glycolic Acid: A User's Guide

For your skin to reap the full benefits of a glycolic acid product, it must be used correctly, says Dr. Clark. Here's how to choose and use these products, whether you get them from the corner drugstore or a dermatologist.

Test the waters. Try an over-the-counter product before consulting a dermatologist, suggests Dr. Price. You may find that using a lower percentage of glycolic acid will give you the results you want.

Get the right formulation for your skin. Both over-the-counter and dermatologist's-office glycolic acid products come in creams, gels, and liquids (sometimes called serums). Generally speaking, people with dry skin prefer cream formulations, while those with thicker, oilier skin prefer the gels or the serums, says Dr. Perricone.

Test before you treat. Using glycolic acid isn't without its drawbacks: It can cause some people's skin to sting, itch, or, in rare cases, break out in a rash. So take a skin-sensitivity test before using glycolic acid for the first time, says Dr. Clark. Rub a small amount of the product on the inside of your elbow every day for a week. If there's no redness or irritation in this time, chances are that the glycolic acid won't overly irritate the skin on your face, she says. If you do experience irritation, Dr. Clark suggests that you try using the product only every other or every third day. If that doesn't work, try a lower concentration.

Apply it at night. After you apply glycolic acid, it takes at least 15 minutes for it to penetrate the skin. So if you have only minutes to spend on your morning skin-care routine, smooth on your product before bed, suggests Dr. Clark. Applying moisturizer or makeup immediately after glycolic acid can reduce its effectiveness, she says. Be sure to avoid getting glycolic acid products in or around your eyes.

Use sunscreen. The use of glycolic acid products can make skin more sensitive to the sun than it was before. So without fail, apply a sunscreen with a sun protection factor (SPF) of at least 15 before going out for the day, says Dr. Fusco. Or use one of the many moisturizers or foundations that contain SPF 15 sunscreen.

Quit if your skin cries "ouch!" Stop using glycolic acid *immediately* if your skin becomes intensely red, irritated, or inflamed, says Dr. Clark. While such severe reactions are rare, they do occur, especially in women with sensitive skin.

The "A" Team: Retin-A and Renova

When the acne medication Retin-A was introduced in 1969, women with severe acne cheered. But in 1988, when a study showed that it could also tackle wrinkles, women everywhere stampeded to the nearest dermatologist.

As we mentioned, the active ingredient in Retin-A (and its spinoff, Renova) is tretinoin. While dermatologists still prescribe Retin-A for acne, they also routinely prescribe it for aging skin. Renova is formulated specifically for the treatment of aging skin.

Like glycolic acid, Retin-A and Renova loosen and remove dead cells on the skin's top layer, making it appear smoother. But research also shows that tretinoin increases the skin's levels of collagen, lightens sun-induced freckles and age spots, and improves skin discoloration.

At the cosmetics counter. Since Retin-A and Renova are drugs, you won't find them at the cosmetics counter. What you *will* find, however, are anti-aging products that contain retinol, another derivative of vitamin A, says Dr. Terezakis.

While retinol sounds like Retin-A, there is no conclusive evidence that it *works* like it. As an antioxidant, however, retinol may offer skin some protection from free radicals, those unstable oxygen molecules that are unleashed by sunlight, smoke, and pollution and that may prematurely age skin, explains Dr. Clark.

At the dermatologist's office. Retin-A comes in cream, gel, or liquid formulations and in varying concentrations of tretinoin. For dewrinkling, most dermatologists prescribe the cream. Renova contains 0.05 percent tretinoin in a cream base.

WOMEN ASK WHY

Why do those anti-aging creams cost so darn much?

There's no *good* reason that purchasing an effective skin-care product should require a woman to take out a personal loan. No product on this earth warrants a $70 or $100—or, in some cases, a $300—price tag.

Still, cosmetics companies have their reasons for jacking up the prices of these anti-aging formulations. First, they have to pay big bucks to package and advertise them. A fancy box and a beautiful glass container often cost more than the product they contain. Second, women are willing to pay high prices to look younger, and manufacturers are happy to accommodate on that account.

Unfortunately, many women still believe that the higher the price, the higher the quality. The fact is that lots of $10 products are just as good as more expensive ones, and it's unlikely that any formulation priced over $25 is worth the money.

That said, some *ingredients* in over-the-counter products can, in theory, help aging skin look better. These include antioxidants, like vitamin C and vitamin E, which fight free-radical damage, and substances such as hyaluronic acid and mucopolysaccharides, which help skin hold on to moisture. Products containing alpha hydroxy acid (AHA) can help by exfoliating the skin.

But even if these products do work—and there is no hard proof that they do get rid of wrinkles—they still can't perform miracles. If you're looking for a "miracle" skin-care product, buy a bottle of sunscreen.

Expert consulted
Paula Begoun
Bestselling author
Professional makeup artist
Owner of a small chain of cosmetic
*   stores*
Author of Don't Go to the Cosmetics
    Counter without Me

Whether a dermatologist prescribes Retin-A or Renova depends on skin type. "People with oily skin tend to use Retin-A, while those with dry or sensitive skin prefer Renova because it has the consistency of a really heavy night cream," says Dr. Clark.

Using either one is a no-brainer. Dr. Clark recommends applying two pea-size drops—enough to cover the whole face and neck—to clean, dry skin, either every night or every other night before bed. Dot the medication on each cheek, your forehead, and your chin. Then rub it into your skin, avoiding your upper eyelids. A 2-month supply of either medication costs about $30.

Many people using Retin-A or Renova notice that their skin feels smoother after a month of treatment, says Debra Jaliman, M.D., a dermatologist in New York City. Research shows that the most significant improvement occurs over 4 to 10 months. And the more damaged your skin, the more improvement you're likely to see.

Using Retin-A or Renova does have a downside. Both, particularly Retin-A, can cause skin to swell, burn, itch, or peel. These side effects normally fade in a few weeks as skin becomes used to the medication. But if the irritation continues, a dermatologist may advise applying the drugs less often, or—in the case of Retin-A—prescribe a lower dosage, says Dr. Perricone.

Using Retin-A and Renova

Retin-A and Renova are *drugs*. So don't apply more than indicated, and don't use them more frequently than your dermatologist recommends. Also, don't use Retin-A or Renova if you are pregnant. To get the most anti-aging bang for your buck, follow the tips below.

Start now. Retin-A and Renova seem to prevent wrinkles more effectively than they erase them. So fill your first prescription before you spy the first crinkle, advises Dr. Fusco. "If you're 35 or 40 and have never worn sunscreen or have a history of burning and tanning, don't wait for the damage to show," she says.

Slather on sun protection. Every single day, apply a sunscreen with an SPF of at least 15 or use an SPF 15 moisturizer or foundation, says Dr. Fusco. Because Retin-A and Renova return the skin to its more youthful plumpness, the newer, fresher skin underneath is vulnerable to sun damage.

Soothe irritation right. To reduce temporary redness, flakiness, and irritation, use a hypoallergenic moisturizer with no added fragrances or preservatives, such as Eucerin or Complex 15, suggests Dr. Clark. Or smooth on a dab of over-the-counter hydrocortisone cream every other day.

Also, consider taking 800 international units (IU) of vitamin E a day. Preliminary studies suggest that vitamin E may reduce the irritating effects of Retin-A and Renova, says Dr. Clark. But be sure to check with your doctor before using amounts higher than 200 IU.

Practice kinder, gentler skin care. While using Retin-A or Renova, avoid using astringents or toners with a high alcohol content, products with scrubbing grains, and clay facial masks. Stay out of saunas and steam rooms, too. Since moisture and heat increase blood flow, they also increase the penetration of medications, which can cause redness. All can further irritate skin, says Dr. Clark.

Double the benefits. Ask your dermatologist about teaming Retin-A or Renova with glycolic acid, suggests Dr. Clark. "When they're used together, both seem to be more effective," she says. Generally, you apply the glycolic acid in the morning and the Retin-A or Renova before bed.

Vitamin C: Future Youth?

Topical vitamin C is the Next Big Thing in anti-aging skin care, according to Dr. Clark. Tiny vials of vitamin C "serums" sell at cosmetics counters for $65 and up, and still we empty cosmetics-counter shelves.

Research suggests that topical C can help protect our skin in several ways, says Dr. Price. "There is definitive evidence that topical vitamin C functions as an antioxidant, thereby helping to protect skin against free-radical damage," she says. "There's also strong evidence that it helps protect skin exposed to the sun: When vitamin C is applied to skin, it gets less burned. And topical C may have a protective effect when used in conjunction with sunscreen."

Sounds good so far. But does it "regenerate collagen," "renew elasticity and firmness," and "promote a smoother, firmer, more youthful-looking complexion," as its major manufacturers claim?

According to preliminary research (much of which, by the way, was conducted by folks who are selling the stuff), L-ascorbic acid can, indeed, promote the formation of collagen. Moreover, some dermatologists, including Dr. Clark, swear that the skin of their patients who use topical C appears fresher, more evenly pigmented, less blemish-prone, and, in some cases, less furrowed.

Other dermatologists say the jury's still out on topical C's crinkle-fighting capacity. "There's little scientific data to suggest that topical C definitely reverses wrinkles and promotes the production of collagen, although it may," says Dr. Price.

What does she tell her patients about C? "I tell them that, at this

WOMAN TO WOMAN
She Wanted to Revitalize Her Skin

Just past her 40th birthday, Diane McCurdy, a licensed aesthetician from Philadelphia, received an unwelcome "gift"—her first fine lines and wrinkles. But she didn't get blue. Instead, she started applying a pea-size amount of one of the new "youth" creams to the fair, freckled skin of her face and neck. Did it work? Here's her story.

I was 41 when I noticed that my skin was looking, well, older. I have my father's Irish skin—fair, freckled, very dry. My skin looked dull and felt parched, and I was seeing my first lines.

I had heard that Renova, a prescription cream that gets rid of fine lines and age spots, was really helpful. I happen to work for a dermatologist and asked him if it would work for me. He examined my skin and prescribed Renova.

I've used this thick, virtually fragrance-free cream for 2 years now, and I couldn't be more pleased. My skin looks brighter and rosier. Its texture is much smoother, and the fine lines around my eyes and the vertical lines above my lips are less noticeable.

The difference in my skin has actually made my makeup look better. If you have any lines in your face at all, you know how foundation and powder can kind of cake into them. Renova sloughs off dead cells from the skin's top layer, so your makeup goes on more smoothly.

Looking younger on the outside has improved my inside. My self-esteem is higher. I have more self-confidence—I feel good about myself.

Renova has definitely helped my skin look younger. But I have to credit my sunscreen habit, too. You absolutely have to use sunscreen. Every single day I use a sunscreen with a sun protection factor (SPF) of 20 that contains zinc oxide or titanium dioxide because it gives a much broader range of protection against ultraviolet A and B rays.

A lot of my friends and acquaintances have noticed the improvement in my skin. My husband's reaction? He got his own prescription for Renova. He has Irish skin, too.

point in time, the best way to protect their skin is to use a broad-spectrum sunscreen that contains transparent zinc oxide. And then, if they can afford to, they should use topical C, because the combination will probably be more protective than sunscreen alone."

Typically, topical C is applied to clean, dry skin once a day. According to the manufacturers of Cellex-C, one of the most popular topical vitamin C products, fine lines will become less noticeable in 3 to 8 months.

Don't Get Lost at "C"

Keep in mind that topical C has not been conclusively proven to reduce wrinkles. ("With topical C going for $70 a pop, I'd put my money on tretinoin," says Dr. Terezakis.) On the other hand, if you want to maximize the effectiveness of your sunscreen, it may be worth buying—if you can afford it. Here's what to look for.

At the cosmetics counter. With some notable exceptions, vitamin C creams are unlikely to work, says Dr. Price. Mostly because vitamin C is extremely unstable and loses its potency rapidly, explains Dr. Clark. There's also no telling how much vitamin C these products contain—or if it's in a form that won't break down as soon as you open the jar or that has already been broken down by other ingredients.

The *only* topical C products that have been scientifically tested for their effects on aging skin contain a 5 to 15 percent concentration of L-ascorbic acid, a specific form of vitamin C. They also have a low (acidic) pH, which helps the skin absorb the vitamin. They're pure formulations that don't contain extra ingredients, such as sunscreen or other vitamins, and they are kept airtight in their dispensers to prevent oxygen from breaking down the vitamin C and turning it brown. These products have been shown to penetrate the skin and protect against free-radical formation.

Currently, several brands of topical vitamin C meet these standards, say Dr. Price and Dr. Clark. And you can find them all in the cosmetics departments of fine department stores, licensed skin-care professionals' offices, and skin-care salons. You can also get them through mail order.

Cellex-C's High-Potency Serum contains 10 percent L-ascorbic acid. Another brand, EmerginC, offers a serum (with 12 percent L-ascorbic acid) and a cream (with 10 percent). The Skinceuticals line features a High-Potency Serum 15 (with 15 percent L-ascorbic acid) and a High-Potency Serum (with 10 percent).

Getting the Most from C

Want to see for yourself whether topical C smooths away your fine lines and wrinkles? To increase your chance for success, follow the expert-recommended tips below.

Store C correctly. To prevent vitamin C cream or serum from breaking down too quickly, store it in a cool, dark place, says Dr. Clark. It's okay if the cream turns honey-colored or amber, she says. But if it turns dark brown or begins to smell funny, toss it.

Use a pump formula. A pump bottle seals out oxygen, which will extend the life of the product, says Dr. Clark.

Use C before Zzzs. It takes a full hour for L-ascorbic acid to properly penetrate the skin, says Dr. Clark. So rather than use a topical vitamin C product in the morning—and waiting to apply your moisturizer and makeup—apply it at night, before bed. If you're also using Retin-A or Renova, or other alternate products, then apply topical C on your "off" nights, she says.

Keep the sunscreen flowing. While topical C seems to offer skin extra protection from the sun, it is *not* a sunscreen, says Dr. Price. So keep slathering on that SPF 15.

Update Your Makeup

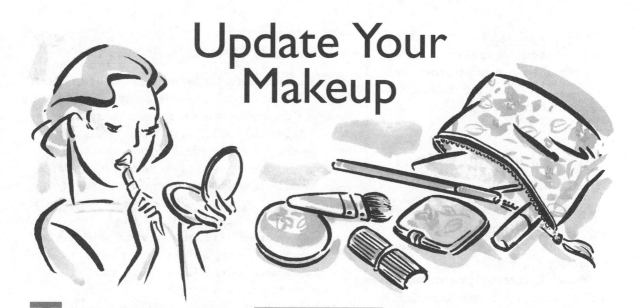

There comes a time in almost every woman's life when, standing bleary-eyed in front of her bathroom mirror, she offers up a brief prayer of thanks:

Thank God for makeup.

Using cosmetics is the simplest way to minimize or conceal age-related skin imperfections—instantly. Foundation softens the appearance of fine lines, brightens skin, and hides discoloration. Concealer erases dark circles under your eyes or broken capillaries on your cheeks. Blusher returns the bloom of youth to a tired-looking complexion, while lipstick gives pale or sallow skin a welcome jolt of color. A touch of powder ensures that makeup lasts longer and colors stay truer.

What's more, makeup has gone high-tech. Today's products are lighter and sheerer. One-shade-fits-all makeups are a thing of the past, and there's a wide selection of cosmetics formulated specifically for dry and aging skin.

If you wear little or no makeup, you may be afraid that starting now will make people think you've developed a sudden interest in a career with Barnum and Bailey. But rest assured, you'll look just terrific. According to Laura Geller, makeup artist and owner of Laura Geller Make-Up Studios in New York City, makeup is virtually goof-proof once you learn the three golden rules: Less makeup is more. Don't be afraid of color, just use it subtly. And blend, blend, blend. Be sure to blend your makeup carefully, particularly in the zones shown in the illustration.

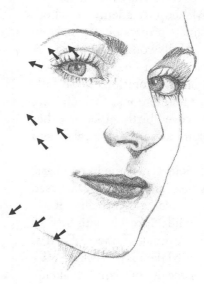

To put your best face forward, try some of these suggestions made by Geller and other makeup artists who are experts at enhancing youthfulness in mature skin.

Foundation: Add Color, Subtract Flaws

Mature skin needs color *and* subtle concealment. The right foundation delivers both. And no one will know you're wearing it but you.

Most flattering formulation: Before choosing a foundation, answer these two questions: How much do you need to hide? And does your skin need more moisture or less?

Foundations come in three weights, or amounts of coverage: sheer, medium, and full. Generally speaking, mature skin is most flattered by a sheer- or medium-weight foundation, says Doreen Milek, director of the Studio Makeup Academy, a school that trains professional makeup artists, in Hollywood, California. "A sheer foundation may not cover blotches or discoloration, while full-coverage foundations, which are meant to cover birthmarks or other serious skin flaws, can look cakey and chalky."

Foundations also come in two basic formulas: oil and water. Oil-based foundations, such as Maybelline Revitalizing Liquid Make-Up with SPF 10 Sunscreen, Almay Time-Off Age-Smoothing Makeup, or L'Oréal Visible Lift Line-Minimizing Makeup,

ARE YOU A MAKEUP ABUSER?

Makeup can help us erase the years—unless we don't apply it correctly. Then it can actually *add* them, says Doreen Milek, director of the Studio Makeup Academy, which trains professional makeup artists, in Hollywood, California. Check the list below to see if you're making these common makeup goof-ups.

Wearing too much makeup. Some of us try to hide the years beneath layers of cosmetics, says Paula Mayer, a makeup artist in San Diego. "The truth is, using too much makeup makes you look older." If your blusher looks more like windburn than a subtle wash of color, if you use a very thick foundation and apply it with a heavy hand, or if your eye makeup reminds you of Cleopatra's, chances are you're looking older than you have to.

Not blending in. Too many of us end our foundation at our jawlines, or don't blend our blusher into our foundation. That's the Tammy Faye Bakker approach to makeup—and it adds years, says Milek. So blend your foundation, blusher, and eye shadow until you can't see where they begin and end.

Wearing those "Groucho" eyebrows. Okay, you don't make your eyebrows *that* dark and heavy, but you get the picture. "Use a powder eye shadow on brows," recommends Mayer. "It gives brows a soft, natural look that brow pencils can't." She uses a deep gray shadow on brunettes and women with gray hair, and a soft brown on blondes and redheads.

Using too much liner under eyes. "It makes eyes look smaller," says Laura Geller, makeup artist and owner of Laura Geller Make-Up Studios in New York City.

Being stuck in the past. We wouldn't be caught dead in the miniskirts we bought in 1968 or the gaucho pants we loved in 1978. But many of us think nothing of applying makeup the same way we did when the Supremes (or Led Zeppelin) broke up.

The point: Makeup styles change, and to look more youthful, we have to keep up. "Not adapting your makeup to reflect the times is aging," says Milek. "Your face has changed, and your makeup should reflect those changes."

Here are some of the ways—subtle and not-so-subtle—that makeup styles have evolved over the years.

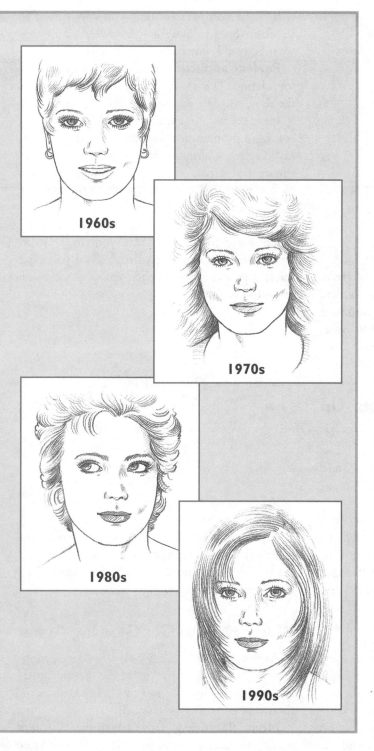

1960s

1970s

1980s

1990s

are best for dry or mature skin, says Geller. Oil-based foundations add moisture to skin, giving it a dewy appearance.

Whatever foundation you choose, select a product that contains added sunscreen, says Milek. It will help fortify your skin against sun damage.

Can't-go-wrong colors: The first step is to decide whether your skin contains more red (ruddy) or yellow (sallow) tones, says Geller. (If you can't tell, hold a piece of very white paper against your skin. It will help you to see these red or yellow tones.)

Yellow-based shades such as gold beige or honey beige are most flattering to ruddy skin, while rosier shades such as rose beige and ivory beige can perk up a sallow complexion, says Geller. Very fair skin is most flattered by shades that look more ivory than yellow, such as alabaster.

Test makeup on your chest or neck, rather than on your hand. "The skin in these areas is a closer match to skin on your face," says Milek.

Perfect application: Apply an oil-based foundation with a wet cosmetic sponge, says Milek. "It goes on more thinly and evenly that way." Sponge on a bit more foundation on areas of discoloration—for most of us, the cheeks and the sides of the nose.

Don't use too much foundation under your eyes. "A thick layer of foundation in this area will draw attention to crow's-feet and skin that's gotten a little mottled like crepe paper," she says.

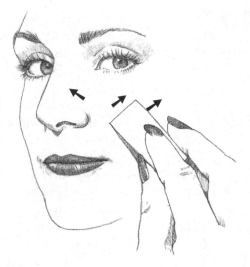

Tips and tricks: To get the look of flawless skin without using a ton of foundation, use your fingers to smooth a small amount just over your cheeks or the sides of your nose, suggests Geller. Blend well so that you can't see where the foundation begins and ends.

Concealer: The Great Cover-Up

Remember when concealer had the consistency and color of Spackle? Not anymore. These days, concealers are lighter and creamier, and they come in almost as many shades as foundations do.

Most flattering formulation: Choose a creamy concealer that comes in a pot or with a wand (such as Almay Extra Moisturizing Undereye Cover Cream or Almay Time-Off Age-Smoothing Concealer). They're sheerer and lighter than stick formulations, so they won't look thick or chalky when you wear them. They're also easier to blend than stick concealers and won't drag across the thin, delicate skin under the eyes.

Can't-go-wrong colors: Choose a concealer one shade lighter than your skin tone, says Geller. To find a perfect match, go to a store where samples are available, then dab a bit on your cheek and head outside (or to a window)

with your compact so that you can view the shade in broad daylight. (As awkward as this sounds, you'll only have to do it once.)

Perfect application: Apply concealer *after* foundation. "This way, if your foundation covers the flaw, you can skip it altogether," says Geller.

Here's how to camouflage dark circles, a common problem for women with mature skin, says Geller. Using a small, soft brush or your finger, dot a tiny amount of concealer under each eye, from the inside corner to the middle. (Don't extend it to the outside of the eye because it will eventually seep into crow's-feet.) Then blend the product into your foundation with your finger or a tiny brush until you can't see it anymore. Blot off the excess with a tissue or cotton square.

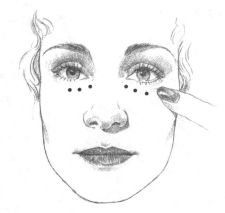

Tips and tricks: If the skin under your eyes is very dry, pat on a light eye cream before you apply concealer, says Geller. It will make even a sheer concealer sheerer.

Blush: How to Get Glowing Again

As we get older, skin often becomes more sallow. But no one has to know. Properly selected and applied, blusher can help mature skin recapture the rosiness of youth.

Most flattering formulation: Blushers come in cream, powder, and cream-powder formulations. Cream formulations, such as Revlon Colorstay Cheekcolor (which comes with a sponge rather than a brush), or creampowder blushers are most flattering to dry or mature skin. "Powder blushers accentuate lines and wrinkles," says Milek. For sheer, "barely there" color, try a gel, such as Origins Pinch Your Cheeks (available in some department stores).

Can't-go-wrong colors: Warm shades of blush that contain more yellow than red are more forgiving of mature skin. "Virtually any woman looks beautiful in warm shades of peach and pink," Milek says.

If you have gray hair, use shades of pink, rose, plum, or mauve. "They complement gray hair beautifully, no matter what your skin tone," says Geller.

Perfect application: If you need to minimize lines and wrinkles, apply blusher to the apples of your cheeks only, says Geller. (To find this point, smile broadly, then find the swell with your fingers.)

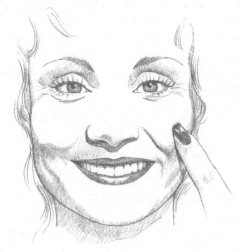

GETTING THE LIPS YOU WANT

As we age, we may lose pigment in our skin and lips. Some women also notice that their upper lips get thinner.

To counteract the effects of time and get fuller-looking lips, choose light- to medium-colored lipstick and a matching lip liner. Keep in mind that lighter colors tend to make lips appear larger and fuller, while darker colors will shrink them. The same goes for lip liner, says Pat Ely, a makeup artist in Walnut Creek, California. "A lot of women like to use a dark liner to outline their lips, thinking it will make them stand out, but darker colors will only make lips look smaller."

Instead, match your liner to your lipstick, adding a spot of glossy color to your bottom lip for a fuller effect. Outline your mouth with lip liner and fill in with a matching lipstick. If you're not happy with the natural shape of your mouth, says Ely, apply the lip liner slightly outside of your natural lip line.

To make your bottom lip look fuller, use a lighter shade of frosted or glossy lip color in the center of your lower lip.

To apply cream blusher, place a dime-size dot on each cheek with a finger or a cosmetic sponge, says Geller. Then blend, wiping off excess color with a piece of tissue or a cotton square. To apply cream-powder blusher, touch the bristles of the brush to the product, tap off the excess color, and apply lightly. Blend until you can't see where the color begins or ends.

Tips and tricks: While powder blushers are beautiful, many contain intense pigment and end up looking too dark, says Milek. To tone down the color of your favorite powder blush, dip your blusher brush into a little loose powder (baby powder is fine), then apply the blusher itself.

Powder: Set It and Forget It

Despite what you may think, using powder will *not* draw attention to your every line and wrinkle, says Milek. "Used correctly, powder sets makeup and gives it a polished look," she says.

Most flattering formulation:
Powders come in two formulations—
pressed or loose—and both can be used
on mature skin, says Milek. Pressed
powder comes in a compact and is applied with a dry sponge. Loose powder
comes in a container and is brushed on
with a large, fluffy brush.

Whichever formulation you choose,
buy a product made specifically for
mature skin: They contain added moisturizers. Two to try are Revlon Age-
Defying Pressed Loose Powder and
Maybelline Moisture Whip Loose
Powder.

Can't-go-wrong colors: Select a
powder three shades lighter than your
foundation, says Milek. If you don't
wear foundation, dust your face with a
sheer, tinted, loose or pressed powder
to hide flaws and give skin a more polished appearance, suggests Geller.

Perfect application: To apply
pressed powder, "tap" the powder into
your makeup using the puff that comes
with the compact, says Milek.

Dust on loose powder with a big,
fluffy makeup brush, whisking off the
excess. Once a week, clean your powder
brush in warm, soapy water. A clean
brush slips across your skin better than
one permeated with facial oil, says Milek.

Before you touch up your makeup,
blend foundation that has seeped into
the lines around your eyes and mouth
with a dry sponge or a piece of tissue,
advises Milek. "If you don't, your
powder will set those creases," she says.

Tips and tricks: For special occasions, dust
a lightly frosted powder over your cheekbones,
suggests Geller. "It will give your skin an
added glow."

REAL-LIFE SCENARIO

*She's Never Worn Makeup and Doesn't
Know Where to Start*

**Marti had one of those "peaches 'n' cream" complexions
when she was younger, firm and unblemished, with lively,
impish green eyes and full lips that seemed to curve up at
the edges, as if she were smiling at a secret. Her mother
would never let her wear makeup. Someone so fresh,
healthy, and full of color didn't need it. Only now that she's
in her forties, she does need it. Her eyes, once so bright,
seem washed out. Her complexion has become pale and
dry. Her lips have grown thinner. Her friends have encouraged her to start wearing a little makeup, but when she tried
applying foundation, lipstick, eyeliner, and rouge, they made
her look even older. She's not discouraged yet, but she
doesn't know what to try next. Is there a good place for her
to start?**

The truth is, applying makeup is a
skill, and as with any skill, practice makes perfect. Marti will
need to experiment with makeup until she hits upon products that suit her skin and she finds her own unique
makeup style.

Marti will save money and learn more quickly if she ex-
periments with one or two cosmetics at a time. Lipstick
and mascara are makeup basics, so she should focus on
them first.

Finding the "right" lipstick is a matter of trial and error,
even for women who've used cosmetics for years. But in
general, cream lipsticks in soft, warm shades soften the look
of aging skin and play down lines around the mouth.

If Marti has tiny vertical lines around her mouth, using a
colorless (nude) lip pencil will keep her lipstick from
bleeding. Nude shades are virtually invisible, so they're most
forgiving of shaky fingers.

Eye Makeup: Pump Up
Your Peeper Power

A soft smudge of liner around your eyes and a
coat or two of mascara can make your eyes ap-

As for mascara, Marti should avoid the "thickening" formulas. Many contain fibers that can make lashes look clumpy and messy. To thicken her lashes, she can dust them with powder first, then apply mascara.

Blush comes next. Because Marti has dry skin, she should opt for a cream blush that closely matches the shade of her lipstick.

Finding the right foundation can be tricky, but once Marti finds it, chances are she'll never have to do it again.

An oil-based foundation makes dry skin look fresher and gives it a dewy appearance. To find the right shade, Marti should match the foundation to the skin on her neck—in natural light, if possible.

Sometimes, makeup-shy women don't like the feel of foundation on their skin. To get the look of flawless skin without feeling as though she's wearing a mask, Marti can apply foundation only to areas of discoloration—on most women, the cheeks, around the nose, under the eyes, and the chin, blending until she can't see where the foundation begins and ends.

Makeup novices often end their foundation at their jawlines. If Marti wants to use foundation all over her face, she'll need to use it on the entire front of her neck, too. Using a makeup sponge moistened with water will help her blend flawlessly and give her foundation a sheer, "barely there" look.

Marti can tackle eye shadow and other eye makeup later on, when she's mastered the basics. It shouldn't be long until she's using makeup with confidence and looking more youthful.

Expert consulted
Paula Mayer
Makeup artist
San Diego

age. Cream-based eye shadows and pencils will nourish this delicate skin while they camouflage crinkles.

Eye shadow. Eye shadows come in two basic formulations. The cream shadows (such as Revlon Age-Defying Eye Color) are usually applied with a wand. Powder shadows come in a cake and are applied with a sponge-tip applicator or a brush. If your skin is very dry, opt for cream-based shadows, says Geller. "They're easy to apply and long wearing," she adds. And like cream blushers, creamy shadows soften the appearance of wrinkles.

Also, select a shadow with a bit of shimmer to it—in makeup artist jargon, a "low-pearl" shadow. Yes, you heard right. "Most women think that frosted shadows will accentuate aging eyes," says Geller. "In fact, a softly shimmering shadow can soften them." Be sure to avoid Las Vegas–showgirl frosts, however. Very sparkly, glittery shadows spotlight every droop and wrinkle.

Eyeliner. Opt for pencil liners, recommends Geller. Wax-based eye pencils are fine, but the softer ones may smudge, and the extra-hard ones will drag across delicate undereye skin. So she recommends using powder eyeliner pencils (such as Elizabeth Arden Smoky Eyes Powder Pencil or Revlon Softsmoke Powderliner). "They make the eyes look smoky and soft, and they're easy to apply," she says.

What *not* to use: liquid liners. "If you have lines on your face, you don't need to paint on more," says Milek.

Mascara. Choose a fiber-free mascara. Most mascara is fiber-free, but if not, the packaging

pear bigger and brighter. And if you have droopy lids, a subtle application of the right eye shadow can help bring them out of hiding.

Most flattering formulation: The skin around our eyes becomes thinner and drier with

will be labeled "with fibers," Geller says. Mascaras that contain fibers tend to cake, clump, and look goopy, which draws attention to aging eyes.

Can't-go-wrong colors: Afraid you'll use the wrong shade of shadow or pencil and end up looking like, well, your eccentric Aunt Matilda? You won't if you use muted hues that flatter your hair color and skin tone.

Eye shadow. Those of us with dark hair and medium to dark skin can wear virtually any shade of shadow. "Brunettes look particularly good in bronze or champagne, which is a very pale pink," says Geller. Blondes with ruddy skin look best in shades of taupe, beige, and charcoal brown, while blondes with more yellow in their skin are flattered by shades of violet, slate, and gray-brown. If you have gray hair, you'll always look great in shades of taupe and soft gray, she says.

Eyeliner. Darker shades of navy and hunter green flatter any skin tone and make the whites of the eyes appear brighter, says Geller. For a more subtle effect, use shades of brown or khaki (a soft greenish brown). If you're using black liner, toss it immediately: "Black is much too harsh for mature skin," she says.

Mascara. Black for brunettes, brown for blondes and redheads, says Geller. To give your eyes an extra sparkle, try navy mascara. "It adds just a hint of color and will make your eyes appear brighter," she says.

Perfect application: Applying shadow, liner, and mascara to your best advantage can be tricky, but using the tips below will make the job much easier.

Eye shadow. To apply a cream-based shadow, smudge it on with a clean pinky finger, says Milek. "It's easier to control your finger than an applicator, and the color will be softer and more subtle," she says.

Stroke on powder shadow with a small eye brush. "A brush distributes the color more finely and evenly than a sponge applicator can," says Geller. Brush a V-shaped arc of shadow from the outer corner of your eye, extending one side of the V so that the shadow covers any drooping area over the lid and brushing the other side into your lashes.

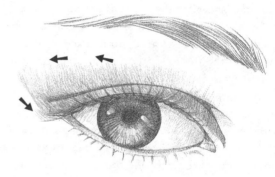

Eyeliner. If you have shaky fingers, apply eye makeup sitting at a table, using a mirror placed at eye level, suggests Geller. Rest the elbow of the hand holding the eye pencil on the table. Then anchor your elbow with your other hand.

Mascara. For clump-free lashes, wipe off the wand before applying mascara, says Milek. To thicken skimpy lashes, dust them with powder before you apply the first coat.

Tips and tricks: Curling your lashes will make them appear thicker and your eyes bigger and brighter, says Milek.

Dig out your metal eyelash curler—the one you swore you'd never use again—and hold it under your blow-dryer for 5 to 10 seconds. The heat will help your lashes hold their curl, says Geller. (Use common sense, please: Test the metal against your hand before touching it to your eye area.)

Lipstick: The Bare Essential

"Every woman should wear lipstick, regardless of her age," says Geller. "But if you have mature skin, the right lipstick can brighten up your entire face, making your skin appear more youthful."

Most flattering formulation: Lips get drier with age. To keep them moist and supple, choose cream lipsticks, which contain added moisturizers (such as Revlon Moon Drops Moisture Creme and Lancôme Hydra-Riche Hydrating Lip Colour), advises Geller. As a bonus, cream formulations soften the appearance of mature skin and draw attention away from lines and wrinkles, she says.

If you prefer a more natural look, try lip gloss. "It provides just a hint of color and a faint shimmer," says Milek.

Can't-go-wrong colors: If you're a fair-skinned blonde, opt for soft shades of mauve (warm pink), says Paula Mayer, a makeup artist in San Diego. Blondes with darker skin look great in warm browns, such as sand, or orange-based reds. Olive-skinned brunettes look best in shades of peach, orange-red, wine, and burgundy. Fair-skinned brunettes should favor bright fuchsias or softer shades of pink. Redheads with freckles look best in cinnamon and terra cotta colors.

Shades of mauve, apricot, and copper will

HOW TO BE A SMASH AT YOUR CLASS REUNION

Class reunions are a time for fond memories, greeting long-lost friends . . . and worrying about how you're going to look to these people, now that you're 20 or 25 years older. How to look your best? These tips will help you stand out from the crowd around the punch bowl.

Flash a smile in drop-dead red. A woman in red lipstick demands attention, says Laura Geller, makeup artist and owner of Laura Geller Make-Up Studios in New York City. And chances are, it will complement whatever you plan to wear. Red matches especially well with neutral colors such as black, brown, navy, gray, and, well, red. Forget the red lips, though, if you plan to wear an unusual color, such as purple or orange.

Shape up those brows. Now is a perfect opportunity to have your eyebrows professionally waxed and shaped, says Geller, especially if they're on the bushy side. "Neat, well-groomed eyebrows emphasize your eyes," she says. Depending on where you live, this little luxury could cost you less than $15.

Be perfectly polished. As long as you're getting your brows done, treat yourself to a professional manicure, too, says Judith Ann Graham, vice president of the Association of Image Consultants International in Washington, D.C. "You'll be holding and hugging people, and your hands will be on display."

Sport a jacket. Consider wearing a pantsuit with a jacket. "Wearing a jacket makes a statement: 'I'm powerful, in control,'" says Graham. That's not to say you should wear your interview suit. "An elegant, feminine pantsuit in a color you love can make you look powerful, yet still approachable," she says.

"cool down" ruddy skin or deemphasize broken capillaries, adds Milek.

All of us can wear what's called a true red, which contains an equal amount of yellow and blue. "True red lipstick looks particularly striking on women with gray hair," says Milek. Another foolproof color, according to Milek: Natural Mist Cream, made by Sally Hansen. "It's not brown, it's not peach, it's not pink, but a combination of the three. And it works on every woman," she says.

Whatever color you choose, stick to soft shades. "Lips get thinner with age," says Geller. "Very dark colors make them look even thinner."

Perfect application: Most of us slick on lipstick straight from the tube. Perfectly fine, says Geller. But if your lip color seeps into tiny creases above your lips, enlist the aid of a lip pencil, she advises. "The wax in the pencil acts as a barrier, keeping lipstick from feathering or bleeding," she says. For a soft, natural look, use a nude lip liner.

Tips and tricks: To plump up thin lips, choose a lip color with just a hint of frost. "Soft frosts reflect light, which makes lips appear fuller," says Geller.

To keep lipstick off your teeth, do what models do: After you apply lipstick, put your index finger in your mouth. Then draw it out slowly, with your mouth closed. "Whatever ends up on your finger would have ended up on your teeth," says Geller. Or you could just swab a little petroleum jelly onto your front upper teeth to keep the lipstick off, she adds.

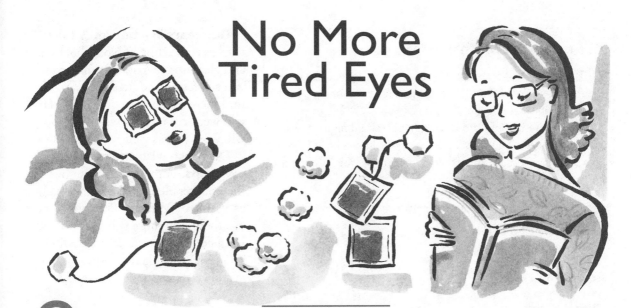

No More Tired Eyes

Of all six senses, we rely on vision the most. In fact, a full 80 percent of the information that we gather from the world around us passes through our eyes.

With that kind of activity, our eyes are entitled to get a little tired and sore from time to time. But these days, eye problems seem more prevalent than ever. That's because we're devoting more time to what optometrists call near-point tasks—things such as gazing at computer and TV screens and reading the tiny type in stock reports and on food labels. Unfortunately, human eyes weren't designed for this kind of up-close work.

"Most common eye conditions—including bloodshot eyes and eyestrain—can have a functional cause, meaning that they occur because of the way we use our eyes," explains Anne Barber, O.D., director of program services for the Optometric Extension Program Foundation, an organization based in Santa Ana, California, that promotes vision education. "They're characteristic of a visual system that isn't functioning as efficiently as it should."

Regular exams are your best eye insurance because they'll catch any vision changes—as well as serious conditions such as cataracts, glaucoma, and macular degeneration—early on. Dr. Barber suggests that you see an optometrist or ophthalmologist every two years until you reach age 55, then every year thereafter. "If we catch a problem early on and start treating it right away, we stand a better chance of saving vision. So be sure your vision care provider does a full series of near-point vision tests and provides vision therapy to take care of functional problems or refers you to an office that does," she says.

For more run-of-the-mill eye conditions, proper self-care is usually sufficient. Eye doctors share these favorite natural remedies for keeping the eyes and eye area healthy.

Bloodshot Eyes

As eye problems go, bloodshot eyes are easy to self-diagnose. You just have to look in the mirror. To bring those blood vessels down to size and get rid of the redness, follow this advice.

Clear your eyes with cold. Wrap ice cubes in a clean washcloth and lay the compress over your eyes for 30 minutes.

EYEDROPS MADE EASY

The tough thing about putting in eyedrops is that you can't see what you're doing. More drops end up running down your face in the opposite direction!

Here's the no-fuss, no-drip way to self-administer eyedrops, from Anne Sumers, M.D., an ophthalmologist in Ridgewood, New Jersey, and spokesperson for the American Academy of Ophthalmology.

Tilt your head back or lie down on the couch. Pull your lower lid away from your eye so that it forms a little pocket. Then, squeeze the eyedrop into the pocket. Do not let the dropper touch your eye or eyelid. Bacteria can contaminate the eyedropper if it touches you. Contact with the dropper can also scratch your cornea.

Do the second eye immediately after the first. Then, after the drops are in, close your eyes for a minute or two and press your index fingers next to the corners of your eyes where they meet your nose. Keeping your eyes open or blinking will send the drops into the drainage duct between your eye and nose. If that happens, your eye won't benefit from the drops at all. In fact, if you're using a type of prescription drops called beta-blockers and it goes down into that duct, you could experience a slow or irregular heartbeat, says Dr. Sumers. But closing your eyes and pressing against them with your index fingers closes that duct so that drops stay in the eye where they belong.

Before opening your eyes, wipe away any lingering moisture from your closed lids. Finally, if you don't think the drop got into your eye, do it again. You can't overdose on eyedrops, says Dr. Sumers.

Buy tears in a bottle. Artificial tears ease the sting of bloodshot eyes and clear up the irritation that made you see red in the first place. You'll find these products in drugstores. (If you wear contacts, rewetting drops will work just as well.)

Dispense with the medicated eyedrops. Funny thing about over-the-counter medicated eyedrops such as Visine or Murine: The more you use them, the more you need them. It's a condition that doctors call rebound hyperemia. So reserve medicated eyedrops for occasional use.

Crow's-Feet

The first signs of crow's-feet usually appear when we reach our late twenties. At that point, the tiny lines are visible only when we squint. They gradually deepen over the years and become prominent once we reach our forties.

The sooner you take steps to prevent crow's-feet, the younger the skin around your eyes will remain. But even if you already have lines, you can minimize their appearance.

Fade lines with AHAs. Alpha hydroxy acids (AHAs)—natural acids derived from foods such as fruits, sugarcane, and sour milk—diminish crow's-feet by sloughing off old skin cells and exposing younger cells underneath. AHAs also plump the skin and restore its ability to retain moisture. Look for an eye cream containing 5 percent AHAs. (Be careful to avoid your eyelids when applying.)

Switch from alpha to beta. If you have sensitive skin, use a product containing beta hydroxy acids. They reduce fine lines and wrinkles just as well as AHAs but with less irritation.

Invest in cool shades. Always wear wraparound sunglasses in bright or hazy outdoor light. Sunglasses may help prevent crow's-feet by stopping you from squinting.

Stop rubbing your eyes. The skin around your eyes can stretch and wrinkle in response to repeated rubbing.

Dark Circles

Go ahead and blame Mom or Dad for those dark circles under your eyes. Contrary to popular belief, heredity—not lack of sleep—typically paints that bluish black or brownish tinge on the skin. While fatigue doesn't cause dark circles, it can certainly make them more pronounced. So can excessive sun exposure, as the sun's rays break down collagen and elastin. Allergies, illness, menstruation, and even pregnancy can also aggravate existing dark circles.

Medically speaking, dark circles under the eyes are harmless. Still, if you have them, you probably wish they were a little less noticeable. They can be, if you follow this advice.

Count on chamomile. Chamomile helps minimize dark circles by constricting the blood vessels, including those under the eyes. Place a steeped, chilled chamomile tea bag under each closed eye for 10 to 20 minutes in the morning, while you're waiting for the coffee to brew.

Note: Some pollen-sensitive people may be allergic to chamomile tea. Discontinue use if you experience any negative reaction.

FOLK REMEDY: DOES IT WORK?

Cucumber Slices on Puffy Eyes

The old saying "cool as a cucumber" is probably what sparked the idea that putting cucumbers on your eyes can help reduce puffiness (much like an ice pack can reduce swelling).

"Puffy eyes are induced by things like crying, menstruation, or any other factor that may cause the body to retain fluid," says Mary Ruth Buchness, M.D., chief of dermatology at St. Vincent's Hospital and Medical Center in New York City. So even something as cool as a cucumber isn't going to take the fluid away.

The problem is that cucumbers may even make your eyes feel worse. They contain a substance that can cause an immediate reaction in the form of hives in some women.

RECOMMENDATION: Forget It

Let witch hazel do the work. As an alternative to chamomile, soak cotton balls in witch hazel and lay them on the skin under your closed eyes for 20 minutes.

Keep them hidden. To cover dark circles, use a yellow-based stick concealer. Yellow neutralizes pink, red, and purple hues in the skin.

Eye Irritations

Unless you wear protective goggles 24 hours a day, you're eventually going to get something in your eye. It could be a speck of dust, grit, or makeup. The longer it stays put, the more red, scratchy, and swollen your eye will become.

But foreign objects aren't the only things that irritate eyes. Smoke, pollen, and chlorine (in swimming pools) do the job just as well. If you have removed an irritant yet you have discharge coming from your eye or other abnormal symptoms, see your ophthalmologist. Irritation can also arise from a bacterial or viral infection.

Whatever its cause, eye irritation can usually be treated at home with simple self-care techniques. Here's what to do.

Flip your lid. If something is in your eye, you can use your eyelids to gently push the particle down and out. Grasp the eyelashes of your upper lid between your fingers, then pull the upper lid over the lower lid. This allows the lower lashes to brush the speck off the inside of your upper lid. If the particle moves to the corner of your eye, remove it with the corner of a moist tissue.

Let the water flow. Ordinary tap water can flush a foreign object from your eye. Go to the sink, lean down close to the faucet, and splash water into your eye.

Be bold with cold. For irritation caused by an allergy, lay a washcloth soaked in fresh cold water over your eyes for 5 to 10 minutes.

Make a shampoo solution. Eye irritation sometimes results from blepharitis, a condition in which the eyelid margin (the thin edge of skin between your eyeball and eyelashes) becomes swollen from excess oil production. To treat blepharitis, add two or three drops of no-tears baby shampoo to one-third cup of water, dip a cotton swab into the solution, and run the swab along the bottom eyelid margin while your eye is open. Then close your eye and run the swab over the top eyelid margin where the lid meets the eyelashes. Use this remedy once or twice a day.

Pinkeye

Feel as though a mosquito is permanently lodged underneath your eyelid? Are the whites of your eyes so irritated that they've turned pink or bloodshot red? Odds are that you have pinkeye.

REAL-LIFE SCENARIO
She's "Contacted" an Eye Problem

When Marie moved to Tucson, Arizona, last year to get relief from her allergies, she decided it was time for a total makeover. She took up exercise, got a new hairdo, started wearing makeup, and traded in her glasses (which she had been wearing since she was 5) for contact lenses. At 35, she never looked better in her life, but she's having problems with her contact lenses. Even though she switched to makeup formulated for sensitive eyes, her eyes feel itchy and dry by the end of the day. She doesn't want to go back to wearing glasses but is worried that the contacts will ruin her eyes.

The reasons why Marie is having problems with her eyes are multiple, but they're not too big to overcome.

To begin with, most women's eyes tend to dry a bit after age 35, which is complicated even more by living in a dry climate such as Tucson. And if she takes antihistamines to control her allergies, they can make a dry problem even drier. Plus, eyes can be sensitive to makeup. So it's no wonder that her contacts are irritating her eyes. This doesn't mean, though, that she must go back to wearing glasses.

First, she should talk to her ophthalmologist about

Typically, pinkeye results from an allergy to pollen, pet dander, or certain chemicals or from a bacterial or viral infection. In fact, the same viruses that cause the common cold can also cause pinkeye. And like the common cold, infectious pinkeye is extremely contagious and easily spread by hand-to-eye contact.

Bacterial pinkeye is the most serious type, and unless it's treated with prescription medication, it can lead to loss of vision.

Seeing a doctor at the first sign of pinkeye is important. She can decide whether you require a prescription or you can manage the condition with self-care alone. Then use these strategies to help relieve the immediate symptoms and prevent the spread of germs.

switching to a lens with a lower water content to prevent her eyes from dehydrating. She can also try over-the-counter moisturizing eyedrops, or artificial tears, which are especially helpful at the end of the day. And since she lives in a sunny climate, she should always wear sunglasses when outside. Sun is irritating on the eyes, too.

At home, Marie can create a more humid environment for her eyes by using air-conditioning less, running a humidifier, and keeping plants in the bedroom. Most important, she should give her eyes a rest and take her contacts out when she's in for the night. When she cleans her lenses, Marie should use a preservative-free solution, as preservatives can irritate sensitive eyes.

Marie's makeup may be adding to her problem, but it's probably not the main cause of her itchy eyes. Her eyelids would be itchy, red, and uncomfortable all day long if that were the case. But using a good makeup remover for sensitive eyes—baby shampoo is a good one—is still wise. The key, of course, is to get it all off.

Expert consulted
Anne Sumers, M.D.
Ophthalmologist
Ridgewood, New Jersey
Spokesperson for the American Academy
of Ophthalmology

Remove your contacts. If you wear contacts, take them out at the first sign of redness and irritation. Otherwise, they'll only exacerbate your discomfort and, if you have infectious pinkeye, they'll trap the germs in your eyes.

Run hot and cold. Alternating hot and cold compresses stimulates circulation and draws infection-fighting white blood cells to your eyes. Soak a clean washcloth in very warm water, wring it out, and hold it against your eyes for a minute. Then soak the cloth in cold water, wring it out, and hold it against your eyes for a minute. Repeat this process two or three times.

Check out chickweed. The herb chickweed helps fight infection, yet it's mild enough to use on your eyes. Brew a pot of chickweed tea

and let it cool until it is comfortable to the touch. Then dip a clean cloth into the tea and hold the cloth against the affected eye while it's closed. Continue rewetting and reapplying the cloth for up to an hour.

Get goldenseal. If you have bacterial pinkeye, an eye bath of goldenseal tea can soothe your eyes and fight the infection. To make the eye bath, put one teaspoon of dried goldenseal into one cup of freshly boiled water. Steep for 10 minutes, then strain the mixture and allow the liquid to cool. Use an eyedropper to squirt two drops of the liquid into the affected eye.

Leave your eyes *au naturel*. Avoid wearing eye makeup while you have infectious pinkeye. Replace your mascara and liner. If your mascara wand or liner becomes contaminated, you'll just keep transferring the virus or bacteria from one eye to the other.

Sties

Each of your eyelids contains eyelash follicles. Sometimes one of these follicles becomes infected, perhaps because it's clogged with dandrufflike scales or you have used a germ-laden mascara brush. Eventually, a painful red lump with a white head of pus sprouts at the base of the eyelash. This is what's known as a sty.

If you have a persistent or recurrent sty, see your doctor. It could be a sign of diabetes or a cyst. Also see a doctor if your sty doesn't get better or gets worse after two days.

As with a pimple on your face, a sty should never be popped. It may rupture beneath the surface of the skin, aggravating the inflammation. Instead, heed this advice.

Hold a hot potato. Wrap a warm, damp washcloth around a hot baked potato (the cloth will retain the heat longer). Then hold the cloth against the affected, closed eye for five minutes. Repeat four times every day for two weeks. This will gently coax the sty to break open and heal.

Give your eyes a break. Stop wearing eye makeup until the sty heals. This means all eye makeup—mascara, eyeliner, and shadow. Otherwise, you may end up with several sties.

Tired Eyes

Tired eyes, while uncomfortable, are seldom cause for alarm. Still, if your discomfort persists, you should see an ophthalmologist. You may need eyeglasses when you do close work.

To perk up tired eyes, try these tips.

Look around. The moment your eyes begin to bother you, look up from your work and into the distance. This lets your eye muscles relax.

Put your palms to work. Rub your hands together to warm them up a bit. Then gently position your palms over your closed eyes. Hold for five minutes, breathing easily while you do. This should rest and rejuvenate your eyes quite nicely.

Squeeze out fatigue. Take a deep breath while raising your shoulders and squeezing your eyes and fists as tightly closed as you can. Then exhale and relax all of the muscles at once. By tightening and releasing the voluntary muscles in your shoulders and fists, you can trick the involuntary muscles in your eyes into releasing as well.

Under-Eye Bags

Women and women doctors alike often talk about baggy eyes and puffy eyes interchangeably. But there is a difference between the two.

Baggy eyes develop with age. As you grow older, the muscles under your eyes weaken, and the skin becomes less elastic. Fat tissue pushes through and around the muscles, giving the skin a swollen appearance. Once bags develop, you can't do much about them other than concealing them with makeup or having cosmetic surgery.

Puffy eyes, on the other hand, are temporary. They occur when something prompts your body to collect and retain fluid under the eyes. That something could be almost anything, including crying, lack of sleep, allergies, menstruation, or eating salty foods. If you awaken and find one eye swollen three times greater than the other, call your physician. This could be a sign of an allergic reaction to an insect bite, or hives. In addition, visit your doctor if your eyes don't close all the way (it could indicate thyroid disease).

As with baggy eyes, you can use makeup to mask puffy eyes. But to get rid of the puffiness for good, try these strategies.

Spoon on relief. One of the fastest, easiest, and cheapest ways to reduce puffiness around your eyes is with a glass of ice water and four metal serving spoons. Chill the spoons in ice water, then place one over each eye. When the spoons become warm, switch them with the others chilling in the glass of water.

Make tea bag compresses. Tea contains tannins, natural astringents that pull skin taut and reduce puffiness. Wrap two steeped tea bags that have cooled in tissue (so they won't stain your skin), then lay the bags over your closed eyes for two to five minutes.

Dry out with dandelion. A natural diuretic, the dandelion herb helps your body eliminate excess fluid. Drink a cup of dandelion leaf tea or take one-half teaspoon of dandelion leaf tincture three times a day. You can buy herbal tinctures, dried herbs, or teas in health food stores.

Note: Women who are taking diuretics, such as for high blood pressure, should not drink dandelion tea. And if you have gallbladder disease, do not use without your doctor's okay.

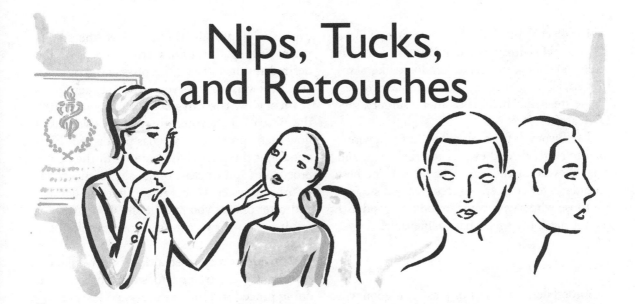

Nips, Tucks, and Retouches

If we all stayed indoors our whole lives and never used our faces to convey emotions by smiling, laughing, or crying, our faces could probably withstand the rigors of age and weather much better than they do.

But that's not reality. We go out into the sunshine, we show our feelings, and the years take their toll. By the time we've reached our thirties or early forties, the first signs of aging have begun to appear, and they show up on every part of our faces. Here's how they develop.

The eyes. Fine lines develop at the sides and underneath the eyes. Puffy upper and lower eyelids may begin to make you seem tired, even when you've been getting your Zzzs. Your eyebrows may seem lower than they once did.

The mouth. Vertical lines develop around your mouth, the corners of which may begin to turn downward in an expression of perpetual unhappiness. Your teeth may look dull, like a dingy wall in need of a fresh coat of paint.

The cheeks. Your cheeks, once full and rosy, may lose their color and their form. Excess skin may seem to drape down from your cheekbones to form jowls. If you've exercised all your life and

kept your weight in check, you may look gaunt: hollow-cheeked, with eyes that seem to sink into your face.

The nose. Your nose may seem larger, its tip thicker and lower than it was in your youth.

The neck. Your neck may begin to look stretched in the center and saggy at the sides, giving you that dreaded turkeylike appearance you may remember from the old ladies in the church choir.

What You Can Do

Granted, those wonderful women from your church were enthusiastic hymn singers and casserole makers. But they weren't sexy, didn't seem athletic, and wouldn't even think of competing on a professional level with younger women or men. In today's world, women lead active lives into their sixties, seventies, and even their eighties. They want their faces and bodies to reflect their youthful outlook on life, says Paul Carniol, M.D., a cosmetic, laser, and reconstructive plastic surgeon in Summit, New Jersey.

A woman whose face looks drawn and wrinkled at 45 can't be magically made to look like a 20-year-old swimsuit model. But she can definitely take steps to make her look like a refreshed, vibrant, energetic woman in her forties. Those steps may include cosmetic surgery, says Dr. Carniol.

"I tell women to think about how they look for their age, how they feel for their age, and what they do at their age," he says. "The best candidates for cosmetic procedures and surgery are those who say, 'I want to look as good as I can for me at my age.' That's achievable."

Where to Begin

A good dermatologist or plastic surgeon will sit down with you to discuss *your* areas of concern and not presume to know what's best for you.

"If a woman were to come in with a frog on her nose, I would still ask, 'What brings you here today?'" says Patricia S. Wexler, M.D., a cosmetic dermatologist in New York City.

Don't let a physician talk you into having your eyelids done if the thing that bothers you most are acne scars that seem more prominent on your cheeks as you age, she counsels.

Here are some ways to make certain that your first trip to the doctor's office is a fruitful one.

Dig into your photo album. A cosmetic consultation isn't like a haircut. Don't bring a picture of Cindy Crawford and ask to be made into her. Instead, select a few photographs of yourself as you've aged: one from your high school years, a few from your twenties, maybe one showing your face in your early thirties. This will help the physician see what elements of your face may be hiding in the background as you age, says Dr. Carniol.

Talk results. Some patients arrive at the office with a certain procedure (a face-lift, for example) or technology (lasers or ultrasound) in mind. Sometimes, however, a less invasive, less expensive approach would achieve the results you're seeking, notes Dr. Carniol. Focus on the desired result, but ask the physician's opinion about the various ways you could get there.

Interview the physician. Ask how much of the practice is devoted to cosmetic work and how many procedures she has performed. Find out about the physician's training in the newer procedures and whether or not she teaches them to other physicians. Be aware that the before-and-after photos you may be shown reflect best results, not your surgeon's average results, says Dr. Carniol.

Consider cross-specialties. In general, dermatologists are trained to work on the skin, doing procedures such as peels and laser resurfacing and using fillers such as collagen and fat. Plastic surgeons are more associated with face-lifts, brow-lifts, and blepharoplasty (eyelid tucks). In the cosmetic surgery world, however, the barriers have begun to blur. Dermatologists have been among the pioneers of liposuction. Most plastic surgeons have become adept with lasers.

In any case, be sure that your physician is board certified in a relevant field. You can use two reference books found in many public libraries to find board-certified plastic surgeons listed by state and city: *The Directory of Medical Specialists*, published by Marquis Who's Who, and *The Compendium of Certified Medical Specialists*, published by the American Board of Medical Specialties.

Factor the risks. Weighing the risks and benefits of surgery is even more important in cosmetic surgery than in medically necessary operations, since these are procedures simply designed to help you feel better about yourself, not to correct a health problem. Serious complications of anesthesia can be deadly. Infection, scarring, and a temporary or even a permanent loss of feeling are all possible with cosmetic surgery. Your doctor should be the one to bring these up, and you should sign a form indicating that you understand these risks before undergoing even the most minor cosmetic surgery procedure, says Dr. Carniol.

Make plans. You should leave the physician's office with a step-wise plan that addresses your concerns and reflects the amount of time and money you are willing to spend, says Dr. Carniol. The physician should also explain to you potential complications, recovery times, and care required as you recuperate.

Exploring the Possibilities

These days, cosmetic surgery offers a huge array of options to patients who want to appear youthful and more energized. From the top of your forehead down to your neck, there are choices to make about which of your features you want to enhance, how invasive a procedure you'll tolerate, how long a recovery time you can afford, and how much you're interested in spending.

To keep from getting confused or overwhelmed when you're making plans with your surgeon, get to know about some of the possibilities she may suggest before you even get to her office.

Pack your bags. Blepharoplasty is minor surgery to remove excess skin and fat from the upper and lower eyelids. The incision is hidden in the fold of your eyelids. If your vision is impaired because your eyes have become obscured by puffy lids, insurance may pay for this proce-

---

THE PRICE OF BEING CHER

While Cher has admitted to only a few cosmetic procedures, including a rhinoplasty (commonly known as a "nose job"), a breast-lift, and laser removal of two of her tattoos, gossip columnists and tabloids speculate that much more work has been done on that beautiful bod.

Without knowing details, it is difficult to estimate an exact price tag for Cher's new body, but here's a wild guess, based in part on 1997 average surgeon's fees compiled by the American Society of Plastic and Reconstructive Surgeons (ASPRS).

❧ Rhinoplasty	$3,428
❧ Breast-lift	$3,480
❧ Laser tattoo removal	$3,000*
❧ Liposuction	$1,842
❧ Face-lift	$4,783
❧ Abdominoplasty (tummy tuck)	$4,050
❧ Cheek implants	$2,083
GRAND TOTAL	$22,666

*Prices are difficult to estimate for laser tattoo removal. At the Laser and Skin Surgery Center in New York City, sessions cost $300 to $800, but many sessions may be needed, depending on the colors and size of the tattoo, type of ink used, and length of time since the tattoo was done.

---

dure, says Sterling Baker, M.D., an ophthalmologic surgeon in Oklahoma City. The average cost for blepharoplasty of the upper and lower eyelids is about $3,000.

Frown no more. One of the most revolutionary developments in cosmetic rejuvenation in recent years has been the growing popularity of Botox, a highly diluted form of botulinum toxin A. Injected into the deep furrows ("frown lines") of the mid-forehead and crinkly crow's-feet at the edges of your eyes, Botox temporarily paralyzes certain muscle groups that prod facial expressions into wrinkles.

The injections have to be repeated every 4 to 6 months and may cause some bruising. Despite the scary things you may remember about botulism, Botox uses extremely tiny, safe doses. The most serious side effect, says Dr. Wexler, is a drooping of the eyebrow, which is rare. You can expect to pay $400 to $600 per treatment of Botox injections.

Lift a little. Using tools that require minimal incisions, surgeons can reach under the skin to tighten muscles or lift the skin of your forehead, brows, and even the center of the face or neck without subjecting you to the rigors of a full face-lift. In many cases, this may be enough to address your cosmetic concerns. A minimal excision/endoscopic face-lift costs about $5,000.

Lift a lot. A full face-lift, called a rhytidectomy, tightens loose skin from the jowls, jaw, and neck. Scars are hidden around the ear or in the hairline, and the results are often combined with liposuction, laser resurfacing, or both to correct the problems a lift can't help, such as excess fat in the face and neck, surface wrinkles, and blotchy, sun-damaged skin. A traditional face-lift costs about $4,800.

Opt for the big fill. Whereas women once went for extreme face-lifts that pulled their skin up and back so tightly that they looked like they were in a wind tunnel, today's surgeons are responding to calls for a less radical look.

In many cases, that means using fillers to fill in hollowed-out regions of the lower face that have lost their youthful fullness. Generally, these include the deep creases that run between the outer edges of your nostrils to the edges of

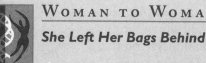

WOMAN TO WOMAN
She Left Her Bags Behind

Jaimie Keyser's friends thought she looked fabulous. After a crushing divorce 5 years before, the Oklahoma City mother of two had dieted and exercised her way into shape, gotten a new hairstyle, and landed a new job. But the beautiful, round, brown eyes that had been her most pronounced feature during her twenties told a story of stress, sun, and genetics. Then, with her 40th birthday approaching, she decided to do something about it.

After my divorce, I knew I had to recover and move on, so I went on a major program to lose weight and tone my body. I also changed the style and color of my hair. My body looked good, and I felt as if I had my soul back. But whenever I checked the mirror, I saw a set of eyes that could have been my mother's. No doubt about it, I looked old.

When I was younger, I had huge, round, brown eyes. People used to comment on them. But as I got older, they just seemed to disappear behind heavy, drooping upper eyelids—just as my mother's had. I had crow's-feet, too. I became more and more self-conscious about my eyes, especially when I went to PTA meetings, where all the other moms looked 25.

Fortunately, I knew I could do something about the situation. After years of managing early childhood education programs, I had decided to change careers and had recently taken a job as a practice coordinator with Dr. Sterling Baker, an ophthalmologic surgeon in Oklahoma City. He specializes in cosmetic surgery, so I would watch all these patients come through the office and leave looking years younger.

Finally, I decided it was my turn.

First, I had Botox for my crow's-feet. Botox is made of

your lips (the nasolabial folds), perhaps your thinning lips or pinched chin, or the mid to outer cheeks.

"A lift lifts. It doesn't fill," says Dr. Wexler, who often uses fillers to restore fullness to the cheeks.

toxin from the organisms that cause botulism, a fatal type of food poisoning, but it's very diluted. It temporarily paralyzes and relaxes the muscles around wrinkles. That was really fun to watch. The lines just disappeared.

Then I turned 39, and I had one of those midlife-crisis things. It led to a decision: I really didn't feel old, so I wasn't going to go on looking old. I talked to Dr. Baker and decided to have upper lid blepharoplasties to tighten the skin above my eyes and take out the fat pads at the edges.

The whole procedure took about 45 minutes. I had an IV, and I was put to sleep for about 10 minutes, during which time I got injections to numb the whole area. After that, I was awake and asking questions. There was no pain. All I could feel was tugging.

For that first day, I let my friends take care of me. Mothers hardly ever get babied, so I decided I was going to lie back and enjoy it. They brought me ice packs and I took extra-strength Tylenol. The next day, I was good to go, although I didn't drive for another 24 hours.

The most fun was when I went to church a week later. We're always late, so we came bustling in, and this older woman who was really supportive during my divorce turned around to give me a hug. She said, "You look great today!"

Then I noticed she kept peeking at me all through the service. Afterward, she took my hands and said, "You must love your job and your life, because you are simply glowing!"

Some people thought that I lost weight. And one friend told me, "You have your daughter's eyes." That really meant a lot to me.

I guess there are people who think this is vain. But I think you should make the most of every moment of your life, and to me, looking my best is part of being the best I can be.

When it comes to fillers, the choice is ever widening. Dr. Wexler often selects the safest, simplest alternative: the patient's own fat. For this, she performs a two-in-one procedure that liposuctions a woman's own fat from her hips, thighs, or abdomen and uses a bit of it to fill areas that could use a little plumping up.

What can't be used at once is frozen securely for monthly injections. After a year of treatments, Dr. Wexler guarantees 30 percent of the injected fat will remain permanently, which is almost always enough to fill grooves and pits. The average price for an office visit for fat injections in the face and neck is about $1,000.

Get cheeky. Ironically, it is often the women who stayed in the best shape throughout their youth who suffer the ravages of age earliest, says Dr. Wexler. That's because as we age, muscle tone and fat are lost in the face, and the skin doesn't retract but hangs on the facial bones like a half-dismantled tent sagging from its poles.

When more bulk is needed, physicians turn to a variety of products, many of which can be cut or rolled to fit the depression to be filled. Gore-Tex makes one such material; another is AlloDerm, a natural product derived from sterilized human skin cells treated to remove all cells that would transmit disease, leaving only the structural network of skin.

AlloDerm can be rolled to fill lips or folded over to level out an acne or chicken pox scar. One form of Gore-Tex comes in threads to fill a long wrinkle line. Other fillers are derived from bovine (cow) collagen or collagen grown from samples of your own tissue in a special processing laboratory. Both the cost of fillers and their placement vary widely. Collagen injections cost an average of $325 per site.

Peel away the years. Physicians or aestheticians (skin specialists trained to perform some of the less-involved procedures such as laser hair removal or light chemical peels) may recommend that you have a chemical peel, which comes in many forms. Glycolic acid, trichloracetic acid (TCA), salicylic acid, and phenol peels are applied to the face and perhaps the neck, chest, and hands for a brief period of time. Fans, ice packs, and sometimes local anesthesia will be used to reduce the immediate irritation; your skin will crust and then peel over the ensuing days to give you a smoother skin surface. The average charge for a chemical peel is $1,600.

Laser those lines. Entranced by *Star Wars* and planetarium light shows, many women believe laser beams are virtually magic, able to blaze through a person's wrinkles in a flash, without going through the trauma of plastic surgery.

The truth is that lasers come in many different forms. The Erbium-YAG laser can smooth fine wrinkles close to the skin's surface and even out irregular skin tones, producing results similar to those of a medium-strength peel. The more powerful carbon dioxide laser can erase deeper wrinkles and photodamage, but at a price. The burn left by such a laser takes weeks to heal, and the redness that follows can last up to a year. Full-face laser resurfacing costs about $2,800.

Go lightly. A new technique, microdermabrasion, has recently arrived on the American cosmetic scene from Europe. Known by such names as the Parisian Peel, Power Peel, and Derma Peel, this is a way to gently buff the skin with a machine that blows purified abrasive particles against it, then vacuums them away. Virtually painless, microdermabrasion can be performed quickly and without anesthesia. You'll

REAL-LIFE SCENARIO
She's Going After Liposuction for All the Wrong Reasons

In two weeks, Marguerite is turning 40, and she's going to give herself a birthday present: beautiful legs. She's been telling herself forever that she's going to get rid of the extra padding on her hips and thighs—especially those cellulite dimples—with a strict program of diet and exercise. But Marguerite doesn't take to strict programs of anything very easily, and beach season will be here before she knows it. She's already purchased a gorgeous new bandeau she wants to show off, but she absolutely will not wear it if her legs aren't perfect, especially in front of her husband, who she fears is losing interest in her. So she's off to the plastic surgeon to get those dimples vacuumed away through liposuction. All the stars do it. Why shouldn't she? It's as easy as one-two-three. Or is it?

Marguerite is off to a great start with her diet and exercise program, and if she sticks with it, she'll definitely improve her look. But for several reasons, she isn't the kind of liposuction candidate that most surgeons like to treat.

Chronically overweight people are not likely to achieve wonderful and permanent results, simply because their

be a bit pink, but you can return to work or your normal activities immediately. A series of five or more sessions is generally performed on a weekly or biweekly basis, followed up with monthly sessions. Microdermabrasion costs vary. You can expect to pay $100 to $200 a treatment.

Farther South

Aging doesn't stop at the face, of course, and sometimes the aging problems that most affect our appearance are well south of the chin. Cosmetic surgeons can also help you in those areas.

Sculpt your curves. Has your bikini spent the last decade stuffed deep in your pajama

weight is likely to soar after the procedure, and the fat will come back—usually in nearby areas, although it may return even to areas previously liposuctioned. The worst candidates are those whose weight yo-yos.

Marguerite has another problem: She has a hard time following strict programs. Liposuction is a surgical procedure that demands strict adherence to a doctor's orders, before, during, and after the surgery. Not doing so could compromise Marguerite's health.

Marguerite may also be unhappy with the results. Liposuction can smooth stubborn lumps of fat and provide a nicer contour to the figure, but it's not always effective at getting rid of cellulite, which is a normal and natural phenomenon in women over 30.

The biggest flashing "error" light in Marguerite's story, though, is her hope that liposuction may reignite her husband's interest in her. Removing fat off her thighs will not give her a happy life. At best, it will give her self-image a little boost.

Expert consulted
Patricia S. Wexler, M.D.
Cosmetic dermatologist
New York City

drawer? Even with exercise and a healthy eating style, most women notice that their weight begins to settle in problem areas as they approach middle age. Liposuction can help to smooth stubborn bulges in your hips, upper thighs, flanks, abdomen, and upper back.

"Liposuction won't replace weight loss, but it will contour you. It will give you back your curves," says Dr. Carniol. "It can significantly improve the contours of people who are moderately overweight and have not been able to lose weight through diet and exercise."

You should seek out an experienced liposuction surgeon who aims for a three-dimensional,

whole-body approach. Otherwise, if you gain weight, it will settle in areas you didn't have liposuctioned, says Dr. Carniol. Liposuction of a single body area costs about $1,800.

Erase your spider veins. Even if your legs are in great shape, you may be reluctant to wear shorts because of tiny red or purple lines lying close to the surface of the skin. A physician can inject these with a special solution to make them fade, in a procedure called sclerotherapy.

The process will require you to wear support stockings even after your dressings have been removed. Sclerotherapy costs an average of $300. Some physicians are using special lasers to target the pigment in spider veins; this will probably cost more, closer to the $500 range.

Recapture Your Smile

You're not a smoker and you brush, floss, use mouthwash, and see the dentist twice a year. So why the dingy smile?

"Teeth will darken with aging," sympathizes Stephen H. Fassman, D.D.S., a dentist and attending surgeon at the New York University Medical Center in New York City.

To brighten your smile again, you may want to consider bleaching your teeth. If you do, here's the way to go about it.

Skip the drugstore. No matter what they claim, companies aren't allowed to sell over-the-counter products strong enough to significantly whiten teeth, says Dr. Fassman. True teeth-bleaching formulas are considered drugs by the Food and Drug Administration. They have to be dispensed by a dentist, he says.

Start fast. In a single visit, your dentist can paint a bleach on your teeth that will lighten your teeth by a half to one full shade.

Bleach at home. You'll be fitted with soft plastic mouth guards that fit over your teeth, top and bottom. For 1 to 2 hours a night for 2 to 4 weeks, you'll fill the guard with a white, sticky gel that you get from your dentist and fit the guard snugly over your teeth.

"Within a few days, the change will be very apparent. Your teeth should be at least three shades lighter by the end of the second week," Dr. Fassman says.

"At-home bleaching is usually the method of choice," says Dr. Fassman, "but some people like to combine an in-office bleaching with the gel you use at home." The total cost for whitening your teeth will be $450 to $1,000, depending on the methods you use.

Making Your Decision

So now that you know the possibilities, how will you choose the ones that are right for you? Here are some factors to consider.

Mix and match. You may find that you can't meet your needs with just one procedure. Often, a combination of approaches is more effective, says Dee Anna Glaser, M.D., assistant professor of dermatology at St. Louis University. She weighs many factors when it comes to deciding which approaches to use on a woman's aging face.

If your deepest lines run vertically over your upper lip, you may want to consider having a laser treatment just there and using a medium-strength TCA peel on the rest of your face and neck to even out your skin tone and give you a smooth, bright, and youthful appearance, Dr. Glaser says.

High and low maintenance. A peel requires care during phases of oozing and crusting. "Some women are going to be grossed out or don't want to follow a lot of instructions," she says. For them, a laser rejuvenation may be best, even though the healing time is longer, since a synthetic dressing is applied to the entire face afterward and a nurse changes it in the office.

Putting aside time. A laser resurfacing procedure generally requires 2 full weeks of recuperation, during which you won't want to be seen in public. Many plastic surgery procedures also require hefty amounts of time spent "lying low" as bruises and scars heal enough to be covered with camouflage makeup. Some women would rather commit to numerous small procedures such as microdermabrasion, Botox injections, or light peels until their lives slow down enough to consider a more dramatic step. Others want to have everything done at once. "They might want to get it all done quickly in time for a daughter's wedding," Dr. Glaser says.

What you can afford. A face-lift, upper and lower blepharoplasties, and a full-face laser resurfacing with a peel of the neck, chest, and hands would make Grandma Moses look like a glowing beauty. But they would add up to almost $12,000.

"Before you do anything, ask yourself, 'What do I really want? What's really going to make me feel better?'" suggests Dr. Carniol. It may be that cosmetic surgery will give you a rejuvenated look that is well worth the price. On the other hand, it may turn out that what you really want is a relaxing cruise in the Mediterranean.

Secrets of Thick, Shiny Hair

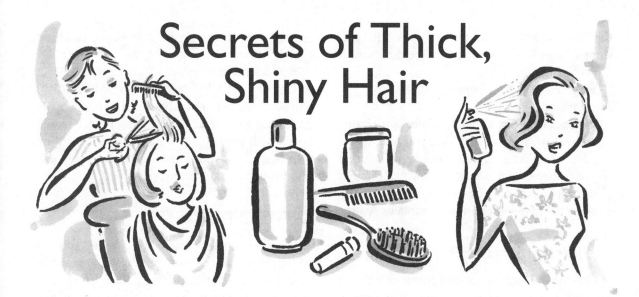

Good cuts, bad color, strange or expensive products—most of us have lived through a whole gamut of experiences during our quest for the perfect 'do. Then, just when we thought we'd won the battle, our hair started to change. During or just after our thirties, "the grays" began their assault. To make matters worse, our hair started growing more slowly and becoming finer.

So now what?

So now it's time to update the 'do, to give it back the shine, resiliency, color, and shape that looked so great just a few short years ago.

Finding Your New Look

Every woman feels a little anxiety, as well as a little excitement, when she's on the verge of changing her hairstyle. And for no small reason. She may enter the salon as one person and come out looking like someone else altogether. People will react to her a little differently than they ever have before. And when she looks in the mirror, she'll meet a new person, whom she hopes she'll like.

It can end up being a very good experience or

a very bad one. Here are some ways to tilt the odds in your favor.

Assess from head to toe. Your hair is part of a package, so selecting a style that suits only your face can undermine your entire look. Not only should you consider the shape of your face, but also your height, weight, what your day-to-day life is like, and how handy or not you are with styling, says Victoria Meekins, vice president of Kenneth's Salon/KEB Associates at the Waldorf-Astoria Hotel in New York City. The key to a great look is homing in on the styles that best suit the total you.

Be open to change. Committing to a hairstyle isn't like taking an oath of allegiance. "It's only hair; it'll always grow back," says stylist Alex Ioannou, co-owner of Trio Salon in Chicago. On average, hair grows ½ inch a month. So experiment, try new things. If it doesn't work, there's always next time.

Define yourself. Even a hairdresser who knows you well isn't psychic. Without specific examples, she may not understand what you mean by an updated or youthful new hairstyle.

"What you think is attractive and what I

think is attractive may be two very different things," says Keith Ayotte, creative director for Vidal Sassoon in Atlanta.

So give the subject some thought *before* you see a stylist.

Collect images. Whenever you see a picture of a model with a hairstyle that you like, tear it out. Start a collection. Don't worry about whether any of the styles will look good on you. "Pictures give me a better idea of what you're looking for. Making the style work is my job," explains Ayotte.

Building a Better Partnership

On-the-job experience and constant training help professional stylists develop a keen sense of what's right—or wrong—for a client. Your role in this transaction isn't passive. Whether you've seen the same stylist for decades or you're searching for someone new to help you update your look, there are steps stylists say that you can take to ease the process.

Book a consultation. You don't have to get your hair cut and styled every time you step into a salon. It'll probably feel weird walking out without a cut, but getting an expert opinion is a great first step to giving your image a fresh new edge.

Fire a warning shot. When you're ready for an update, put your hairdresser on alert. Call a couple of days before your appointment and tell the pro that you want to try something new. Your stylist will probably be excited by this creative opportunity and love the idea of having the time to research some great options.

Pick and choose. There are many different types of salons. Go to one that caters to contemporary style without being too avant-garde. The people at the modern salon are more grounded. They are the ones who know how to make a trend wearable.

Shop with care. Look for an experienced stylist. If in doubt, a salon receptionist can offer background on the stylist that you're thinking about visiting.

Build a relationship. Once you've chosen a stylist, stick with her. Someone who knows you will be much better at advising you than a complete stranger would be. Whenever you become bored with your current cut and color, she'll be your best ally in choosing a new look. And you'll know that you can trust her judgment.

Do's and Don'ts

We live in an era of fashion flexibility. You can go long or short, curly or straight without incurring the wrath of the fashion police. Yet it's still possible to end up with a "don't" when you're updating a 'do. Here are some suggestions to keep you on the right track.

Be true to you. "I don't think that sticking with the latest trend is what makes you look younger," says Ayotte. It's fine to pay attention to the popular length, style, and color, yet these shouldn't dictate your choices. Regardless of the look that others are touting, go with what works for you. "You'll look beautiful, and when you look beautiful, you'll look and feel younger," he says.

Cut the curl. Meekins spent the 1960s with her locks wrapped in juice cans, and the 1970s using chemical straighteners. No matter what this New York City resident tried, controlling her frizzy hair was a struggle, so she went natural. Doing her hair became easier, but there was something about her look that she just didn't like.

Finally, she asked her stylist about it. The candid answer was an eye-opener, "Your tight, short curls make you look old." Taking her cue from the expert, she grew her hair almost to her shoulders and started straightening it again. But this time she's getting a professional blow-dry styling every 3 to 4 days, instead of chemical treatments.

Try longer locks. It's tempting to solve an image dilemma by cutting off your hair. In fact, some women think that chopping their locks is a rite of passage. "It drives me crazy that so many women buy into the myth that they have to go shorter as they get older," says salon owner and stylist Frank Shipman of Technicolor Salon and Day Spa in Allentown, Pennsylvania. "Shoulder-length hair can look fabulous if it suits you."

Accept your hair. Long, short, thick, thin, straight, curly—whatever your hair's characteristics—it's more than likely that you want to change something about it. But the grass isn't always greener on the other side of the salon. Find a style that works with your hair's texture and growth patterns. You'll be happier with the result. Ioannou says that working with, rather than against, your hair eliminates the passé habits of setting, spraying, and teasing.

THE PAGEBOY: SMART CHOICE

Whether you call it a Dorothy Hamill cut, a China doll bob, or a pageboy, new variations of this hairstyle crop up time and again, and they always look modern and fashionable. No matter what the shape of your face, there's a good chance that some version of this versatile cut will look smashing on you. The classic one-length style can end at your ears, chin, or a bit lower. You can have long or short bangs, no bangs, or bangs that are longer than the back of the hairstyle.

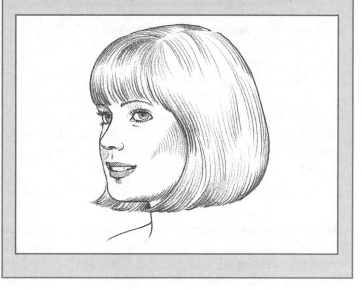

Hairstyles That Complement Glasses

First came the shock of discovering that you need bifocals—or that your eyes have weakened over the past year. Now you have to sort through a huge array of eyeglass frames to find a shape that works with your hair, the shape of your face, and your personality.

Ayotte explains where to start.

Balance the act. The main consideration is balancing the volume and shape of your eyeglasses with your hairstyle. Identify the strongest elements of your hairstyle and then choose a frame that matches.

Combine classics. A classic hairstyle, one that needs minimal styling and is one length all over the head, is best suited to frame shapes that have also stood the test of time. Simple round or square eyeglasses are good options.

Measure the extreme. A strong, trendy style demands eyeglasses that can hold their own. For example, bangs that are little more than a high fringe require eyeglasses with strong lines. Ovals, squares with triangular edges, even the good old cat's-eyes, like the ones you might have worn as a kid, work wonders.

Pull back your hair. A classic chignon or ponytail at the nape of the neck gives you many choices for eyeglass frames. Merely choose a style that suits the shape of your face.

AGE ERASER
An Instant Face-Lift

A good stylist can direct attention away from problem areas merely by changing the shape of your hair, according to Frank Shipman, owner and stylist at Technicolor Salon and Day Spa in Allentown, Pennsylvania. "Weight lines," which establish strong horizontal "edges," can do wonders. A weight line is the place on your hairstyle that draws attention and appears to have the most visual weight or volume.

A weight line can add definition to your face. Consider, for example, a jawline that's softened by a double chin. To remedy this problem, one option is a bob that's slightly raised in the back. Another option is putting more visual weight near the temple to give the illusion of a narrower jaw.

Another great use of a weight line is in deflecting attention from a less-than-perfect neck. In this case, shift the weight line higher so that the thicker hair is closer to the crown, drawing attention away from your neck.

Repeat the geometry. Continue the circular motifs of curly hair in your eyeglasses. Round or oval frames look beautiful. Square frames, on the other hand, are too much of a contrast. Since even short curly hair has movement, choose frames that don't have a lot of detail.

Show your face. Large eyeglasses cover quite a bit of the face. This isn't a problem, as long as you keep your hair under control. Otherwise, people will ask, "Who's hiding behind those glasses and all that hair?" One simple step is cutting off long bangs.

Colorful Options

All our lives we've been led to believe that gray hair marks the end of our youth. By our early thirties, we're diligently seeking and plucking those harbingers of "old age" and worrying about

what's around the corner. True, some of us look on those first few grays as a badge of honor. But over time, concern mounts as more and more appear.

As we age, the cells in our hair produce less pigment, explains Ivan Cohen, M.D., associate professor of dermatology at Yale University School of Dermatology. First, the hair shifts to a lighter color, then to gray, and then on to white. This process varies—and sometimes stalls—depending on your genetic heritage.

Sooner or later we all start wondering if it's time to add color. This isn't an all-or-nothing decision. In fact, most women ease into the process with a variety of subtler treatments: demi- or semi-permanent color, highlights, low-lights, blending, foils. The greatest thing about color is that you can always change it, although you can never take it back to natural.

Blend away the gray. You've probably already seen foils in action at your favorite salon. Women receiving this treatment have clumps of hair sticking out at all angles, with what looks like strips of aluminum foil wrapped around the base of each section. Don't laugh—remember how we used to look in skullcaps, with thin strands of hair sticking out everywhere? Foils don't jab at our scalp like the "crochet" hooks did.

Rather than applying color to single strands, foils add color to larger groupings. Color is closer to the base, so touch-ups aren't as frequent, and there's more control over the color placement. According to Meekins, foils also allow the colorist to apply two, three, sometimes even four colors to the hair for a more natural effect.

Face reality. Reverting to the color of your teens and twenties is a mistake. Your skin color has lightened, so you may not be able to carry the stronger color. Use it only as a reference point for going one or two levels lighter, suggests Shipman. Also keep in mind that warm hair colors are usually more flattering. The tones reflect on the face to give it a glow, rather than washing out the complexion as cool colors tend to do.

Go for broke. When it's time to take the plunge into total coverage, consider the benefits. You'll have softer, shinier hair that gives your face a glow. "Allover color isn't a horrible thing. It can be really quite an esthetic experience," says Shipman.

Remember your past. Highlights and low-lights give the illusion of more shape and a youthful appearance, says Meekins. The sun-kissed color that your hair turned during the summers of your youth suggests wonderful highlights for your current hair.

Shine on. If you're still debating the merits of coloring your gray, consider the hidden benefits, Meekins suggests. Color processes add body, dimension, shine, softness, and texture—all the things that are missing in gray hair.

Try a teaser. When the gray strands first appear, try using processes that cover gray rather than remove pigment from the hair. You won't get total coverage, but the gray is camouflaged. It now blends into your natural color. A semi- or demi-permanent does just that, depositing color on the hair. At first, you might just want to add a bit of color to brighten the base.

WOMEN ASK WHY

Why don't women get bald like men do?

Some do, but they're few and far between. Male hair loss is an effect of dihydrotestosterone, a by-product of the male hormone testosterone. Since women have low amounts of testosterone, baldness isn't usually an issue. When there is genuine hair loss, called androgenic alopecia, it's usually at the front. A drop in estrogen and an increase in male hormone in the body causes this genetic condition. Minoxidil (Rogaine) may stop the hair loss and thicken the remaining hair.

For most women, the female hormone estrogen helps hair grow healthy and strong. But as women approach menopause, estrogen production wanes, and more bad hair days start happening. Even if hair retains its color, it becomes finer because the follicle (the cavity containing the hair root) for each strand shrinks. Hair no longer grows as long either, because its growth cycle shortens as we age. Hair on a 40-year-old may grow for 3 years before shedding but will shed after 1 to 1½ years when the same woman hits 60.

Women of all ages may sometimes notice a few too many hairs in the bathtub drain. Don't worry. Any kind of stress, such as that resulting from a divorce, rapid weight loss, pregnancy, illness, disease, or medication, can cause temporary hair loss. Called telogen effluvium, it's completely reversible and requires no treatment.

Expert consulted
Ivan Cohen, M.D.
Associate professor of dermatology
Yale University School of Dermatology

"This is kind of like a tease, to ease you into permanent hair-coloring processes," Ayotte says.

Graying Gracefully

Coloring your hair isn't the only way to reenergize your appearance, especially if gray or

WOMAN TO WOMAN
She Jumped Off the Chemical Seesaw

Valerie Hoffman, a lawyer in Chicago, started to gray during her college years. She loved the effect when she was young, but as her other features matured, she thought that coloring her shoulder-length hair might give her a younger look. It took a great haircut and reverting to her natural, white hair for Valerie to discover that long, colored hair wasn't her path to the fountain of youth.

When I was growing up, my hair had always been a light brown color, but when I went to college, it started turning gray. What a surprise that was! I actually liked the effect, and when I became a lawyer, the mature look that it gave me helped to foster my clients' trust in me.

By the time I reached 28, however, I started to feel that I was looking too old for my age. Naturally, I figured that dyeing my hair back to its original color would help. Unfortunately, my hair wasn't willing to go along with the plan.

Every 6 weeks, I'd go to my stylist to dye it. But in between appointments, I would spend a lot of time playing outdoor sports, and the exposure to the sun would fade the brown to a washed-out blonde color. The changes were obvious and not at all flattering.

It was no use. It was time to stop the dye jobs and I wanted a quick transition that didn't involve stripping out the color. My stylist convinced me that the way to do that was to cut my hair very, very short.

It was a scary suggestion. I love long hair, and I was afraid I'd end up looking like a boy. But I hated the coloring so much that my decision was clear-cut. When my stylist was finished with me, my hair was about an inch long.

How did I feel when I looked into the mirror?

My hair looked fabulous, and now at age 45, it still does. Its length and pure white color are a great combination. I no longer look dowdy, and my small features don't disappear under a mop of hair.

All in all, I'm really happy with my look now. And I wish the same for other women. Take the bold step—it can make a huge difference.

white hair is the perfect color for the lighter complexion you've gained in recent years. This doesn't mean that you're doomed to looking older than you feel. Shiny, healthy gray or white hair can make you appear full of vitality.

Blue clues. The yellow cast and dullness that affect gray or silver hair can be washed right out of your hair. Meekins says that shampoos with a violet or blue base maintain your hair's vibrancy and clarity.

Use protein. Conditioners with protein and vitamins add instant volume to your tresses. Hair absorbs protein, then swells so that it looks thicker. The effect won't last forever, says Meekins, but it's a wonderful way to add volume. Spritzers and other styling products that include keratin, which is a protein, give strength and shine. Keratin also helps with the breakage problem that crops up with processed hair, she adds.

Products with silicone bases also give your hair shine, but not as much as keratin. You might also want to consider a salon application of glosses and intensifiers.

Wash 'n' wear with care. Brush, shampoo, and wash your hair gently. Wet hair is fragile. Towel it dry carefully, and brush it without tugging. It's preferable to use a brush with bristles that don't have sharp ends. Meekins suggests that when your hair is dry and you head out the door, you put on a hat, wrap a scarf over your hair, or keep to the shade.

Best Bets for Beautiful Nails

The computer revolution has had at least one unexpected and as yet unexplained health benefit for women. All that tap-tap-tapping on computer keyboards appears to make fingernails grow faster and stronger.

Even if you're not computer-crazed, any activity that has you striking your nails against a hard surface—from playing the piano to drumming your fingers—can stimulate growth, according to Diana Bihova, M.D., a dermatologist in New York City and author of *Beauty from the Inside Out*. So can menstruation and pregnancy. "Weather is a factor, too," she says. "We don't exactly know why, but fingernails grow faster in summer."

Hard as Nails

Of course, moving to warmer climes isn't the most practical way to get longer, stronger nails. Thankfully, you have more sensible options. The following strategies can keep your nails looking their best.

Trim after you bathe. Cutting your nails while they're dry leaves them vulnerable to damage. Instead, plan your manicure for after your bath or shower, when your nails are soft.

Avoid cutting corners. When trimming your nails, leave them square at the corners. This maximizes nail strength.

File away flaws. Keep an emery board in your purse or desk drawer. At the first sign of a nick or chip, use the board to smooth out the unevenness and prevent further damage. Always file in the same direction.

Slather on moisturizer. Apply moisturizer to your hands every time you wash them. Take a moment to massage the lotion into your skin and nails.

Be prudent with polish remover. Frequent use of nail polish remover can dry out your nails. So use remover sparingly, preferably no more than once a week. Look for an acetone-free product, which is less drying. Apply a small amount to a cotton ball, press it against the nail for about two seconds, then gently rub off the polish.

Protect your mitts. Whenever you wash dishes or use household cleaners, wear protective latex gloves with separate thin cotton gloves underneath. The cotton gloves help absorb perspi-

A MANICURE FOR HEALTHY NAILS

Some manicures—French manicures or sculpted nails, for example—are designed to make your nails look great. Others are designed to make your nails look great and healthy. Here's the best way to buff and shine your nails to perfect health, according to Ida Orengo, M.D., associate professor of dermatology at Baylor College of Medicine in Houston.

➤ First, place your hands in a small dish of warm water mixed with mild detergent for five minutes to remove dirt and bacteria. "This will get your nails fresh and clean and avoid the possibility of pushing any bacteria under your cuticles while giving yourself a manicure," says Dr. Orengo. Dry your hands gently with a soft clean towel.

➤ While they're still soft, gently cut or clip your nails to about one-quarter inch in length. Hard, dry nails can crack or split when you cut them. One-quarter inch is the perfect length for strong nails. Anything longer can break, split, and chip more easily.

➤ With an orange stick wrapped in cotton, gently push back your cuticles. Cuticles should never be cut, says Dr. Orengo, because they protect your nails against bacterial and fungal infections.

➤ File your nails with an emery board. This also needs to be done while they're soft and pliable. Otherwise, they could split. File in one direction, from side to center, until they are squared off at the top. Filing in a back-and-forth motion can weaken and damage the nail, says Dr. Orengo. Filing nails to a point will also weaken your nails and cause them to break easily.

➤ Rub your nails with a nail moisturizing lotion. The lotion will hydrate your nails and prevent them from drying and cracking. "Rub the lotion liberally into your hands and nails," says Dr. Orengo. Wipe off the excess. Wait two or three minutes for the moisturizer to soak into your nails.

➤ Before applying color, brush on a clear pre-coat polish. The clear polish will prevent your nails from turning yellow.

➤ To prevent your nails from drying out, remove polish with a non-acetone remover no more than once a week, says Dr. Orengo.

ration. That's important because sweat makes hands soggy, further weakening nails.

Brittle Nails

It's doubtful that any woman will get through life without getting brittle nails. Some of us are born with them. Others get them after years of submerging their hands in water or harsh household detergents. Getting older takes a toll, too: Almost everyone's nails become thinner with age.

So what can you do to restore moisture to your nails and keep them healthy and strong? For starters, try these tips.

Offer 'em olive oil. Immerse your fingertips in one-half cup of warmed olive oil and soak for 15 to 30 minutes.

Break open the bath beads. As an alternative to olive oil, break open three or four bath-oil capsules and empty their contents into one-half cup of warm water. Soak your fingertips in the diluted bath oil for five minutes.

Make bedtime a formal affair. Before going to bed, coat your nails and hands with a thick layer of petroleum jelly. Then slip on a pair of white cotton gloves to protect your hands overnight. You'll love the way this treatment makes your nails look.

Go for a quick fix. To salvage a split or broken nail, apply a very small amount of nail glue to the tear. Reinforce the tear by covering it with a small piece of tissue from a tea bag. Let the glue dry completely, then use a fine buffer to even out the nail surface. (Be sure to leave the tissue in place.) Finally, apply a top coat over the tissue.

Hangnails

A hangnail forms when a small piece of skin tears away from your finger right by the nail bed. Even though it's tiny, it can be quite painful and even bleed.

If you get a hangnail, don't pick at it or try to bite it off. It can actually become infected. To remove a hangnail the right way, use this three-step technique.

Start by softening. Never cut off a hangnail while it's dry. Instead, soften it by soaking it in warm water and olive oil.

Clip it cleanly. Use nail scissors or nail clippers to remove the hangnail. Cut it as short as you can without damaging the skin around it.

Apply the finishing touches. After clipping the hangnail, massage the skin around your nail with moisturizer, cover it with an adhesive bandage, and leave it alone.

Sore Cuticles

That tiny rim of near-transparent tissue at the base of each nail is there for a reason. It serves as a barrier, protecting the nail against infection.

FOLK REMEDY: DOES IT WORK?

Gelatin for Soft Nails

Since gelatin is made of protein extracted from the bones and skins of animals, the theory goes, ingesting gelatin has to be good for the protein we know as our fingernails. So for decades, women have been eating gelatin or taking gelatin capsules to strengthen weak and brittle nails.

Truth is, it does little, if any, good, says Diana Bihova, M.D., a dermatologist in New York City and author of *Beauty from the Inside Out*. Gelatin is the only animal protein that lacks the important amino acid tryptophan, which is needed to absorb the protein. So gelatin merely travels through the body without even a howdy-do to your nails.

RECOMMENDATION: Forget It

To repair damaged cuticles and keep them problem-free, add these steps to your nail-care routine.

First, soak them. Before you do anything to your cuticles, soften them in warm sudsy water for several minutes. This prevents drying and cracking.

Then give them a gentle push. Wrap the tip of an orange stick in cotton gauze. Then use the stick to gently push back each cuticle.

Finish with petroleum jelly. After pushing back your cuticles, massage them with a thin layer of petroleum jelly to seal in moisture.

Flatter Your Face and Figure with Color

Back in the early 1980s, you could walk into almost any clothing shop and find a woman scouring the racks for colors that matched her "season." It was the era of color revolution in fashion, launched almost single-handedly by a book called *Color Me Beautiful*.

That book brought color theory to the masses, showing how wearing the right colors can make anyone look fabulous. By assessing skin undertones, a reader could categorize herself as a winter, spring, summer, or autumn color type, and then learn to use image-enhancing hues to her best advantage.

The concept is sound. Color can bring energy and vitality to your appearance. And once you know how, you can apply the concept to your entire wardrobe.

Complements of the Season

If you've ever "had your colors done," as the expression goes, then you already know that using the right colors near your face is like getting an instant face-lift and chemical peel all in one. But if the colors you're wearing aren't flat-tering, any imperfections you may have are going to be magnified. Even in shorts, the wrong color will emphasize skin flaws on your legs.

In *Color Me Beautiful*, author Carole Jackson categorized people into four groups, named after the seasons and based on an assessment of skin undertones, hair color, and eye color. Each season has a palette of colors that suit it. Think of the dominant colors in each season of the year, and you'll have a good idea of which colors belong to its group.

It's a model that image consultants like Donna Fujii, who trains beauty consultants in San Francisco and Tokyo, follow to this day, although many have created subcategories within the seasons and developed new groups. Her award-winning book, *Color with Style*, expanded color theory to embrace the diversity of skin tones for African-American, Asian, and Hispanic women.

If you haven't already, take the time to read both books. They're great primers for doing your colors. But if you want to start right now, here are some tips from Fujii and other fashion experts that will point you in the right direction.

Identify your undertone. Even experts use a trial-and-error method. Pieces of fabric from each season are draped around the client's neck, one at a time. If the skin looks washed out or sallow, the color is wrong. After several colors are tested, a pattern becomes clear. Skin that has blue undertones (summer and winter) looks best in cool colors; so orange-yellow fabrics aren't flattering. Skin with yellow undertones (spring and autumn) needs warm colors. Vibrant blue-violet, for example, brings out the worst.

As you assess your skin, keep in mind that the coolness or warmth of skin tones has nothing to do with the light or dark quality. Darker skins do tend to be warmer, but this isn't a hard-and-fast rule.

Check the contrast. It's not enough to know if you can wear warm or cool colors. The contrast between hair and skin is also a consideration. High-contrast women—brunettes with fair skin, for example—can wear stronger colors, whereas women with gray or salt-and-pepper hair are low-contrast and need to tone things down. A low-contrast person can, however, get away with stronger colors in evening light.

Lower the contrast. Having your colors done isn't a one-time event. As we age, our hair and skin lighten or dull, so the color value and intensity that we can wear may soften a notch or two. If, for example, you usually wear black and other dark colors, charcoal gray and winter white may now be more suit-

COLORS THAT HIDE

You can use the colors in your wardrobe to get thinner instantly.

Stop laughing. It's true.

It's simply a matter of optical illusion, of drawing attention to your assets and away from your liabilities. In wardrobe color theory, it's called color blocking, and whether you realize it or not, you already know the basics, says Jan Larkey, an image consultant in Pittsburgh and author of *Flatter Your Figure.*

Every time you combine separates you're working with color blocking. When you try on a dark blouse with pastel slacks, for example, you instinctively know something is wrong. You look off-balance because, visually, light colors make areas look larger while dark colors have the opposite effect.

To fix the imbalance, all you have to do is put on a jacket or sweater of the same color as the pants. Now there's proportionally less of the dark color visible. The one-color silhouette creates a long, tall vertical, and, if you leave the jacket or sweater open, the lapels form two more slimming vertical lines down the center front.

Any outfit in a single, darker color takes off pounds. Don't sabotage the effect by adding a belt in a contrasting color that chops you in half. Shift the contrast higher—to a yoke on a blouse, for example—and voilà!—instantly wider shoulders. This is a great way to balance a larger lower body. Shift the contrast to a color band around the hips, on the other hand, and you're in trouble, unless you have a small derriere and hips.

To develop a keen sense of color blocking, start by honestly assessing your body. Create vertical color blocks over any body parts you wish were taller or slimmer, and horizontal color blocks on the parts you wish were wider. Now make a point of never placing colors in a manner that draws attention to trouble spots. When all else fails, you can create a winning look by combining medium-color separates with a flattering scarf at the neck.

Is Basic Black for Everyone?

Colors go in and out of fashion, but like an old, steadfast friend, black is always there for you. Sometimes it steps aside for brown or blue among your wardrobe basics, but no other color switches from serious business to casual daytime to evening wear so effortlessly.

Unfortunately, there's a problem: Few women look good with black next to their faces. Hardly any of us can pull off the stunning effect that black creates on a silver-haired woman who has taken the time to define her eyebrows and apply a strong lipstick color. But does this mean we have to give up all the black hanging in our closets? Not at all.

In her book *Quickstyle: How to Expand, Enhance, and Update Your Wardrobe with Accessories*, fashion guru Christine Kunzelman espouses the tremendous benefits of wearing a basic black collarless dress but suggests adding accessories and layering it over with other clothes.

Her idea is to place your most appealing colors nearest your face. Consider downplaying black with color in a loose-buttoned overblouse, an open or closed jacket, a turtleneck underneath a black collarless garment, a sweater draped over the shoulders with the sleeves tied together in front, or a scarf.

Combine your colors with care, however, as your choices can pack on the years. For the most up-to-date look, mix black with brown, khaki, or other neutrals.

black is beautiful, brown looks dowdy. A year later the entire scene can totally reverse. Don't take trends too seriously, says Fujii. Study them, use what appeals to you, then find your own way. Here's some advice to help you.

Remain neutral. For your clothes, combine neutrals. Dress simply and spice up the look with interesting shoes, says image consultant Diana Kilgour of Vancouver, Canada. In any case, it's a good idea to keep your shoes current.

Oust the old combos. Seek out interesting new ways to combine your separates and accessories, suggests Kilgour. A continental, European effect might mix winter and summer colors, mix neutrals, or add baby blue, black, brown, or charcoal to navy blue. For a suit, combine black and brown rather than black and emerald green.

Pick and choose. "In every trend—in every season—there's going to be more than one color palette," says Fujii. Home in on the colors that work for you. Pick three, maybe four, but never more than five. Even within a single color trend, there's a range of tones, so you should be able to find one that works with your complexion.

Context counts. The environment in which you plan to wear an outfit is just as important as color suitability. For example, if you're wearing peach and people around you are in black, you'll look too young, says Kilgour. So plan ahead and try to fit in with the crowd.

able. Salt-and-pepper hair might look better in sand, taupe, or pearl gray.

"I'm wearing colors today that I couldn't wear several years ago," says 49-year-old image consultant Pat Newquist, owner of Wardrobe Image in Tempe, Arizona. To be safe, consult an expert every 5 years.

On the Edge of Trends

Every few months, there is a flurry of activity as designers and fashion experts announce the season's colors: bright pink is in, pastels are out;

Face Up to Colors

Our natural skin tones, hair color, and clothes aren't the only colorful things about us, of course. We also wear makeup. And where enhancing our facial features is concerned, it's tough to let go of old habits. In fact, most of us tend to wear makeup the same way for 10, even 20 years, says Newquist.

When we do this, we're walking away from a wonderful opportunity. With new application methods, colors, and products, we can shed years. In fact, makeup expert Linda Stasi of New York City, former beauty editor and columnist for *Cosmopolitan*, *Elle*, and *New Woman* magazines and coauthor of *Boomer Babes: A Woman's Guide to the New Middle Ages* says that the effect of reworking eyebrows is as dramatic as a face-lift.

Pat Newquist, Linda Stasi, and Donna Fujii, who has her own line of makeup and skin treatments, offer more advice.

Correct and conceal. Dark circles under the eyes need a color corrector and a concealer. Apply the corrector first. The color you select depends on your skin tones. Although there are huge color variations within ethnic groups, you can narrow your color choice by considering your background. African-Americans can choose yellow or amber, Asian skin needs pink, Mediterranean is best suited to yellow, and Scandinavian selects a whitish product. Blend the edges of the corrector, then apply concealer that is almost the same color as your skin.

Go lightly. Skin tones lighten or dull with age, so it makes sense to go a little lighter on the makeup. Use colors that aren't as intense as those you used before. For example, shift from black to brown eyeliner. Choose soft, sheer makeup that's blended with brushes rather than your fingertips. Ensure that the color doesn't sit on top of your skin, and wear neutral eye shadow. Your blush should match the color that your cheeks get when you're working out. Apply blush below the cheekbones.

Update regularly. Lipstick may last a year or more, but it's still a good idea to reevaluate your makeup colors at least once a year. What you see may inspire you to make a bold change, drop the eyeliner, or buy a new lipstick that's a few shades lighter or darker than the one you're using. Splurge. After all, lipstick costs less than dinner and a movie.

Secrets of Dressing with Style

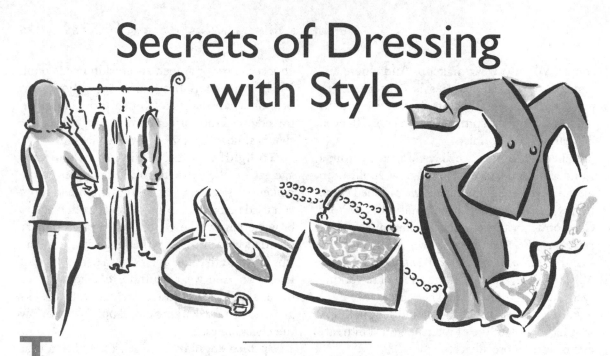

The wish: You walk into a party, and the room lights up. Everyone is smiling in your direction. You look fabulously youthful, vibrant, stylish. People are happy just to be with you.

The fear: You walk into a party and people cover their eyes and mouths to hide their embarrassed looks and snickers. You look outlandish or silly in clothing that's too young or too wild for you.

The reality: You walk into a party and nobody notices. You look the same as you always have because you're afraid to wear a style that's new or different.

Nothing can take years off your look faster than the right clothes, but changing the way you dress is risky business. We're all a little afraid of making fashion mistakes. So we end up dressing as we always dressed and dating ourselves a little bit at a time.

The great news is that there's really no need to be so timid. In fact, with a little bit of knowledge and a few tricks up your sleeve, you can "loosen up your look" (that's image consultant lingo for dressing in a more youthful way) and turn your wish into reality, while leaving your fear behind you.

Avoid Wearing the Right Things the Wrong Way

So many department stores and so little time. Where do you begin?

Tips from image consultant Pat Newquist, owner of Wardrobe Image in Tempe, Arizona, will help you hunt for the silhouettes, garments, and accessories that instantly update a wardrobe.

Evolve gradually. Like a big-game hunter, use a cautious approach. Newquist often tells clients of her 16-year-old company, "If you don't know how to wear it, you'll look too young." At first, stick to classics and add only a few trendy items. Proceed one step at a time. That way, even if you make a mistake, it will be a small one.

Spot the trends. A great way to dress for a youthful look is to pay attention to what's hot, says Newquist. But it takes a bit of work to identify worthwhile trends. The best place to start is in the fashion magazines. What are the models wearing? Notice details of color and cut. What styles do you think might look good on you?

Also pay close attention to ads and watch what the stars are wearing on the fashion, music, and movie awards shows. These people are in the business of keeping an up-to-date, attractive image.

Study brands. Look for labels that create a womanly interpretation of junior trends. For example, a few years ago, the younger crowd was wearing fitted, waist-length leather jackets. Designer Dana Buchman offered her customers leather jackets that still looked fitted but weren't quite as tight and had lower hemlines than clothes made for young women.

Shopping Savvy

Developing a flattering, age-defying collection of clothing starts with careful shopping. Newquist gives her clients specific guidelines to follow when they're ready to hit the stores.

Dress up. "When you plan to try on clothes, get dressed up really nice," says Newquist. Wear good-looking undergarments and slip on brand-new panty hose so that you're more comfortable with the image staring back at you.

Window-shop. Spend a weekend browsing through clothing stores. Don't take any money, just try things on. It's important to go alone so that you're free of influence from others. Be playful: Try on whatever catches your fancy.

Fit loose. "It's better to wear your clothes

SHOES THAT SHINE

Both by the way they look and the way they feel, a pair of shoes can either age you or put a youthful spring in your step. Once you own a pair of classic pumps and flats in your basic wardrobe color, you can start exploring some other options.

Accessory guru Christine Kunzelman writes in her book *Quickstyle: How to Expand, Enhance, and Update Your Wardrobe with Accessories* that every wardrobe should include ankle boots, ballet flats, colored tennis shoes, espadrilles, lace-up brogues, loafers, riding boots, spectator pumps, strappy high heels, and strappy leather sandals.

Pat Newquist, owner of Wardrobe Image in Tempe, Arizona, says it's also very important to keep your shoes current. Just buying one or two up-to-date styles every season gives your wardrobe a fashion edge. Shoe stores are so full of eye candy that you're certain to home in on footwear that works with your updated image.

But remember: It's hard to project an energetic attitude when your tootsies are aching, so to make sure you get a good fit, follow this advice.

- Feet grow with age; have yours measured regularly.
- Measure both feet and fit the largest.
- Allow $\frac{3}{8}$ to $\frac{1}{2}$ inch of space between the end of the shoe and your longest toe.
- Accept only a minimum amount of slippage at the heels.
- When you're trying on shoes, position the ball of your foot in the widest part (ball pocket) of the shoe.

---

loose rather than snug," says Newquist. "They'll make you look 10 to 20 pounds thinner. You should be able to insert two fingers into a waistband. Pants and skirts are too small through the hips if you can't pinch out 2 inches of fabric."

The Wrinkle Check

Your face stares back at you from the mirror, and for the umpteenth time this week, you see that new wrinkle at the corner of your mouth.

Scrutinizing your face while applying makeup is a rite of passage that we all go through. But there's a whole other set of wrinkles, not on our face, that age us and are visible from many feet away from the mirror.

The next time that you dress, look for diagonal, horizontal, and vertical wrinkles. These, says international fit and sewing expert Sandra Betzina, point to fit problems. Host of the television show *Sew Perfect* on the cable channel Home and Garden Television and author of the *Power Sewing* book series, Betzina gives thousands of women advice and guidance on garment fit.

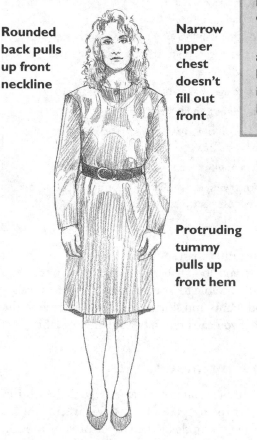

Rounded back pulls up front neckline

Narrow upper chest doesn't fill out front

Protruding tummy pulls up front hem

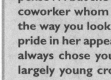

Forward-pitched, sloping, or uneven shoulders. Diagonal wrinkles travel across the shoulders and neck. Try shoulder pads, says Jan Larkey, an image consultant in Pittsburgh and author of *Flatter Your Figure*. Place the blunt end of the pad just beyond your sleeve seam to hide rounded shoulders. If one shoulder is higher than the other, use a thinner pad on that side of the garment. Larkey pushes her own pads toward the back to compensate for a curved spine.

Full high hips. There are small horizontal wrinkles immediately under the front and back waistband. Wear garments that hang from the widest part of your lower body, particularly if your hip fullness starts almost immediately below the waist.

Makeup is part of the problem. A consultant can show Andrea how to choose and apply subtle, attractive colors. As for her hair, she should shift the ponytail to the base of the neck and twist it into a chignon.

Her pleated skirt can work in her favor, so long as it fits properly. Pleats should hang straight, without opening, so if Andrea's skirt is fluffing at the hip, there's a problem.

The tight sweater and ankle socks are big mistakes. Clothing that reveals your figure is wrong for the office at any age; and ankle socks with a skirt and business shoes are always inappropriate.

Andrea's overall look, particularly the sweater, is more "social casual," than "business casual," which means it would be appropriate only on "Casual Friday." Even then, a better option is a twinset (jewel neckline pullover and matching cardigan) paired with tailored slacks.

Expert consulted
Jan Larkey
Image consultant
Author of Flatter Your Figure
Pittsburgh

Protruding tummy. Side seams pull forward, skirts hike up at center front, and pants are tight through the crotch. Waist darts emphasize your roundness. Instead, choose garments that hang straight from the fullest part of the tummy. Look for hidden tummy panels that control the potbelly.

Rounded or full upper back. The neckline pulls down in back and up in front. If the garment was made with a center back seam, a dressmaker can let it out for you.

Bodywork

Clothes that used to look fabulous on us now look frumpy. Why? Our bodies change with age: weight shifts, shoulders slope, backs round, hips and thighs get fuller. Although we may still be the same size we were 10 years ago, we notice that our clothes have become too loose in some places and too tight in others.

To fit and flatter our new bodies, the styles we wear should change through the years. This isn't a matter of dressing our age—it's about dressing our *shape*.

Betzina offers suggestions for each age group in her home sewing pattern collection called "Today's Fit by Sandra Betzina." She developed the collection, which is based on extensive research of body shapes and measurements, in collaboration with Vogue Patterns.

Ages 24 to 34. This is the time to celebrate your youthful body. While a bit of padding may be creeping onto your hips, tummy, and thighs, there's no need to run for the cover of extra fabric. In fact, you can continue wearing fitted clothing.

But this is the time of life, cautions Betzina, when you have to acknowledge that your body is

Full upper arms. Diagonal wrinkles cross the upper arm near the shoulders and grow steeper along the lower arm. Some well-known designers insert a vertical seam along the top of the sleeve. It can be let out for nicer fit.

Low or flat bottom. "Frowning" horizontal wrinkles form under the back crotch, and the pants' waist pulls down at the center back. Invest in body-shaping undergarments that lift a low bottom or pad a flat derriere.

Narrow upper chest. The shoulder seams drop off the shoulder, and there are horizontal wrinkles across the upper chest. This figure problem is very difficult to fit in ready-to-wear garments. The best solution is to hire a dressmaker.

changing. If this means switching to a larger size for the lower half of the body, then so be it.

Ages 34 to 44. Your braless days are over, your waist is thickening, and a potbelly is starting to show.

Although you no longer have the body of a 20-year-old, you can continue wearing the same styles as a decade earlier by making a few concessions to your evolving shape. Experiment with wearing clothes that are looser in areas where you're not as full. A wrap top over a shaped skirt, for example, is figure-flattering yet still has enough room to skim fuller arms and other trouble spots.

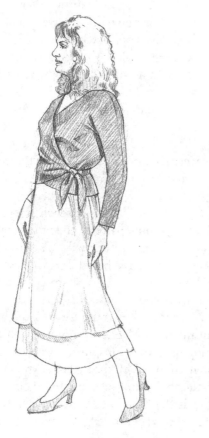

A POINT ABOUT BRA FIT

"A sagging bustline adds 10 pounds and 10 years to a woman's figure," writes image consultant Nancy Nix-Rice in her book *Looking Good: A Comprehensive Guide to Wardrobe Planning, Color, and Personal Style Development.*

To perk up your appearance, look for a bra that lifts the bust point to a more youthful location, midway between the base of the neck and the waist. Look for a bra that has built-in support: underwires, nonstretch straps, push-up pads, and other shapers.

Strap and band fit are equally important. The front and back elastic should wrap around the body in the same place, neither drooping nor pulling up in any spot, says Jan Larkey, an image consultant in Pittsburgh and author of *Flatter Your Figure.*

While on inspection, make sure that the elastic isn't stretched out. You should be able to slip a finger under the elastic. Now face front. If you have a bulge at each front arm crease (between the underarm and top of the shoulder) you need a larger cup.

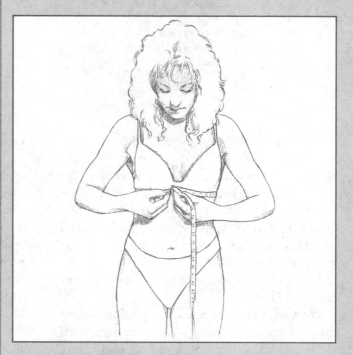

First, measure around your rib cage directly beneath your bust and add 5 to the measurement. This is your bra size.

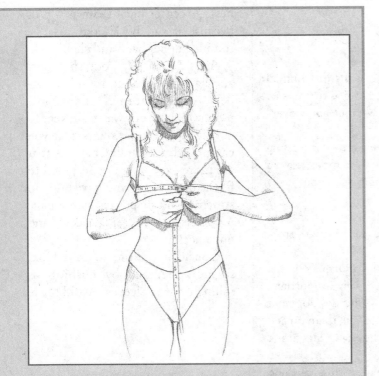

Then, measure the circumference around your full bust. The difference between the rib-cage and full-bust measurements indicates your cup size.

Difference	Cup Size
½ inch	AA
1 inch	A
2 inches	B
3 inches	C
4 inches	D
5 inches	DD or E
6 inches	DDD or F
7 inches	FF or G

Ages 44 to 54. Now your tummy measurement is beginning to exceed the circumference of your hips, so it's most important that garments drop straight from the fullest part of your lower body—usually the waist or high hips.

In pants, this translates into the classic trouser shape that Audrey Hepburn wore.

You can pull off a great suit look if the pants are topped with a longer jacket that has set-in sleeves (the top of the seam that joins the sleeve to the jacket is positioned at the upper arm/shoulder hinge).

Since there may be rolls between the bottom of the bra and the waist, garments that skim the body are

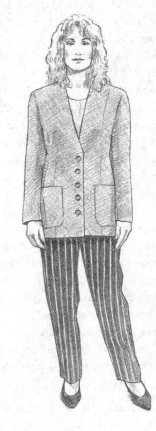

JEANS FOR COMFORT AND FIT

Many people feel that few things can give them a youthful look the way jeans can. The key is to find a style that tips its hat to the trends the kids are wearing without going overboard.

For example, when the twentysomething crowd is wearing an oversize and sloppy look, you can opt for a more relaxed fit and a low-rise waist that rests just below your belly button.

While it's easy to decide on a style that flatters your body, fit is harder to pin down. Some of us like jeans that are snug, while others prefer a looser feel.

"There really isn't a standard," explains Norma Willis, a design manager at the Lee Apparel Company in Merriam, Kansas. When a new style of jeans is in the development stage, however, a Lee fit model is asked to pull them on and move around: sit, bend to ensure that the upper legs aren't too tight, and walk a bit.

You can apply these same criteria the next time you shop for jeans. If the pants' rise is too short, the crotch will "cut" you when you sit.

As to choosing high-quality jeans, here are some tips.

Check seams. The best-made jeans have a lot of double-needle construction. Look for seams that have two lines of stitching, except along the outer leg/hip seamline. Here, single-seam construction does a better job over womanly curves.

Be a metal detector. A metal zipper is best because the chain teeth last longer.

Test bands. In a lightweight jean fabric, make sure that the waistband is stiffer so that it doesn't roll.

Look over hems. The best hem, featured on basic jeans, is rolled over double, which lasts longer than the wider, one-layer hem of fashion jeans.

Bring out the inner jean. At home with your new purchase, you can preserve the new color by washing the jeans inside out. Then let your pants drip-dry so that they don't shrink as much.

best. A center back seam is a plus because it can be let out to fit a rounded upper back and shoulders.

Ages 54 to 64. Your shoulders and back continue to round, a potbelly often becomes more pronounced, and your waist thickens.

Buy the best garments that you can afford. Generally, clothes that are more expensive are designed to fit the body better and have built-in structure and shape that camouflage problems. Opt for set-in sleeves and open necklines.

Consider a more relaxed look, suggests Betzina, by pushing or rolling up your sleeves. Avoid tuck-

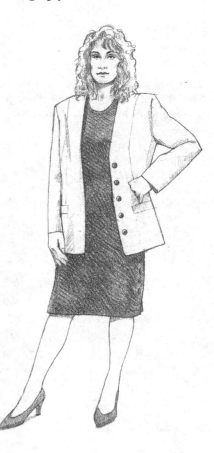

ACCESSORIZE WITH STYLE

Classic or funky, your choice in accessories can define an outfit. A gold chain worn with a classic black dress is elegant. Now take off the necklace and put on an oversize watch to be instantly sporty.

These little touches—pins, necklaces, earrings, belts, and scarves—can make getting dressed so much fun. And once you have the basics, you can play with trends without taking a big bite out of your budget.

Bring a guide. Some image consultants advise you to shop alone so that you'll develop your own style. Princess Jenkins, image consultant and owner of Majestic Images International in New York City, suggests the opposite. Shop with youthful friends and family members. They know the trends, and they'll let you know when you've stepped over the line.

Think smaller. Image consultant Donna Fujii of San Francisco suggests borrowing a popular print, color, or motif that the twentysomething crowd is wearing in garments and buying yourself a belt or scarf with the same theme.

Out with the old. If you don't see young people wearing a particular kind of jewelry, then you shouldn't either, says Diana Kilgour, an image consultant in Vancouver, Canada. A lapel pin, for example, isn't popular now, so tuck your piece in a memory box rather than the jewelry box.

in looks because these emphasize a thick waist or tummy bulge.

Instead, consider an overshirt with narrow pants, or a T-shirt dress in a fabric that has drape without cling.

If you want to camouflage certain trouble spots, slip on a jacket with set-in sleeves.

The best way to determine what works for you is to experiment. In our teens, many of us spent hours trying on clothes. Soon, life got in the way, and there was little time to play with clothes.

It's time to start having fun again. "Don't get preconceived ideas of what looks good on you and what doesn't look good on you," says Betzina. "Try on different styles once a year, just like you did when you were young."

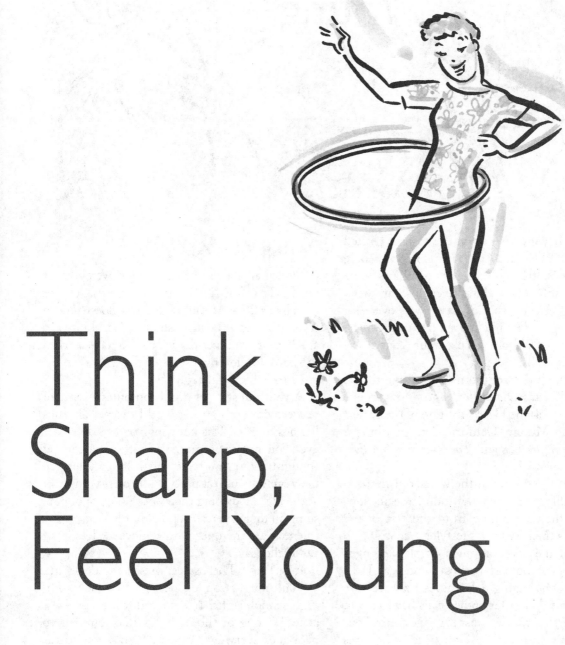

PART THREE

Think Sharp, Feel Young

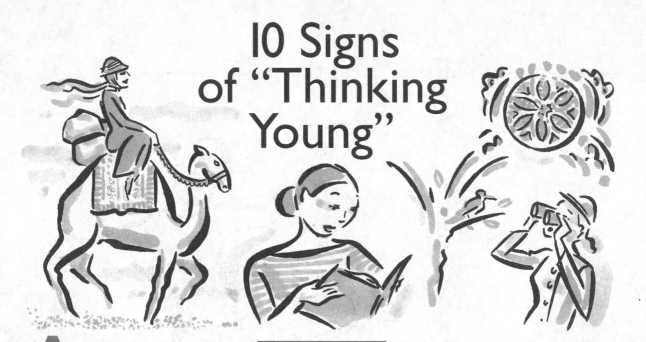

10 Signs of "Thinking Young"

As a boy growing up in the eastern United States, John Deller, M.D., saw plenty of people around him retreat to their rocking chairs while they were still in their middle years. That's what you did after your working career was over—or so he thought. Then he moved out to the West Coast, where 80-year-olds play tennis and organize charity balls.

"Everybody in southern California thinks they're 25," says Dr. Deller, who's now an endocrinologist at the Heart Institute of the Desert in Rancho Mirage, California, and author of *Achieving Agelessness* and *The Palm Springs Formula for Healthy Living*.

Is there something in the water out there in sunny California? Have they found a secret supplement they are hiding from the rest of us? Maybe it's the laid-back lifestyle? According to Dr. Deller, the answer is much simpler: Aging is part biological, but also part psychological. How we *think* about aging determines how well we will actually do it. Our bodies' cells have a say in the matter, but for the most part, we control our relationship with Father Time because aging is mostly just a state of mind.

Acting Your Age

Just what is a youthful attitude? We all know what it isn't: It isn't behaving like a teenager—or even like a 20-year-old. It certainly doesn't mean trying to keep up with fashion fads of kids who are 20 years younger than you. You have worked too hard developing a sense of maturity over the years to fall into that trap.

A youthful state of mind combines a sense of self-esteem with a sense of all the possibilities life has to offer. It is knowing you can do whatever you put your mind to without a second thought about how many birthday candles you blew out at your last party. "The ones who work at the idea of keeping their options open, of pursuing all their interests, and of not looking at the calendar are the ones who achieve agelessness," Dr. Deller says.

It isn't easy. There's peer pressure to deal with.

You thought you left peer pressure behind in high school, right? Not so, unfortunately. Like acne, it's one of those things that happens to people of every age. It just gets more subtle as you get older.

People around you may have some pretty set-in-stone ideas about how you are supposed to behave at any given age, and without even realizing it, they may pressure you to slow down just when you feel like sprinting. Or you may apply the pressure yourself.

"You think because most people who are this age do or don't do this, you should, too. Being in a youthful state of mind means not giving too much of a damn what other people think. Don't be restricted by other people's stereotypes," says Albert Ellis, Ph.D., president of the Albert Ellis Institute for Rational Emotive Behavior Therapy in New York City and coauthor of *Optimal Aging* with Emmett Velten, Ph.D.

10 Attributes of a Youthful Mind

People in a perpetually youthful state of mind come from many different backgrounds, but they all possess personality traits that transcend age. Here are 10 qualities you'll find in youthful people, no matter what their chronological age.

Humor

"I was born in 1962. True. And the room next to me was 1963 . . ."—Joan Rivers. Age and getting older have always been the butt of jokes. Why? Because laughter puts things into perspective. If you can laugh at something, it can't be all that bad.

On the other hand, what kind of person comes to mind when you think of the word

---

SAY WHAT? WORDS THAT GIVE AWAY YOUR AGE

Maybe your appearance doesn't give away your age. And your attitude is more youthful than that of the kid who mows your lawn. So just what could tattle on you when it comes to how old you really are? Your mouth. Just one word or phrase from a bygone era can date you as fast as a paisley shirt and a pair of bell-bottoms. Here are a few to watch out for.

➤ Dungarees	➤ Jumping jacks
➤ Bermuda (as in shorts)	➤ Going steady
➤ Nifty	➤ When I was your age
➤ Icebox	➤ Gal or fella
➤ Brassiere	➤ Calling everyone "Hon"
➤ Typewriter	➤ Coed
➤ Record player	➤ Hi-fi
➤ Album	➤ Far out
➤ Rouge	➤ Heavy
➤ Put on my face	➤ Hip
➤ Hanky	➤ Necking
➤ Lady-friend	➤ Here comes the judge

Make up your own list. Your kids will be happy to point out new entries as they fall over laughing when you say them. In the meantime, "Peace and love!"

---

crotchety? You got it—humorless. Remember, a sense of humor got George Burns past 100. (Well, it certainly wasn't his cigar smoking that did it.) "Not only do older people who utilize humor seem younger in attitude, they actually look younger to me. On the other hand, when you see someone who is depressed and sullen, they look old and haggardly," says Steve Sultanoff, Ph.D., adjunct professor of psychology at Pepperdine University in Malibu, California, and president of the American Association for Therapeutic Humor.

No need to take pratfalls on banana peels.

WOMEN ASK WHY

Why does time seem to go by faster as I get older?

Perhaps no one told you just how busy the middle years would be. You are potentially at the peak of your career, your children and your parents rely on you, and you are trying to fit a social life and extracurricular activities in as well. So you have a lot to do and not enough time in which to do it.

That sense of being rushed creates a feeling that time is fleeting and that life is moving at a rapid pace. And that's the way your brain actually registers it. Why? Handling too many tasks at once interferes with the brain's ability to accurately measure time. When you think back years ago, it is not that time went slower, you just had a lot less to do.

The natural process of aging may also alter your sense of time passing. Each of us has what experts call an internal clock. This clock enables you to reasonably measure time in your head. Therefore, your perception of time relies heavily on two processes in the brain: memory and attention, both of which slow down a bit as you get older, throwing your perception of time off track.

This natural slowdown combined with managing a hectic schedule and numerous responsibilities knocks your internal clock a bit off center. Your brain handles all these factors in a way that makes you feel like time whizzes by faster than before.

Expert consulted
Deborah Harrington, Ph.D.
Research scientist
Veteran Affairs Medical Center
Albuquerque, New Mexico

tain comedian, slapstick humor, or funny props? Some people never take the time to seek out different brands of humor and just assume they are laughing-impaired.

Surround yourself with laughter. Once you have identified what humor you like, keep it around. Buy movies and books by your favorite comedians and pull them out when you need to laugh. Tack hilarious cartoons or quotes around your home or office. Carry clown noses or silly props with you and yank them out. "I carry Groucho glasses and clown noses everywhere I go," Dr. Sultanoff proudly admits. This is not a requirement, however.

Look for humor in serious situations. Your teenager has just come home an hour past curfew. You mete out a punishment. You're angry; she's resentful. And that adolescent attitude is just about to send you up the wall when . . . a fly lands on her nose, she crosses her eyes, and she smacks herself trying to get it.

Dr. Sultanoff says that a good laugh could be what you need during a tense moment to bring in a new perspective.

Hang out with children. Children, in their innocence, are inherently funny. Spend some time with children and learn to laugh and play like them, Dr. Sultanoff says. If children aren't in your circle of friends, just hang out with funny people or even furry friends that make you laugh.

Give yourself permission. Afraid people will laugh at you? Well, that's the point, Dr. Sul-

There are simpler ways to get the humor rolling. Here are just a few.

Find humor you enjoy. Does Robin Williams make you laugh or make you sick? Identify what types of humor you like, Dr. Sultanoff says. Do you enjoy jokes, cartoons, a cer-

tanoff says. In order to delight in humor, you must allow yourself to be funny. Some people get so wrapped up in the seriousness of life that they won't permit themselves the enjoyment of humor. Give yourself the green light, and you will feel lighthearted and younger, he says.

Optimism

Just think about what it means to be a pessimist: You believe that bad events are all your fault, that misfortune will follow you always, and that life will consistently turn out for the worst. No wonder it ages you.

Martin E. P. Seligman, Ph.D., a leading expert on optimism and author of *Learned Optimism*, says in his book that optimists age better, live longer, catch fewer infectious diseases, and have stronger immune systems than pessimists. Studies have also shown that pessimists give up more easily and get depressed more often. An optimist has a firm grip on reality but also recognizes that just about any event—good or bad—has advantages. Here's how to look on the bright side of anything.

Argue with yourself. According to Dr. Seligman's groundbreaking book, dispute your pessimistic beliefs. For example, let's say that you hand in a report and the boss doesn't like it. Your first reaction is that you will be fired. But cross-examine your thought processes. Will you really be fired for one not-so-hot report after years of good work? Can't you go back and make the revisions she wants? Often, you'll realize that you blow negative events out of proportion.

Turn bad events into good motivators. An optimist views a negative event as an opportunity, Dr. Ellis says. If you don't like your job and think you will be miserable forever, use that as a catalyst to find a new job. If you are sad because family or friends moved away, use your newfound free time to find new interests or meet new people.

Seek out the silver lining. Perhaps you just got a new job. A few weeks after you start, your car breaks down, your dishwasher blows up, and your roof needs repairs. Now you can think: What terrible luck I have. I've just started earning a decent paycheck, and all my money's gone out the window. Or you can think: These things were going to happen eventually, so it's really lucky that they happened now that I have a new job, when I can afford the repairs. A simple change in perspective can make your life a lot more enjoyable, Dr. Ellis says.

Curiosity

Spend any amount of time with a 4-year-old, and the word you're likely to hear most often is *why*. Spend the same amount of time with a 44-year-old, and *why* may be the word you hear least. "If you look at children, they are curious about the world. Unfortunately, we lose that as we get older," says William Strawbridge, Ph.D., an epidemiologist at the Public Health Institute in Berkeley, California.

Why? Perhaps we felt foolish too many times for asking "silly" questions, or maybe we just stopped caring about the hows and whys of life and began taking it at face value.

To recapture that sense of wonder and inquisitiveness is to recapture part of your youth, Dr. Strawbridge says. As a bonus, curiosity leads you to other interests in life such as new hobbies, new experiences, and possibly even new careers. Want to know how you can recapture that precious part of yourself?

Ask why. It is such a simple question, but one that people often don't ask, Dr. Strawbridge says. Start to ask yourself and others why. Why is the sky blue? Why do I want this job? Why can't I take up a new hobby?

Don't accept "just because." It's easy to take someone else's word for something, but you will miss out on the excitement of your own discoveries. It's better to do your own homework, Dr. Strawbridge says. Ask if there is a better way of doing things at home, at work, or even at play. Albert Einstein based his success on simple curiosity: "The important thing is not to stop questioning."

Dig into things. If something intrigues you, look into it, Dr. Strawbridge says. Want to know how a computer works? Tinker with one. Then read books and newspapers and get on the Internet to learn more about the subject. You can take the same approach with any interest from sewing to botany. Get hands-on experience and immerse yourself in some research at the same time.

Adventure

In 1998, Sister Clarice Lolich celebrated her 80th birthday by skydiving out of an airplane. Not that this type of adventure was new for this nun and former aerospace education specialist with NASA: She has also bungee-jumped, parasailed, and whitewater-rafted.

She never lost her sense of adventure, an important key to staying young, says Dr. Ellis. Emotionally healthy people take risks. But as some people get older, they become more cautious. By regaining that sense of adventure, you are very likely to feel younger and more alive, he adds.

You don't have to jump out of an airplane or take a trip to the Amazon to partake of an adventure (unless you want to, of course). A trip to a new restaurant, a new job, or a new vacation can fill that bill very well. "You can take many risks, both large and small," Dr. Ellis says. Here are some places to start.

> ## MAKING THE MOST OF MIDLIFE CRISIS
>
> The term *midlife crisis* comes to us from art history. In studying the careers of some of the world's most famous artists, one author noticed that they all had shown a dramatic change in their work after age 35. They seemed far more concerned with images that reflected their own sense of mortality than with pictures that celebrated the past.
>
> You know you've hit a midlife crisis when you start to reevaluate just about everything around you—your job, your relationships, your achievements. "You no longer feel secure with the status quo, but you aren't exactly sure how to proceed. What you are sure of is that life doesn't last forever and that you need to make some decisions about how you will proceed with the rest of yours," says Leonard Felder, Ph.D., a psychologist in Los Angeles and author of *The 10 Challenges*.
>
> Many people reach this midlife point and reflect on the mistakes they have made over the years. Instead, they should be contemplating their futures. "Most women that I see go back and beat themselves up for some decision they made years ago and think that will help them get through a midlife crisis. It is not about finding a guilty party. It is about making excellent choices," says Dr. Felder.

Eat exotically. Take your tastebuds on a trip to another country by dining at an ethnic restaurant, Dr. Ellis says. Eating new foods can be an exciting escapade.

Change your travel plans. Do you go to the same vacation spot year in and year out? Pick a different destination, Dr. Ellis says. You don't need to travel to Bali or Australia. Simply navigating your way in a new city or locale can bring out the adventurer in you.

Introduce yourself. Meeting people often turns into an adventure, Dr. Ellis says. Introduce yourself to new people at work or join a special-interest group or social club. Unless you

What triggers a midlife crisis? It can be the illness or death of someone your own age, watching younger people climb past you on the ladder to professional or personal success, or simply feeling that there has to be something more to get you out of bed each morning. Each of these events provides the perfect opportunity to make positive changes. Here's how Dr. Felder says you can make the most of a midlife crisis.

➤ Make small changes first. "People often bolt from a job or a relationship that wasn't really so bad. Then they regret leaving when it is all over," he says. Identify what you don't enjoy about your job, your relationships. Then change that aspect of your life. Small changes make a world of difference.

➤ Seek fulfillment elsewhere. Perhaps your job and relationships are healthy, but you feel that you're still missing something. Take classes in subjects that interest you, volunteer, get active in your community. "Find those activities and values you've put on hold," he says. Many times those deepening activities offer the fulfillment you've been looking for.

➤ Look way into the future. Maybe it is unrealistic for you to quit your 9-to-5 job and become a gourmet chef right now. But who is to say you can't do that when you retire? Use your midlife crisis to figure out what your dreams are, then start laying the groundwork now for your later years.

live on a desert island, new people are everywhere you look.

Maturity

It's a scientific fact: The older you are, the happier you are. A study of 2,700 people from ages 25 to 75 conducted at Fordham University in New York City found that happiness increases with age. "The typical stereotype of the older, depressed individual is just that—a stereotype," says Daniel K. Mroczek, Ph.D., assistant professor of psychology at Fordham University and study author.

Dr. Mroczek attributes this increase in well-being to a number of traits you develop as you mature: experience, a better attitude toward life, a greater sense of living in the moment. "As you get older, you know yourself better. You know what makes you happy. And you are better able to do these things that make you happy," he says. So in order to be happy and youthful, embrace your maturity—don't hide it. "A lot of women try to act young. Why deny that valuable experience, knowledge, and know-how?" he says.

Share your life experience. Share your knowledge and wisdom with friends, family, and coworkers. If you know how to do something better, speak up.

Value what you have done. Think about all you have already accomplished in your life, he says. Enjoy those achievements instead of thinking about what you could have, should have, or would have done—or what you still have to do. You still look toward the future, of course, but don't forget to cherish your past as well.

Savor the moment. In studying age and happiness, Dr. Mroczek found that older people report a greater sense of well-being because they enjoy the moment at hand and worry less about the future. "They stop and smell the roses. They look at sunsets, enjoy the blue sky. They are less future-oriented," he says. Enjoy each day and what it brings, he advises. Good advice at any age.

Knowledge

Henry Ford perfectly captured the secret of staying young when he said, "Anyone who stops learning is old, whether at 20 or 80. Anyone who keeps learning stays young. The greatest thing in life is to keep your mind young."

Research has discovered the role for learning in healthy aging. A study at the Public Health Institute found that people with 12 years or more of education were healthier in their later years than those who had less schooling. But the study's author, Dr. Strawbridge, takes his results beyond classroom experience. Building knowledge is a lifelong endeavor. "Learning follows you all your life. If you are 45, you are not going back to high school. But you can certainly do things to learn and improve your mental activity," he says. Here's how to increase your knowledge as long as you live.

Get back to class. There is a plethora of ways to go back to school now: community colleges, adult education centers, night learning classes, summer programs for adults, Dr. Strawbridge says. And now, unlike in high school, you can take whatever courses you want.

Read, read, read. Being a voracious reader makes you a voracious learner. Beyond books, newspapers, and magazines, the Internet opens up a whole new world of knowledge, Dr. Ellis says.

Use the tube. The television set doesn't always have to numb your mind. Used the right way, this medium is a form of education. Instructional videos can lead to new hobbies or activities. Educational programming such as that on PBS can teach you about science, nature, history, and the arts.

Enthusiasm

A reporter once asked fashion designer Gabrielle "Coco" Chanel about her age during an interview. Chanel, then 86, replied, "I will tell you that my age varies according to the day and the people I happen to be with. When I'm bored, I feel very old, and since I'm extremely bored with you, I'm going to be one

thousand years old if you don't get out of here at once."

Boredom—and surrounding yourself with boring people—can age you instantly. Having an enthusiastic outlook on life means being interested in life, in hobbies, in having fun, and in other people. According to Dr. Ellis, most people are healthier and happier when vitally absorbed in something other than themselves. To grow younger as you age, you need a creative interest as well as daily meaningful interaction with others.

Discover or revisit hobbies. Midlife is a great time to find new interests and hobbies. Rediscover creative activities that you loved to do in the past but lost touch with over the years because of a lack of time, Dr. Ellis says. Even something as simple as a hobby gives you a reason to be enthusiastic about life, and that keeps you ageless.

"It has to be something that is genuine, that you want to do. It can't be 'Now I should basketweave.' You need to really feel charged up about this," Dr. Deller adds.

Keep up with friends and family. As life moves on, sometimes you lose touch with friends and family, or you don't make many new friends. But you want to work on those ties that bind.

According to a study of 65- to 95-year-old people by Dr. Strawbridge, those who had five or more people with whom they had close contact were twice as likely to "age successfully," meaning that they led healthy and active lives well into older age. These close relationships build an instant support system and naturally keep you active and enthusiastic about a world other than your own.

Spend time with friends and family of all ages, Dr. Deller suggests, to keep in touch with all aspects of life.

Get involved in your community. Becoming active in your community kills two birds with one stone: It gives you an interest and provides a way to meet people, Dr. Ellis says. Join local organizations and school boards or attend government meetings.

Compassion

Empathy and understanding may be hard traits to develop, but they often reap benefits for both the giver and receiver. To be able to care, offer help, and show concern for others generates a joy that subtracts years off your age. "You do it because you get joy in doing it. I think that is really quite a healthy attitude," Dr. Sultanoff says.

Being compassionate doesn't mean that you compromise your ideals. "You don't have to accept what they do, but you accept them. When you do that, you actually enjoy helping others instead of criticizing others," Dr. Ellis says. You also fulfill the most basic human desire: to feel wanted and needed.

Become a volunteer. Find a cause you believe in and donate your time and energy, Dr. Strawbridge says. Studies show that volunteering benefits both your body and mind. A national survey of 3,330 volunteers found that they experienced a "helper's high," a sense of euphoria after helping others. They also reported an increased sense of self-worth and better perceived health, which is a predictor of future health and longevity.

Donate your skills. Maybe volunteering for an organization isn't your style, so contribute what you do best. "If you are an accountant,

WOMAN TO WOMAN
She Never Says No to a New Experience

Sylvia Palkowski, 62, a retired secretary from Fort Walton Beach, Florida, is always surprised to see an older woman looking back at her in the mirror—because she doesn't feel any older than 40. She finds all sorts of ways to retain her youth, from doing crafts to tap dancing. Here, she tells how fulfilling a lifelong dream made her feel like a kid again.

I think you're never too old to dream. And we all have dreams we haven't realized. I always wanted to be in a beauty pageant as a young girl but never really had the chance. Then about 10 years ago, I heard about the Miss Senior Okaloosa County Pageant here in Florida.

Being in the pageant turned out to be all I had imagined it would be—and more. Everything leading up to it was so much fun: meeting the seven other contestants, being interviewed by the judges, and walking through the dress rehearsal.

The night of the pageant, we all gathered backstage to primp and prettify before it was our turn to go out on the stage. I felt all aflutter like I was 18 again.

When it was my turn, I went in front of the microphone and summed up my philosophy of life, which I based largely on a prayer by St. Francis of Assisi. For the talent portion, I performed a comedy takeoff of an Erma Bombeck routine. Then it was time for the evening gown competition. We paraded onstage decked out in our most elegant attire. I wore an exquisite turquoise dress with a full skirt and beaded jacket.

The most memorable part of the pageant for me was what went on backstage. The camaraderie. Everybody helping everybody else with that zipper that wouldn't zip or that seam that came undone. Comforting the woman who goofed and encouraging the one about to go on.

I wasn't crowned the winner, but I didn't care a whit about winning. I did it just to do it. To be a part of it. To see what it's like. And it was just wonderful. I made lots of memories—and friends. And when I found out that one of the contestants was 90 years old, I felt like a spring chicken. No matter what our ages, we all made our childhood dreams come true. No one should ever give up a dream. Not ever.

help people with their taxes. Use your skills to help others. It doesn't have to be heavy involvement," Dr. Strawbridge says.

Get a pet. People aren't the only creatures that deserve love and affection; furry and feathered ones do, too. A pet large or small brings out the kindness in you. "You care for another being that totally relies on you," says Dr. Sultanoff.

Open-Mindedness

Nothing can make you feel older than being stuck in a rut. Same cereal for breakfast, same route to work, same vacation every year, same laundry day. Although this monotonous routine sounds terrible, some balk when faced with doing something different. The rut may be boring, but it is safe and comfortable.

If you want to maintain a youthful outlook on life, Dr. Ellis says that you need to be open-minded. "Healthy and mature people tend to be flexible in their thinking, open to change, and accepting in their views of people. They do not make rigid rules for themselves or others," he says.

Change your daily routine. Little changes spice up a routine and slowly get you used to trying something different. Take a different route to work. If you usually brush your teeth then brush your hair, switch. Try a new shade of eye shadow or lipstick. "Do things that aren't very important to you, but that at least break the mold of your everyday life," Dr. Sultanoff says.

Look for alternatives. There is always another way of doing things, another point of view. Don't discount them, Dr. Ellis says. In fact, seek them out. "People think they must do X and Y,

and they don't realize there are always alternatives that are often better," he adds.

Don't make absolutes. Perhaps you always go to your sister's house for Thanksgiving. But you can't stand her husband, other family members nag you to death, and you'd rather be anywhere else. Then why not be anywhere else? Dr. Ellis asks. There is no law that says you have to do something. "You have flexibility and the power to choose," he says.

Faith

Even science has gotten into the act of faith. Experts from Georgetown University School of Medicine in Washington, D.C., and Duke University Medical Center in Durham, North Carolina, who were reviewing studies on religion and health found that religious commitment may prevent many medical problems such as illness, depression, substance abuse, and even early death.

In many cases, faith provides a sense of being cared for, loved, and valued—all feelings that enhance your well-being and feed your youthful outlook. Spirituality also embraces the wisdom that comes with age. "Religion helps you to understand that growing old is not a bad thing," Dr. Strawbridge says.

Get involved. If you are a member of a faith or interested in becoming one, get involved in a church or temple. You become more active in the faith itself, and it often leads to social activities and volunteer work, Dr. Strawbridge says.

Find your own spirituality. Organized religion is not the only avenue to faith. Find your own way to celebrate your beliefs, Dr. Strawbridge says. Perhaps sitting quietly in a natural setting gets you in touch with your spiritual side.

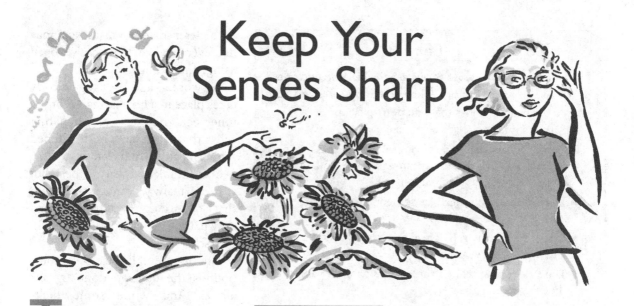

Keep Your Senses Sharp

There are two fundamental facts that life teaches us as we age: The dosage information on cough syrup bottles is entirely too small to read, and teenagers mumble so much that you can never understand them.

Either that or our eyesight and hearing are starting to go.

Keen eyesight and precise hearing are important to us—our senses, after all, are our links to the world around us as we beautify our homes, clarify our career goals, pursue interests that we may not have had time for during our twenties, and watch our children grow toward adulthood.

So it makes good sense to keep our senses sharp and youthful.

Hear Ye, Hear Ye

How old were you when you went to your first amp-shaking, rip-roaring rock concert? How often have you been startled by a blast of volume when you slipped on your headphones at the start of your daily walk or jog? Can you count the times you've had to raise your voice to converse with a friend in city traffic?

As we go about our twenty-first-century lives, the tiny cells in our inner ears take a daily battering from amplified sound waves. Add the racket from snowblowers or lawn mowers on the weekends to the relentless engine revs and brake screeches of city streets, and the "Sounds of Silence" that Simon and Garfunkel once popularized seem like pure nostalgia.

But even before life got so loud, our ears didn't necessarily age gracefully. Age-related hearing loss is quite literally an age-old problem. It just happens to be one that we think won't ever happen to us.

Perhaps that's why women rarely come on their own volition to see John W. House, M.D., president of the renowned House Ear Institute in Los Angeles.

"Quite frankly, it's usually the husband or the partner who makes an issue of hearing loss. He'll have been saying, 'You know, I don't think your hearing is as good as it used to be,'" Dr. House says. She tags along reluctantly, hoping to prove him wrong.

It's very tempting to pretend it's not happening.

on a defense mechanism you may not even realize that you've been using: lipreading.

As women age, a change slowly takes place in a certain region of the inner ear, the cochlea, when hair cells that pick up high-pitched sounds begin to deteriorate.

You'll think that you can hear, but you don't always understand, and that's because you're actually hearing only part of a word spoken, says Dr. House.

Environmental noise only compounds the damage done by age alone. And while some lucky people—including Howard House, M.D., John's father and the founder of the House Ear Institute—hear perfectly into their nineties, by the age of 65, one in three women will suffer age-related hearing loss.

Can You Speak a Little Louder?

Even though age-related hearing loss generally begins in a person's fifties, it may happen sooner if hearing loss runs in your family or you've been exposed to excessively loud noises.

Still, if you're like most women, compensation and denial may prevent you from seeking help, says Dr. House. "They'll say people are mumbling or not speaking clearly, or they'll blame it on noisy restaurants."

As it turns out, noisy places are some of the most likely settings for age-related hearing loss to rear its unwelcome head. High-pitched conversation noise and rattling dishes will steal the words of your companions, and distractions may make it difficult for you to rely

Preventing Hearing Loss

Whether you can still discern every word of every conversation or you've already noticed some loss of clarity, there is lots you can do to keep your hearing sharp and healthy.

Shhhhhhh. The most important thing that you can do to preserve your hearing is to protect yourself from loud noises, says Dr. House. Wear ear protection if you're mowing the lawn, riding in a noisy motorboat, or going to a monster truck rally, he advises.

Buy the CD. Fun as it is to go and see your favorite stars on their nostalgia tours, be aware that the volume at concerts has gotten no less ear-splitting than what you remember. "We've seen people who suffered permanent hearing loss from one exposure at a concert or disco," says Dr. House.

Be smart on the job. Habitual exposure to noise is worse than the occasional blast of jet engine noise you hear as you climb the steps to your commuter flight. If you work in an area where people routinely have to raise their voices to be heard, you're at risk. Wear ear protection, and wear it consistently, says Dr. House.

Target Hearing Loss Early

If you have a hunch that you've begun to suffer mild hearing loss, get it checked out. You won't stay young if you miss out on conversations at parties, lines in movies and plays, and directions at work.

What's more, hearing loss is not only a sign of age. "There are all kinds of causes of hearing loss, and sometimes they are treatable with surgery or medications," says Dr. House.

Otosclerosis, the hardening of bones within the ear, is a condition that is 90 percent curable with delicate surgery, for example. Other mimickers of age-related hearing loss include Ménière's disease, which is treated by medication or surgery, or even a benign tumor on a nerve that lies within the ear. Even though such tumors aren't malignant, they need to be detected early. Besides causing hearing loss, they can grow, causing pressure on the brain.

Begin at the beginning. The best specialist to see is an otolaryngologist, once known as an ear-nose-and-throat doctor, or an otologist, a medical doctor who specializes exclusively in diseases of the ear. Don't start at your local hearing-aid store, recommends Dr. House. "You can always go back and get a hearing aid if you

---

SHADES THAT WON'T FADE: YOUR GUIDE TO BUYING SUNGLASSES

Sure, sunglasses look great. What star would go out without them? But if you're serious about saving your sight, protection should be your number one priority when you go shopping for shades. Sunglasses will help to stave off crinkly little wrinkles around your eyes, but more important, they have been shown to reduce your chances of developing cataracts. They may even help to prevent age-related macular degeneration, a devastating condition in which elderly people lose their central sight, leaving them with only peripheral vision, explains Wayne Fung, M.D., an ophthalmologist at the California Pacific Medical Center in San Francisco.

Lenses should filter out at least 99 percent of the ultraviolet light and be made of impact-resistant material. Make sure that the lenses don't have sharp, unprotected edges that could cut your eye in a fall or sports-related injury, notes John B. Jeffers, M.D., an ophthalmologist with the Wills Eye Hospital in Philadelphia.

Ideally, they should be optically ground and tinted a neutral gray or green to block the most damaging wavelengths of ultraviolet A and B light, adds Robert M. Greenburg, O.D., an optometrist and optometric consultant in Reston, Virginia.

It's unlikely that you're going to find quality sunglasses meeting all these criteria on the bargain rack at your local drugstore, Dr. Greenburg explains. A good pair of sunglasses with the features recommended above will cost you about $50. Don't get taken in by the brand-name specialty sunglasses, however. Just because they are more expensive doesn't mean you are getting more or better protection.

need one, but first you need to rule out other problems."

Test it out. Once you've been checked for potential physiological problems of the ear or other hearing-related health problems, you'll probably be referred to an audiologist, a specialist in the testing of hearing. You may take a test in a soundproof booth with special headphones while you use a device to indicate when you hear sounds of various pitches with each ear.

Don't avoid your first aid. Hearing aids have become smaller, more inconspicuous, and vastly more sophisticated than they were even just a few years ago. Many are digital and capable of filtering out peripheral noise, so they selectively amplify the sounds you've been missing and most want to hear, like voices, says Dr. House.

"Often, I'll recommend a hearing aid, and someone will refuse," says Dr. House. "They tell me they're too young. But are they willing to go around saying, 'What? What? What?' and missing half of what goes on around them?" It's hardly a strategy designed to keep you young in body and in mind.

Early use of a hearing aid can help people adapt better to their hearing loss, Dr. House notes.

The Eyes Have It

It may happen gradually, as you slowly realize that it's getting tougher to see which eyebrows to pluck until you back away from the mirror. Or it may happen virtually overnight, as you sud-

SECOND SIGHT

Steamy romance novels. Sunday drives. Watching your grandchildren grow. All of these pleasures can disappear into the darkness of age-related macular degeneration (ARMD), the leading cause of blindness in people over 65.

ARMD affects the macula, located in the center of the retina, the light-sensitive layer of tissue at the back of the eye. Slowly, the light-sensitive cells in the macula break down, causing loss of central vision and making it difficult to read, drive, or perform other everyday tasks. According to some studies, women may be at greater risk than men.

But there's new hope. Recent research conducted by Stuart Richer, O.D., Ph.D., chief of the optometry section at the DVA Medical Center in North Chicago, proposes a whole new way to prevent—and treat—ARMD. Here's the new sight-saving plan, based on his research.

Get tested. When taken together, four common vision tests can uncover the earliest signs of ARMD, says Dr. Richer. Ask your optometrist to administer the four tests in his study: the Amsler grid (which checks for distortions in central vision); contrast-sensitivity (which tests ability to distinguish between different-size objects); low-luminance, low-contrast (which measures ability to see in the dark); and glare-recovery (which tests ability to recover from glare).

Also, tell your optometrist if you are postmenopausal and not using estrogen replacement; have heart disease, high blood pressure, or high cholesterol; use photo-sensitizing drugs; or smoke. You are at higher risk for ARMD.

denly become aware that you need to hold the newspaper at arm's length to read the classified ads.

Our ability to focus reaches its peak when we're around 12, then declines a little bit with every birthday thereafter. By the time we reach ages 35 to 45, many of us begin to notice we're

Make like Popeye. It appears that ARMD can be delayed, or even reversed, with large doses of . . . spinach. In a preliminary study conducted by Dr. Richer, men with the common "dry" form of ARMD who consumed four to seven servings of spinach a week bettered their scores on the Amsler grid, contrast-sensitivity, and glare-recovery tests. Spinach contains lutein and zeaxanthin, antioxidants found in high amounts in the retina. It's thought that they protect the retina, either by absorbing eye-damaging blue light or by preventing free-radical damage.

Sauté spinach in a small amount of olive oil, or eat it with a meal that contains some fat. Fat helps the body absorb, store, and transport lutein, Dr. Richer explains. Also, if you are prone to kidney stones, eat kale instead of spinach. Kale contains lower levels of oxalic acid, which may contribute to the formation of kidney stones.

Take supplements. If you can't or won't eat your greens, take an antioxidant supplement that contains lutein, advises Dr. Richer. Studies suggest that 6 to 12 milligrams a day can benefit eyesight.

Mind your medication. If you're taking a blood-thinning medication, talk to your doctor before megadosing on spinach. The vitamin K it contains can interfere with anti-clotting drugs.

Shield those peepers. Purchase sunglasses that block out all ultraviolet A and B rays, including blue light, advises Dr. Richer. "Blue light is the short-wave, high-energy part of the visible ultraviolet spectrum, and it has been shown to damage the eyes."

Stub out those butts. Smoking constricts the delicate vessels that nourish the eyes, increasing the risk of ARMD.

If you've already noticed your vision getting worse, all is not lost. Here's what to do.

Take a look—close-up. This is obvious, but it still bears repeating. Schedule an eye examination to review the health of your eyes and the overall functioning of your visual system. This includes tests for how well your eyes focus on objects, both far and near, and how well they work together for depth perception, says Robert M. Greenburg, O.D., an optometrist and optometric consultant in Reston, Virginia.

Don't make excuses, like telling yourself you can see okay so long as the lighting is bright enough or you're feeling okay, advises Dr. Greenburg. It is true that your vision may be sharper in the bright light of a sunny day since the pupils constrict and increase your depth of focus. But you also deserve to see well indoors, in the soothing light of your den, or when you're walking the streets at twilight.

Squint no more. If you find yourself distorting your face to clear up blurry letters, you're doing yourself no youthful favors. Constant squinting deepens the lines around your eyes, making you look older. Squinting in bright sunlight is no better. Wear sunglasses to help to preserve the smooth appearance of your face around your eyes. Sunglasses will also help to prevent cataracts, which can be caused by sun damage, Dr. Greenburg says.

Specs on specs. A new pair of glasses or a specially designed pair of contact lenses will restore your ability to see close-up again. Your own best option may be bifocals, bifocal contact lenses, or a pair of reading glasses. Check with

holding reading matter so far away that our arms seem too short.

It's called presbyopia, the age-related vision change that occurs as your once-flexible lens becomes harder and less clear, says John B. Jeffers, M.D., an ophthalmologist at the Wills Eye Hospital in Philadelphia.

your eye professional to see what she recommends.

Eyes Need Exercise

Although not all eye professionals agree, some advocate exercising the muscles in the eyes the same way you exercise the other muscles in your body. Dr. Greenburg suggests these tips for women who want to keep their visual system functioning well.

Keep track. As you go about your daily life, practice tracking moving objects and following things. Computer games help with this, but take frequent breaks.

Be shifty-eyed. Shift your gaze often. Fix your sights on something in one corner of the room, then the other in a rhythmic way.

Look here and there. Focus near, then focus far. When you're reading, look across the room every 2 minutes.

The Life of a Visionary

The very best thing that you can do to keep your eyes young and your vision sharp is to practice prevention. Investing a little attention in your eyesight now will go a long way toward keeping it healthy in the future. Here's what the experts recommend.

Look for yellow, orange, and green. Wayne Fung, M.D., an ophthalmologist at the California Pacific Medical Center in San Francisco, recommends that women munch on fruits and vegetables rich in beta-carotene. The beta-carotene is important for good eye health, and eating fruits and vegetables adds fiber, which is important to your overall health. Good choices include papaya, mango, kale, Swiss chard, pumpkin, broccoli, and spinach, he says.

Check your chance of cloudiness. As your eyes age, the protein material in your lens may begin to cloud—subtly at first, like adding drops of milk to a glass of water, one at a time. Getting annual eye examinations during your middle-aged years will diagnose cataracts early, before they begin to significantly interfere with your driving ability, sports and hobbies, and reading, Dr. Greenburg says.

Don't let blindness sneak up on you. Perhaps the most important reason for regular eye exams is glaucoma screening. When pressure builds behind the eye, damage can occur to the optic nerve, which can lead to blindness. Since there are no symptoms, an examination is your only path to early detection. If you have suffered a significant eye injury at any time during your life, or if you have blood relatives with glaucoma, you're at higher risk for glaucoma developing during middle age, says Dr. Jeffers.

Protect your peepers. As you lead your busy, active life, make sure that your eyes have the protection they need. Wear impact-resistant sunglasses or safety glasses that protect your eyes from injury as well as guard against ultraviolet rays. Wear a wide-brimmed hat while gardening, golfing, or watching sporting events in the sun. And if you're a weekend handywoman, be sure to wear eye protection while you're swinging that hammer.

Entwine with twine. Dr. Fung warns against a common travel-related eye injury from an unlikely source: bungee cords. It seems that women stretch the handy cords tightly around luggage or across skis on their roof racks. If one end snaps loose, it can fly very quickly into your eye, doing significant damage, he says.

Boost Your Memory at Any Age

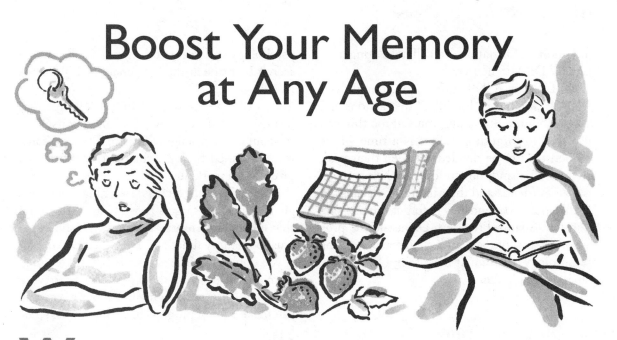

Who ran for vice president of the United States in 1984?

Don't remember? At the time, she was the subject of discussion over nearly every dinner table in America.

Bet you remember now—her face, if not her name.

Our brains are like that: More complex and marvelous than the most powerful computer, and yet we can find ourselves with a familiar piece of information stubbornly eluding us, right at the tip of our tongues.

When you first want that piece of information, you send your memory looking for it among the tons of intelligence stored away in your head. If everything goes right, you have the tidbit you are looking for a few milliseconds later.

Of course, not everything always goes right. And it goes wrong more often as you get older because your memory begins to slow down with age. Many of us have firsthand experience of that irritating little phenomenon. The question is: What can we do about it?

Oh, by the way . . . Geraldine Ferraro.

What's Going On in There?

First of all, relax. Stop worrying about Alzheimer's disease and early senility. Minor memory lapses are common, expected, and easily mended.

We usually begin to experience a gradual decline in memory at about age 30, but we are talking a *very* mild decline, says David Mitchell, Ph.D., associate professor of psychology and director of the Center for Aging Studies at Loyola University in Chicago. "Let's say you make a grocery list, and if you're like me, you forget to bring your list, but you go shopping anyway. When you get home, you're not surprised to find that you forgot to buy two or three items. As you get a bit older, you'll forget three or four," he says.

Aging isn't the only problem. You also have a lot more information to sort through now than when you were younger, and each day you add more data into your memory. With so much to remember, no wonder you forget. "The brain is a finite piece of tissue. Most people in memory research assume that as your system gets more and more information, it will take longer to search," Dr. Mitchell says.

As if a brain full of stuff wasn't enough, you probably also have a life full of distractions and responsibilities. Stretching yourself too thin can also lead to forgetting. "This is a time where women tend to be divided between their jobs, their families, and sometimes even their parents, as well as friends and their interests. Because of all this, there is a tendency to forget things," says Carolyn Adams-Price, Ph.D., associate professor of psychology and chairperson of the gerontology program at Mississippi State University in Starkville.

Keeping the Brain Up and Running

The brain, just like a muscle, needs to work out to stay fit. By challenging and pushing the brain to reach higher and do more, you make it stronger. Studies have shown that animals put into an enriched environment with many opportunities for exploratory activity actually undergo structural changes in the brain, improving their abilities both to learn and to remember, says Molly V. Wagster, Ph.D., program director of the neuropsychology of aging program at the National Institute on Aging in Bethesda, Maryland.

But what may be a challenge one day may be easy going the next. Although mastering any new mental task gets more difficult as you get older (no one knows why), once you have completely mastered a task, no matter how difficult, performing it no longer improves your brain. "We tend to reach plateaus in life. We work at something until we are good at it, then we continue to do it at the same level. But as you continue, the challenge disappears," says Arnold Scheibel, M.D., professor of neurobiology and

psychology and former director of the Brain Research Institute at the University of California, Los Angeles.

In order to keep your brain and memory healthy as you get older, you must constantly seek out new challenges for them. Here are some recommended by Dr. Scheibel that will really give them a workout.

Take a language class. Learning a new language especially targets those areas of the brain that enhance memory. "It is a wonderful stimulus to memory function," Dr. Scheibel explains. If you don't have time to take a class, try learning from audiotapes. Use them as you drive to work each day. "Just work on it a half-hour a day. You can make a lot of progress in a couple weeks," he says.

Make beautiful music. The combination of visual, mental, and physical skills you use playing an instrument invigorates your brain, he says. Music, like many creative pursuits, improves your memory and provides a wonderful expressive outlet.

Seek out the opposite. Work on skills that are the exact opposite of what comes naturally to you. If you are artistic, dabble in the logical world of math or computers. If you are verbal, test out your ability to express yourself visually in painting or drawing.

Calculate in your head. Dr. Scheibel refuses to use calculators or computers to do basic math. Why? Because he found that relying on these timesaving devices soon eroded his ability to do math in his head. Math calculations challenge your brain and keep your memory in good shape.

Switch hands. For about 5 minutes a day, try being a lefty if you are a righty, or vice versa. Write, punch numbers into the telephone, or play tennis with your nondominant hand. This exercise develops the opposite side of your brain.

Surround yourself with interesting people. Dr. Scheibel compares keeping company with intellectually stimulating people to playing tennis. "The very best thing you can do is play with someone better than you because you strive to be better. It is the same thing with people. When you feel, 'Gee, I am just a little bit out of my class here because everyone seems so much brighter,' that makes you extend, and I can't think of a better challenge," he says. Join book clubs, take classes, form discussion and writing groups, or just hang out with people who challenge you in conversation.

Improving Your Everyday Memory

It's the little things that drive you crazy: Where did I leave those papers? What is that guy's name? Did I forget the bread again? What is her phone number? "In the grand scheme of things, they are minor lapses of memory. They may become more frequent and aggravating as you get older, but they are not necessarily a cause for concern," Dr. Wagster says. "It may take you longer to remember a name than when you were 25, but you'll probably retrieve it—even if it takes a few hours."

To keep these petty memory problems from building up into major headaches, try some of the following memory techniques.

Pay attention. You often blame your memory when you can't remember, but many times, it is just as much the fault of your attention span. If you are not paying attention, you are not giving your memory a chance to absorb and store the information, Dr. Adams-Price says. When you are introduced to someone, stop, listen, think about the name, and even repeat it out loud. Do the same when you make an appointment.

Make the unconscious conscious. Make a mental note of all the little things you usually do without thinking, Dr. Scheibel says. For example, if you can never remember where you left your car keys, every time you put them somewhere, stop and make a point of saying to yourself: I put my car keys on the tabletop. "It's a new way of thinking, where you have to reiterate each action that you perform," he says.

Locate with 'loci.' Keep your tomatoes in the bathroom? Sounds crazy, but imagery like that is the basis of an ancient Greek memory system called the loci method. In the loci method, you picture whatever you want to remember as being in a certain place. For instance, say you want to make a mental grocery list. Dr. Adams-Price says to picture the milk on your couch, the bread on your CD player, the apples on the coffee table. Then as you need to remember the item, picture all the things in your living room. As you remember the place, like the couch, you will remember the milk.

Link words with images. Many people remember what they see better than what they hear. So think of what you need to remember as a visual image. For instance, you meet a man named Richard, says Sandra Monastero, a licensed psychologist at Friends Hospital in Philadelphia. In your mind, picture your new acquaintance as Richard the Lionhearted. You see him in your mind as a lion or dressed as a king. It sounds silly, but it works.

Sing your ABCs. If you can't remember someone's name, start reciting the alphabet in your head. "Oftentimes you can cue yourself to remember the name when you come upon the letter it starts with," Dr. Adams-Price says.

Divide and conquer numbers. Cell phones, pager numbers, e-mail addresses, security codes—it seems the numbers you need to remember are infinite. All of those digits easily get mixed up in your brain matter. To make it

GREAT MIND GAMES

Challenging your mind doesn't necessarily mean taking a correspondence course in rocket science. You can have fun doing it. Playing games and solving puzzles, for example, can test your memory, strategic thinking, and other mental skills. Here are six games that can help improve your memory and your mind, according to Carolyn Adams-Price, Ph.D., associate professor of psychology and chairperson of the gerontology program at Mississippi State University in Starkville.

➤ Bridge. It's a game that involves both strategy and memory, providing a total mental workout.

➤ Chess. Although more strategy than memory, chess challenges your brain by forcing you to think several moves ahead.

➤ Cryptograms. Dr. Adams-Price considers cryptograms one of the best games to work your brain. The puzzle involves a lot of thinking and problem solving.

➤ Crossword puzzles. Solving them stretches your vocabulary and memory muscles. Enough said.

➤ Tetris. This video game requires fitting various shapes together at a rapid pace. The game requires spatial skills, which is the ability to visually place objects together. Spatial skills get better with practice, but you don't use these skills often in everyday life. Tetris offers a fun way to get them into shape.

➤ Minesweeper. This is another computer game. You click on grid squares to try to avoid hidden bombs. Play involves a lot of logical thinking.

easier for you, break them down in chunks, Monastero says. Perhaps your automatic teller machine code is 7241. Remember it as "seventy-two, forty-one" instead of "seven, two, four, one." Divide it into two numbers instead of four.

Get Organized

If you are the kind of person who files all your important papers under "S" for "Stuff," you may be one of those people who loses everything from her car keys to her track of time. "Disorganization is part of the problem. People who aren't well-organized are more likely to forget where they put things," Dr. Adams-Price says.

The antidote is the same one you would use to cure a sloppy room: Straighten the place up. You can start here.

Invest in an appointment book. An appointment book can be your central location for information, Monastero says. Use this appointment book for phone numbers, schedules, lists of things to do, appointments, and everything else you need to know. By doing so, you take a lot of stress off your memory. Be careful to divide your book into as few sections as possible. Too many can be overwhelming and defeat your purpose.

Find the best of times. A study at the University of Arizona tested a group of younger people and a group of older people at different times of the day. The researchers found that young people performed better in the evening, while the older group tested better in the morning. It may be that your own circadian rhythms affect how well your memory functions, Dr. Mitchell says. While the study found that the morning was better as people got older, Dr. Mitchell advises you to figure out your own optimal time. "If you have a choice, schedule important things you have to do at that time," he says.

Place things where you will see them. Out of sight, out of mind, right? That's usually the problem, especially in forgetting to take pills, papers, and all sorts of important things. So leave them where you have to see them, Monastero says. Some examples: Put your medications inside your coffee cup, leave documents on your alarm clock. "Make sure that you have to move it to get to something else," she suggests.

Designate special spots. Get into the habit of leaving objects in designated spots. Always keep your car keys on the table by the door; always leave your reading glasses on your nightstand. Monastero also suggests appointing a special location for the next day's work materials. "Have everything for the next day gathered together and put in a central spot the night before. That way, when the morning comes, you don't have to think about where you put things or what you have to do that day," she says.

Color your world. Bright colors help you find objects you often lose. Put your keys on colorful, large key chains. Place a bright-colored string around your reading glasses. With bright colors screaming at you, you won't have to work as hard to find lost items, Monastero says.

Make little ones out of big ones. A big project or an outrageous amount of material to remember can overwhelm you. That sinking feeling leads you to procrastination, which means that you end up doing an awful lot of work at the last moment—and inevitably you forget something. Instead of getting lost in the big picture, break up a large project into smaller discrete tasks, Monastero says. Tackle each task one at a time and complete it. This makes a project more manageable and less overpowering.

Do it now. If behavior guru and Harvard educator B. F. Skinner heard it was going to rain, he got up right then and put the umbrella up against the door so that he couldn't miss it, says Dr. Mitchell. The best way to not forget something is to act upon it as soon as possible, he says.

Make lists. Put information on paper. It takes a load off your mind when it comes to remembering. Lists also force you to organize your ideas. "Even if you forget the list, you took the time to compose your thoughts, which will help you in trying to retrieve the information," Dr. Wagster says.

Living a Memory-Enhancing Lifestyle

Lest we forget, the brain is a part of the body. And just like the rest of your body, it needs the basics: good nutrition and exercise. If you are lacking in these areas, your brain—no matter how well-prepared—will never work at its full capacity. So here are some tips designed to help with the care and feeding of your gray matter.

Get up and go. Regular exercise will help your memory. It's as simple as taking a 50-minute brisk walk three or four times a week, says Robert E. Dustman, Ph.D., research career scientist and director of neuropsychology research at the Veterans Affairs Medical Center in Salt Lake City. In a study of 45 men and women, ages 55 to 70, researchers found that people who started a walking program scored better on visual memory and mental flexibility tests.

"It makes sense that aerobic exercise should be good for the brain, because it's good for the cardiovascular system, and that system is the gateway to the brain," says Dr. Dustman, the study's author.

Toss in strawberries and spinach. Both may help fight the effects of aging on the brain. Recent research shows that giving an extract from either strawberries or spinach to rats helps retard age-related problems of the brain.

"These do have a positive effect on slowing age-related cognitive decline—at least in rats," Dr. Wagster says. Although the findings have

WOMEN ASK WHY

Why is it that I can remember the details of my senior prom, but I can't remember where I had dinner last Saturday night?

For the same reason that just about anyone old enough to remember can tell you exactly what they were doing on the day President John F. Kennedy was assassinated: You have a "flashbulb" memory.

You form a flashbulb memory when you experience an event so significant that you repeat it in your mind for years and years afterward, until you freeze that moment in time.

If you were like many teenage girls, the senior prom—for better or for worse—was a defining moment in your life. For weeks before the big night, you may have painstakingly gone over every detail: your dress, your shoes, your hair, your jewelry.

Afterward, because it was such a significant memory, you replayed it over and over in your mind, probably so often that you'll never forget it.

As for last Saturday's dinner, what was special about it? It probably wasn't much different from dinner the Saturday before, or the Saturday before that. So why on earth would you remember? After all, it wasn't exactly a prom.

Expert consulted
Carolyn Adams-Price, Ph.D.
Associate professor of psychology and chairperson of the gerontology program
Mississippi State University
Starkville

aging. Although you should get most nutrients from a diet filled with fruits, vegetables, and whole grains, you may need to add more of these important antioxidants, Dr. Scheibel says, so take a supplement of 400 international units of vitamin E and 1,000 milligrams of C a day. "The data are more and more pushing in the direction that these two protect the brain," he says.

Get enough of the Bs. The B vitamins thiamin, vitamin B_6, and vitamin B_{12} all play a role in keeping the brain healthy, Dr. Scheibel says. If you are not getting enough of these three B vitamins from your diet, try a good B-complex vitamin supplement, he suggests.

Without enough thiamin, your brain can't use glucose as well. And if that happens, your brain can't perform up to speed. You need at least 1.5 milligrams a day. Good food sources include rice bran, pork, beef, fresh peas, beans, and wheat germ.

Meanwhile, vitamin B_6 helps make neurotransmitters, the chemicals that allow brain cells to communicate. Take at least 2 milligrams per day, from either a supplement or good food sources, such as bananas, avocados, chicken, beef, or eggs.

Last but not least, you need vitamin B_{12} to protect the production of myelin, a fatty covering that insulates nerve fibers. If you don't get enough B_{12}, you may experience memory loss and confusion. You need 6 micrograms a day, either from a supplement or from food sources such as clams, ham, lamb, cooked oysters, king crab, herring, salmon, or tuna.

yet to be confirmed in people, she suggests that individuals eat a balanced diet, which includes foods, such as strawberries and spinach, that are rich in antioxidants.

Supplement with C and E. Because vitamins C and E are antioxidants, they are thought to protect your brain from the normal ravages of

Embrace Change
with Ease

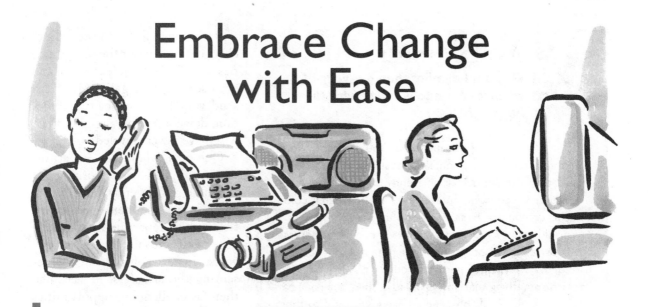

If you were stranded alone on a desert island, which would your first priority be: (a) build a boat to escape in or (b) build a hut to live in?

If you chose (b), you're a survivor. Survivors don't struggle against bad situations. They adapt to them, even thrive in them.

That's the lesson Al Siebert, Ph.D., learned from interviewing people who went through terrible calamities and lived to tell their stories. They survived shipwrecks on high seas. Trapped on mountaintops, they endured days of withering cold. They wandered lost and alone through dark tropical rain forests. In every case, it was the same basic skill that kept them alive: adaptability.

"It wasn't this mythical individual against the sea, the mountain, or the elements. It was the individual *with* the sea, individual *with* the elements. They didn't fight their situations, they adapted to them and thrived," says Dr. Siebert, a semi-retired adjunct professor at Portland State University in Oregon and author of *The Survivor Personality* and *The Adult Student's Guide to Survival and Success.*

So what's the point? Few of us will ever have to survive in an arctic wilderness or find food in a desert. Most of the changes we encounter are far more ordinary: a shake-up at work, for example, or new neighbors or a divorce. But we can still learn from those people who experienced change in the extreme. That's important because, large or small, change is the one thing that none of us can avoid.

An Ever-Changing World

Not all change is sad or difficult. Often it can be happy and rewarding, such as when you have a baby or get promoted. But for some, especially as you get older, it may seem threatening.

"Perhaps people are afraid of change because they don't know where change is going to take them. They may be afraid that there is nothing to fall back on, and the unknown can be scary," says Peggy A. Stock, Ed.D., president of Westminster College in Salt Lake City and a lecturer on change. "Sometimes it just seems safer to stick with what we know."

Safe or not, the benefits of adapting far outweigh the risks. It helps you to cope with what

Why am I dumber than a 6-year-old when it comes to working with the Internet?

The answer is: You're not. Children aren't smarter when it comes to technology and the Internet; they just approach it differently than you do.

Children have two advantages over adults when it comes to using computers. First, they grew up with computers. A 6-year-old has never known a world without Web addresses and browsers and laptops. Navigating the Internet seems as natural to her as finding her way around a playground. Think back to something that you knew as a child but your parents didn't. You probably seemed like a whiz kid to them, too.

Second, kids aren't afraid of breaking things, including computers. You, on the other hand, probably view a computer as a complicated machine—and an investment of several thousand dollars. You tremble with the thought that pressing a wrong button could send that money up in a wisp of cybersmoke. Once you realize that it is practically impossible to actually break a computer by typing on your keyboard or clicking your mouse, you'll lose your fear and feel confident enough to play around on the 'net.

Expert consulted
Alan I. Marcus
Professor of history and a specialist in the history of technology
Iowa State University
Ames

Rather than focus on the risks of change, think about the opportunities it offers. An unexpected and even seemingly negative event can send your life in a positive direction, down a path you might otherwise have never traveled.

One man, whom Dr. Siebert interviewed, had been working for the same state agency for 20 years, when he was suddenly reassigned to another department, then another and another for the next 6 years. Instead of fighting or resenting the transfers, he accepted them as challenging opportunities and decided to learn his new jobs with enthusiasm.

He soon became integral to his new department, acquired valuable expertise about his agency, and jumped up three pay grades. "If you perceive change as a learning challenge, you'll take advantage of your situation and thrive. The people who remain resilient in life and increase their longevity are those who approach change with curiosity. They experiment and explore like playful children," Dr. Siebert says.

Easier said than done, of course. Even people who experience good change, such as buying their dream house or getting married, report increased stress and strain in their lives, Dr. Siebert says. So here are some guidelines to make navigating through a changing world just a little easier.

Revisit your successes. Think back to all the changes you have successfully handled in the past: getting married, having children,

is happening in the moment. The person who resists change will be out of sync with the rest of the world, Dr. Siebert says, and that's no fun. Being out of step with the people and the world around you may lead to a sense of isolation, helplessness, and a feeling that life has gone ahead without you.

moving, starting a new job. Doing so will remind you how often you have triumphed over change. "You'll remember how well you coped and know that you'll handle this situation just as well," Dr. Siebert says.

Talk it over. In his work with women in their forties who have gone back to college, Dr. Siebert learned that they found it extremely reassuring and helpful to talk to other women in similar situations. Find other people who are going through or who have gone through a similar change, he recommends. They can give you advice or just give you peace of mind in knowing that you are not alone.

Stay ahead of the curve. If you see change on the horizon, don't react to it impulsively. Instead, be prepared for it. If it's at work, for example, learn new skills so that you can change careers, if you need to, or make yourself more valuable at your current job, says Dr. Siebert. "If you tell yourself, 'I have to learn all this to be competitive in today's world,' you won't resist the change. But if you're being told you have to do something in order to survive, you'll experience more distress," he says, "and react like a victim instead of a thriver."

Change for the fun of it. Get yourself used to change by making some enjoyable changes on your own accord, Dr. Stock suggests. Try a new sport such as inline skating or golf, read a new genre of books, find

KEEPING UP WITH THE TECHIES

If technology opens up a whole new world, it also opens up a whole new language. This new vocabulary leaves many people feeling lost and confused, says Larry Rosen, Ph.D., professor of psychology at California State University, Dominguez Hills, and coauthor of *TechnoStress: Coping with Technology @ Work @ Home @ Play*.

But just like any other language, you can learn a few key phrases or words to help you communicate with this technological society. Here's a quick primer on some of the most common computer terms and what they mean.

- The Internet: A global network of computers that lets people share information and resources.
- Cyber- (prefix): A person, place, or thing on the 'net. Examples: cyberspace, cyberpunk.
- E-mail: Electronic mail sent over the Internet or an online service.
- World Wide Web: A collection of multimedia documents that are connected. Web documents can include text, pictures, sounds, and video.
- Browser: Software used to navigate the World Wide Web.
- Search engine: A Web site that lets you search the Internet by typing in a keyword or phrase.
- Web address or URL (Uniform Resource Locator): Usually starts with "www." The location of a specific Web site.
- Surf the 'net: Randomly go from site to site on the Internet. Not looking for a specific page, just looking to see what is out there. Similar to channel surfing with your TV remote control.
- CD-ROM: An acronym that stands for "compact disc read-only memory," meaning the audiovisual information stored on a compact disc that you play in the CD-ROM drive (CD player) of a computer. The drive is very much like the CD player you use to play music on your stereo.
- Spam: Not the meat, but unwanted e-mail. Usually junk mail via the computer.

a new hobby. "Change can be fun and rewarding," she says. "It keeps life interesting."

Changing at the Speed of Light

Technology. It can be a scary word. Computers get faster, more powerful, and more intimidating every day. They intrude into everything we do, from reaching a customer service representative on the phone to starting your car. They are in your digital alarm clock, your VCR, your answering machine, the automatic teller machine. Just in one day, the amount of technology you interact with is staggering.

Short of moving into a jungle tree house, there is really no way to avoid it. Technological advancement is one kind of change we are all stuck with. And keeping up with it isn't particularly easy or intuitive. Although we can be extraordinarily adaptable, technology poses a special obstacle for us.

That's because it moves so fast, says Larry Rosen, Ph.D., professor of psychology at California State University, Dominguez Hills, and coauthor of *TechnoStress: Coping with Technology @ Work @ Home @ Play.*

According to Dr. Rosen, throughout most of recorded history, technological advances usually took years—sometimes even decades—to develop, and then took even longer to gain acceptance. All that time gave people the luxury of learning, adjusting, and deciding how this new technology would fit into their lives.

Almost at their leisure, people could grasp the significance of the wheel, the printing press, the automobile, and the television set. But today's technology evolves so quickly that it has eroded away that buffer. People don't have the time to learn, adjust, and adapt to one technological wonder before the next one makes its debut. The result is that we feel intimidated, stressed-out, and fearful, says Dr. Rosen.

The Benefits of Techno-Change

Technology may pose a more daunting façade than other types of change, but it also opens up a world of advantages to us. Here are just some of the many benefits of going with the flow of technology.

New perspectives. Keeping pace with technology prevents your thinking from becoming stagnant. And "by doing something that is so cutting-edge, you get a sense of feeling young at heart," says Alan I. Marcus, professor of history and a specialist in the history of technology at Iowa State University in Ames.

Control. Adapting to new technology gives you control over important aspects of your life: whose calls you receive, when and where you want to work, and how you get your news, travel, drive your car, and protect your home.

Greater access. From new recipes to up-to-the-minute medical knowledge, important information from around the globe is at your fingertips.

Fun. In addition to computer games, technology enables you to make videos of friends, listen to music in your office, and find new ideas for hobbies and creative outlets.

Close connection. Phones, cell phones, answering machines, pagers, and e-mail make contacting someone near or far a breeze. You can send pictures of children or grandchildren via videotape or e-mail pictures. You can use an Internet videophone to see and talk with each other on holidays. "I remember as a child hearing that someday we'll have picture telephones. Well, that someday is now," says Ann Wrixon, president and executive director of SeniorNet, an online community and Web site.

New friends. Whether it is meeting people online or joining a computer class, using technology introduces you to people of all backgrounds and ages. That interaction with a variety of people keeps you active and energized.

Better use of life experiences. The 20-year-old wunderkinds may be the ones inventing these technological marvels, but it is the people 40 and over who know what to do with them. "People with more life experience are the ones who use technology in the most innovative and exciting ways," Wrixon says.

Tackling Technology

It may be good to keep up, but with everything developing so quickly, how exactly can you do that? Where do you go for information? Here are some tips to get you up and running with technology now and to keep pace with it throughout your lifetime.

Read the popular press. Many newspapers now have weekly technology sections that address what's going on and what you can expect, says Dr. Marcus. Popular news magazines such as *Newsweek* and *Time* also have technology sections. The mainstream press keeps things simple and doesn't bog you down in a lot of techno-speak.

Take a class. Public libraries, community colleges, nonprofit organizations, and adult education centers often run classes for people who want to learn about new technology, especially computers. These are often fun, cheap, and designed for adults. Take a class to learn something new or master a program that you already use. Make sure that

THE SYMBOL OF A TECHNO-FEARFUL WORLD

Like many technologies, the VCR is an overly complex machine. "The people who have developed it tried to put everything in it, and because of that it is not easy to do the two things we want it to do—play tapes and record shows," says Larry Rosen, Ph.D., professor of psychology at California State University, Dominguez Hills, and coauthor of *Techno-Stress: Coping with Technology @ Work @ Home @ Play.*

But why has the VCR been ordained the ultimate symbol of the older person's inability to use technology? Mainly, because the VCR is everywhere. Even major technophobes own a VCR. Also, the VCR is in your face. Unlike other technologies that are tucked away in an office, it inhabits the most frequented room in your house, your living or family room.

And that flashing 12:00 is a constant reminder of your failure to master this bundle of bolts.

Because each VCR is different from the next, there are no universal rules about how to operate one. But Dr. Rosen has a few suggestions that will start you on your way to conquering just about any of those little mechanical monsters.

Read only parts of the manual. Some manuals are so poorly written that they don't help much, Dr. Rosen concedes. To make it simpler, read only about what you intend to use. Don't bog yourself down with unnecessary information.

Tape pages to the machine. Photocopy or rip out the pages of the manual that you use most and tape them to the VCR. That way you have them handy when you want to do something, like fix the clock after the electricity goes out.

Practice, practice, practice. Most people wait until they are running out the door or they need to tape something important before they start thinking about how to operate the machine. In their haste, they do it wrong and become even more flustered than usual with their own bumbling fingers. Pretend your VCR is a musical instrument. By practicing regularly when success isn't critical, you will be ready to perform under pressure when you really need to.

the instructor speaks in terms you can understand, Wrixon says.

Practice makes perfect. Just like anything else, using technology takes practice. "You'll get it over time. You don't have to learn it all now," Dr. Rosen says. Whether it be your VCR or your automatic car keys, spend time tinkering with them until you get the hang of it.

Tackle one task at a time. Don't set out to understand the intricate coding of a computer program. You don't need to. Instead, handle one function at a time. "Break it down into small components. You don't need to know everything, just the specifics of what you want to do," Wrixon says. Learn how to send an e-mail, record a show, or access a phone mail message. Once you have mastered one task, move on to another, she says.

Set a goal. Establish a reason you want to learn a certain technology. Do you want to learn how to use the Internet to study your family history or learn how to use a camcorder to videotape your children? This makes learning more fun and gives you a sense of purpose. If you just set out to learn something because you have to, you won't be as motivated, says Wrixon.

Lease or borrow technology. If you are not sure you want or need a new gizmo, you don't have to buy it, no matter what everyone else seems to be doing, Dr. Rosen says. Many stores now offer leasing for computers and technological equipment. Or ask a friend if you can use her devices for a while. That way, "you can decide whether you really like it, and you don't feel the pressure to buy it until you know if you want it," he says.

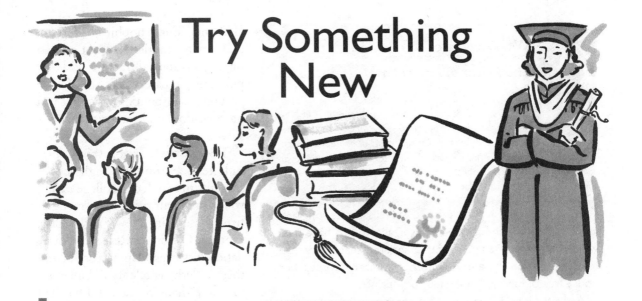

Try Something New

It's been said that the definition of middle age is when you're sitting at home on Saturday night and the telephone rings, and you hope it isn't for you.

By the time we've reached our midthirties, many of us have settled into lives we're comfortable with, which usually includes an aversion to shaking things up.

"People are afraid that if they don't follow the patterns they've established over the years, they'll become strangers in their own lives," says Maryann Troiani, Psy.D., a clinical psychologist with the Mercer Group in Barrington, Illinois, and coauthor of *Spontaneous Optimism*. But expanding beyond our cozy little worlds is just the ticket to staying young, she says. "The more open people are to new experiences, the more they learn, the more passion and energy they have, and the better their quality of life."

So why not take advantage of the many new experiences the world has to offer you? It's been said that it's never too late to be what you might have been, so give it some creative thought. You could take up a sport, travel, volunteer, paint, sculpt, meditate, enroll in classes, get involved in local politics, join a hiking group, become an activist, study astronomy, learn photography, forge new friendships, become a computer whiz, become a better cook, become a better version of yourself. The possibilities are endless.

"The secret to staying young is reinventing yourself with each new decade of your life," says Laura Barbanel, Ed.D., professor and head of the graduate program in school psychology at Brooklyn College of the City University of New York.

Seek and Ye Shall Find

So how do you find the passions that suit you today, knowing that at age 50, 60, and beyond you'll be able to put your energy into whatever matters most to you as time goes by?

If you're not sure where to start, follow these simple steps.

Tap your friends and family. Talking to your family and friends—especially your oldest ones—can help remind you of things that thrilled you when you were younger, says Dr.

WOMAN TO WOMAN
The Power of Puppy Love

Elizabeth Goldstein, 39, was a photographer in New York City a few years ago when she began to sense an internal void that her career couldn't fill. Experiencing recurring bouts of depression, Elizabeth sometimes felt as if her life lacked purpose. But when she began volunteering at a local animal shelter, she discovered the healing—and youth-promoting—power of love.

I have loved animals for as long as I can remember, although I was never allowed to have pets while I was growing up. My father insisted that it was too much responsibility, and my mother wanted to keep her house free of fur balls and muddy paw prints.

As I got older, I found myself grappling with a sense that my life lacked purpose. The years were passing, and in the end, I would be old and stuck with the realization that I hadn't made any difference in the world. I decided not to let that happen. It was time to make some changes.

I started by making one positive change in a small world—that of a homeless animal. I visited a local animal shelter and, at age 31, adopted my first pet: a shy, scrawny black cat. I loved her from the moment I saw her, but I couldn't stop thinking about all the other cats and dogs still caged at the shelter, waiting for someone to come and save their lives.

I began walking shelter dogs, grooming cats, and socializing the animals that had been traumatized by their experiences with unkind people. Soon I joined the shelter's foster program, in which volunteers take very young or sick animals into their homes, give them the care they need, then return them when they are ready to be adopted.

Eight years later, I'm still hooked, still volunteering. And it's given me a payoff that I never expected: I feel younger and more alive now than when I started. There's nothing quite as healing—and renewing—as giving and receiving love. Making a difference in these animals' lives has made all the difference in mine.

Barbanel. Early hobbies, interests, and innate abilities that got stuffed once you started raising kids or pursuing a career can be fertile ground for inspiration now that you have wisdom and maturity on your side.

Take a test. If you think aptitude tests are only for high school students in search of a college major, you're only half right. One research firm based in New York City, Johnson O'Conner Research Foundation, has been helping people find their underlying talents and interests for more than 75 years and has had hundreds of thousands of clients.

A typical test measures musical aptitudes, structural visualization, inductive reasoning, memory, the ability to produce a flow of ideas, and many other forms of manifested brilliance you may be harboring. Other aptitude tests simply help you match your skills with your interests so that you can begin to pursue those things that you're great at and love.

Since some tests can cost $120 or more an hour, you'll want to check around for the best deal. Your phone book or local community college's continuing education office is a good place to start.

Do it yourself. If you'd rather identify your passions on your own and a little writing doesn't scare you, take this three-pronged approach, says Dr. Troiani. First, jot down your best traits, maybe friendliness, honesty, and loyalty—the ones many of us take for granted. Then make a second list of activities that you enjoy, which may include baking, building, learning, and singing. Third and most important, reflect on what you'd like to be remembered for when you're gone and write that down, too. Now, look for common themes and patterns in these three items, such as creativity or a desire to help people. The result is a small but personalized list of avenues you'll want to pursue, she says.

Make it happen. Now that you have a vision of what you'd like to do, how can you make it a reality? Look around you to find out what resources are available. Investigate your public library and local bookstores to learn more about subjects that are new to you. Contact hospitals, children's shelters, animal shelters, and religious organizations about volunteer work. Call local colleges and universities for information about continuing education courses. Check out Web sites to find leads and to make connec-

tions with others who share your talents and interest.

And then, get moving, says Dr. Barbanel. There's no time to waste in our bid to turn back the clock.

LIFE EXTENDER
Get Some Culture

Here's one of the best excuses you'll ever have to go to the theater or opera: It could help you live longer.

That's the word from Sweden, where a large study found that people who frequently attended cultural events such as theater, museums, sports—even sermons—actually lived longer than those who didn't.

It's no surprise that great concerts, plays, and movies can be inspiring. But how could *Les Miserables* help turn back your clock? Swedish researchers suggest that the "vicarious emotional arousal" caused by these events might enhance your immune system and, as a result, help your body fight disease. Just don't watch too many violent films: The study's researchers noted that it might have the opposite effect.

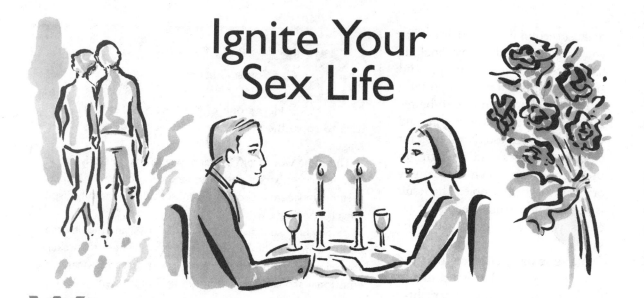

Ignite Your Sex Life

Wish you were in your twenties again? The Sex in America study, which polled more than 3,000 people, found that women in their early twenties reported the least amount of orgasms during sex, while women in their forties and fifties reported the most.

That's right, sex gets better as women get older.

Not only that, but the better it gets, the more youthful we feel. "Women are saying to me that this is a really special time in their lives, that they feel really young. Sex is something that is going to continue in their lives," says Louise Merves-Okin, Ph.D., a clinical psychologist and marriage and family therapist in Jenkintown, Pennsylvania.

But how can that be? Isn't everything supposed to get *worse* as we get older, to break down and fall apart? Whatever is *supposed* to happen, here are three areas of our lives where things definitely improve.

Our bodies. Teenagers aren't the only ones with raging hormones. Many sex researchers believe that because of a hormonal surge, a woman hits her sexual peak in her thirties or later, says

Karen Donahey, Ph.D., director of the sex and marital therapy program at Northwestern University Medical Center in Chicago. By then women also feel more comfortable with their bodies. They know what they like and what they don't like.

And after menopause, the risk of pregnancy is gone. "Many women feel more sexual after menopause because they don't have to worry about birth control," says Alice Kahn Ladas, Ed.D., a licensed psychologist practicing in New York City and Santa Fe, New Mexico, and coauthor of *The G-Spot*.

Our feelings. Women past their midthirties tend to be in secure relationships, advanced in their careers, happy with their children and home life, and generally more confident. When everything else is right in our lives, good sex often follows. "When we're happy with our lives, we're more fulfilled sexually," says Dr. Donahey.

Our circumstances. As we reach our forties and fifties, our family responsibilities fall off a bit. Children move out or are old enough to rely on us less. Now we can focus more of our emotional energy on our love lives. And for a lot of us, that's when the fun really begins.

Of course, not every obstacle to a good sex life moves out with the kids. Everyday life can have a way of getting between you and the bedroom if you let it. But with the right approach, you can keep the sparks flying for the rest of your life. Here's how.

Making Time to Make Love

After a day of errands, chores, cooking, cleaning, and working, sex may not even enter your mind, and if it does, you meet it with a groan. "I hear this more and more in my office. By the time people take a breather late at night, the last thing they want to do is have sex," says Adelaide Nardone, M.D., a gynecologist in Mount Kisco, New York.

As your workload and family responsibilities build up, something's got to give. Unfortunately, what often gives is sex. More times than not, nothing is wrong with your libido, but you run around so much that you're just plain tired, Dr. Nardone says.

So not to worry. Your sex life just needs nurturing. "You put time into things you enjoy. You try to be creative and make important things in your life special. Sexuality shouldn't be any different," Dr. Merves-Okin says.

Need a jump start? Here are some ideas for putting the passion back into your life.

THE BIOLOGICAL CLOCK: IS IT TICKING LONGER?

A woman gives birth to her first child at age 63. A California fertility clinic's *average* patient age is 48. Why are women waiting so long to get pregnant? Has something changed in the biological clock?

Actually, the clock hasn't changed at all. "It's still ticking on its own," says Faith Frieden, M.D., director of maternal-fetal medicine at Englewood Hospital and Medical Center in New Jersey. "But women and medical technology are pushing its limits."

A woman's body works the way it always has. Every month, during ovulation, she releases an egg that can be fertilized. This process continues until she goes through menopause, usually in her early fifties. As long as she ovulates, a woman has the potential to get pregnant.

The quality and quantity of available eggs, however, decline as she gets older, reducing her fertility. Only recently have fertility breakthroughs increased her chances of successfully bearing children later in life. "Women feel like they have more options, thanks to technology," Dr. Frieden says.

Also, women are healthier than their counterparts of years ago. They can expect to live much longer than their great-grandmothers did and remain much healthier through middle age, so many are waiting until their late thirties and forties to have children. In the meantime, many are pursuing careers, says Dr. Frieden.

Unfortunately, with later-in-life pregnancies, there are some risks. A study of 24,000 women at the University of California, Davis, found that first-time mothers over 40 were twice as likely to have a cesarean section and were much more likely to develop pregnancy-related diabetes and high blood pressure. "It is certainly possible, and it is most likely to have a good outcome, but these women should know what they are getting into," Dr. Frieden says. "Unfortunately, late-in-life pregnancies carry a higher risk of fetal abnormalities, such as Down's syndrome."

AGE ERASER

Sex: The Real Elixir of Youth?

Forget that trip to the skin-care aisle. According to investigators in Scotland, the secret to looking younger is right in your own bedroom.

Researchers at the Royal Edinburgh Hospital interviewed 3,500 people who looked and felt younger than they actually were. The survey found that these younger-looking people had sex at a "significantly higher" rate in both "quality and quantity" than the average person.

"Improving the quality of one's sex life can help a person to look between 4 and 7 years younger," says Dr. David Weeks of the Royal Edinburgh Hospital in Edinburgh, Scotland, in his book *Secrets of the Superyoung*. "This results from significant reductions in stress, greater contentment, and better sleep."

Pencil it in. In today's hectic world, nothing seems to get done until it's scheduled. The same goes for sex. "Make a conscious effort to set time aside. It may seem unnatural, but it works. I mean, a tennis game isn't going to suddenly appear. You have to make arrangements for it," says Wendy Fader, Ph.D., a licensed psychologist and certified sex therapist in Boca Raton, Florida. Write it into your schedule. Treat it as you would any other very important meeting, because it *is* just as important.

Set the mood. Light a few candles, grab a bottle of wine, put on a CD of romantic music, even dance with your partner in your bedroom. When you create a romantic mood, things often fall into place. Make sex a pleasurable way to end the day, instead of a chore, Dr. Merves-Okin says.

Wake up early. No matter what kind of day you've had, you're probably too exhausted by 11:00 P.M. to make love. Don't make sex a night-time-only activity, Dr. Nardone says. Get up a half-hour earlier and make love in the morning, or take a lunch break and rendezvous at home.

Attempt a 10-minute tryst. Take advantage of those few spare minutes you have here and there. "There are all kinds of possibilities for sexual interludes," Dr. Fader says. "A 10-minute quickie is just fine. They don't always have to be 2-hour marathon sessions."

Send the kids away. Call a babysitter or ask a relative to watch them while you enjoy a romantic weekend away or even just a relaxing, sensual dinner, Dr. Nardone suggests.

Think about it—all day. "When you wake up in the morning, think about sex. If you think about it all day, it is more likely to happen," Dr. Fader says. Build up a sense of anticipation, and you won't be able to wait until you get home.

Clue him in on your desires. Now that you're in the right mindset, your job is to get him on the same page. "Seduce your mate throughout the day," Dr. Fader says. Leave him love notes that suggest what he'll have waiting for him when he gets home. Or if you are really bold, try the art of seduction over the phone. "That will smooth the way to get the two of you together. It is very titillating," she says.

Tell him that you love him. Sex is the ultimate expression of your love for each other. Unfortunately, as your lives get busy, you sometimes forget to express that love. Without that overall feeling of caring and tenderness, sex often falls by the wayside. "The other person wants to know that you're interested in him and that you love him," Dr. Merves-Okin says. "Start in the morning by leaving him a note that says, 'I'm glad I married you.' Tell him, 'I love you,' every day and tell him the things you love about him."

Wear that little black dress. After a day in jeans and a sweatshirt, you won't feel very seductive. But put on a party dress or teddy, and you may find that looking sexy can make you feel sexy. "Even if it is just you and your husband, put on something nice. You'll feel like a woman," Dr. Nardone says.

Get in touch. Sex shouldn't be the only time you and your mate touch. Hold hands, hug, kiss, sleep in an embrace—every day, Dr. Merves-Okin says. Simple affection often evolves into a caring, wonderful sex life.

Take time *not* to have sex. Your kids aren't the only ones who need quality time with you. Take a walk or set aside 10 minutes a day where you ask each other how your day went. "Get a sense of togetherness," Dr. Nardone says. That sense of connectedness fosters a loving, caring atmosphere where sex can thrive.

Every Night Is a New Experience

A patient of Dr. Nardone, a forty-something single woman, came into the office one day, raving about a new love in her life, a forty-something man. She proceeded to gush that they were having sex twice a day—every day. Where did this middle-aged couple find their inspiration? In the very newness of their relationship. It had spark, romance, and spontaneity—the traits that lead to a great sex life.

What many people perceive as a lack of desire is, frankly, boredom. While spending years with the same partner generates an intimacy and closeness that can enhance sexual pleasure, it also creates a "been there, done that" attitude. "Anything that you do for 15 years is going to be boring," Dr. Fader says. "Even people who say they have a decent sex life find that it is a pretty-mapped-out process. They do it the same way every time. It tends to be humdrum."

Don't worry, you don't have to throw out years of a good, established relationship for someone new to rekindle your sexual passion. In fact, combining your maturity and intimacy with newness and excitement will bring your love life to a whole new level. Making the commonplace new again will take a little creativity and time, but the results will be well worth the effort. Here's how to keep the bedroom sizzling.

Change the scenery. A candle here, music there, some flowers—all these small changes make it feel like a whole new experience. "I would begin with lighting a candle. Make it more inviting," Dr. Fader says.

Indulge in satin. Nothing says let's make love better than satin sheets. Luxurious, soft, and sexy, these silky sheets transform a plain old bedroom into an exotic locale, Dr. Fader says. Put them on when you want to give your partner a hint that tonight's the night.

Find a new location. Always have sex in the bedroom? Why not the kitchen, the dining room, the bathroom? Simply having sex in another room of the house can take it out of the realm of the ordinary, Dr. Ladas says. If you want to go beyond that, rent a hotel room or get away for the weekend and make love in an entirely new setting.

Please each other in new ways. For most couples, sex is goal oriented. Everything leads to one objective: orgasm through intercourse. That takes a lot of the fun out of it, says Beverly Whipple, R.N., Ph.D., professor of nursing at Rutgers College of Nursing in Newark, New Jersey, and president of the American Association of Sex Educators, Counselors, and Therapists. "I like to teach people to climb a 'staircase of pleasure.' Each step is pleasurable in itself and

WOMEN ASK WHY

Why are so many women attracted to older men?

Power is a strong aphrodisiac for many women, and older men often radiate power from the core. That doesn't mean power over the women who find them interesting, but the maturity and experience of many older men often give them control over many aspects of their own lives. Women who long for stability can find these traits irresistible.

Older men are more likely to have climbed the corporate ladder, so they are at a pinnacle in their careers. And unlike their younger counterparts, they're not questioning their life's purpose or career goals, or trying to decide if going to graduate school would be a good idea. Older gentlemen tend to be more confident and self-assured, and they have been around the block a few times, so they know what they want and how to get it. Their established, rock-solid, powerful nature is a definite turn-on to some women who yearn for stability.

In other cases, younger women and older men find themselves in the same stage of life. Say a woman in her late thirties wants to settle down, buy a house, and start a family. A man in that age bracket may not be ready to give up his career or his freedom yet, whereas a man in his forties who feels that he's accomplished what he set out to do in life may be looking for that very thing.

Expert consulted
Louise Merves-Okin, Ph.D.
Clinical psychologist and marriage and family therapist
Jenkintown, Pennsylvania

Learn what else your bodies like. Spend a day touching each other all over, from your toes to the top of your head. Try soft touches, harder massagelike touches. You may find that many other parts of the body—your ears, toes, and knees—can be sensual and erotic, Dr. Whipple says. These discoveries will generate plenty of new ideas for making love.

Reverse your roles. Are you always the seduced and he the seducer, or vice versa? Trade places. Playing the same role every time during lovemaking can become just as much of a rut as doing it in the same old place at the same old time, Dr. Merves-Okin says. Taking on different roles can make it seem like a new experience.

Look for new inspiration. High-quality erotic books and videos can show couples new ways to express their love. One such series comes from the Sinclair Intimacy Institute, which produces the *Better Sex Video Series* and *The Couples Guide to Great Sex over 40*. "These are very good educational films," says Dr. Whipple. But anytime you use erotica, both partners have to agree and be comfortable with it, she stresses.

Dress up for bed. Wearing a negligee or any other garment that seems sexy can make your love life feel a little more extraordinary. "It doesn't have to be a scanty nighty. It can be something that looks pretty and feels nice against your skin. Or maybe just wear a pretty robe. Whatever makes you feel sexy," Dr. Merves-Okin says.

may lead to the next step, but it doesn't have to." Dr. Whipple recommends trying to please each other without intercourse. Experiment and find other things that you enjoy—touching, kissing, cuddling.

Working with Your Changing Body

By the time we reach 50, our lives can be much more open to sexual pleasure. The kids are out of the house, we're more confident in ourselves, and we're not worried about getting pregnant. But our bodies are also going through changes that could get in the way of our sex life. "There are physical changes, but they aren't anything that can't be coped with," says Dr. Whipple.

The biggest change is in our estrogen levels, Dr. Whipple says. Although, on the average, we reach menopause in our early fifties, estrogen begins to decline as early as age 35. Low levels may cause vaginal dryness, which can make sex painful or uncomfortable. "Many women don't associate this problem with estrogen levels because at 35 they're not even thinking about those kinds of changes yet," she says. But left untreated, lack of lubrication can last through and past menopause.

These changes can be discouraging, but those who cope and adapt often find that their sex lives remain satisfying and may even get better than they have ever been. "You have to accept that change is inevitable in all aspects of our lives. What I liked at 25 isn't what I like at 40, but that doesn't mean what I liked at 25 was better. It doesn't mean your sex life is over. It just means it is different," Dr. Donahey says.

Here are some strategies to help you over the rough spots.

SEX SYMBOLS AT ANY AGE

Sex symbol: Two little words that evoke a gallery of images of beautiful and voluptuous young women.

Wait a minute. *Young?*

Plenty of women have shown us beyond a doubt that a woman can be sensuous and sexy at any age. Here's a short list, and there are lots more where they came from.

Mae West. At 43 years of age, Mae West was the highest paid woman in the United States, thanks mostly to the provocative, sometimes downright bawdy roles she played. At age 62, she starred in her own nightclub act (surrounded by muscle men). And in 1978, at the age of 85, she starred in the movie *Sextette*.

Eartha Kitt. Known for her smoldering, slinky performances, a 64-year-old Kitt played a seductress in the recent Eddie Murphy film *Boomerang*. Her 1992 memoir was titled *I'm Still Here: Confessions of a Sex Kitten*.

Raquel Welch. Renowned as much for her beauty and sexiness as for her acting, Welch, at age 57, was named one of the sexiest women in the world in a reader survey by *Shape* magazine and has played everything from bit parts to starring roles in films made both here and abroad. She's also made several exercise videos and has written two fitness books.

Sophia Loren. In her midsixties, the buxom Italian "goddess" is still considered a sex symbol by many and played the object of affection in the 1995 movie *Grumpier Old Men*.

Susan Sarandon. In a 1999 television movie, a 52-year-old Sarandon had an affair with a 25-year-old man. It wasn't the first time Sarandon showed how older women can be sensual and attractive to younger men. She was 13 years older than her love interest in *White Palace*, 12 years older than her boyfriend in *Thelma and Louise*, and 12 years older than her male counterpart in *Bull Durham* (actor Tim Robbins, with whom Sarandon has two children in real life).

Be open to change. For a premenopausal woman, it takes 6 to 20 seconds to lubricate after she is aroused. For a postmenopausal women, it takes 1 to 3 minutes. Instead of fearing these changes, work with them, Dr. Donahey says. You may have to take more time during sex, use sexual aids, or find other ways to please each other. Adapting to these changes can be fun and exciting, she says. Couples who have trouble during this time are often the ones who insist on doing everything the way they always have.

Apply a lubricant. Try some artificial lubrication to keep sex comfortable. Apply over-the-counter water-soluble lubricants (like K-Y jelly, Replens, or Astroglide) right before intercourse. Other products, such as Vagisil Intimate Moisturizer, can be used at any time. You can even make the application of a lubricant a pleasurable part of the sexual experience, Dr. Whipple says, instead of seeing it as something that reminds you of a problem.

Work out your pelvis. There's actually a workout for better sex. Kegel exercises strengthen the pelvic-floor muscles. To find your pelvic muscles, says Dr. Ladas, squeeze your pelvic area as if you were trying to stop the flow of urine. Once you've found them, squeeze, hold for 1 to 2 seconds, then relax. Repeat about 5 to 10 times at first. Try to work yourself up to squeezing and relaxing for 10 seconds each, 10 times in a row. She also suggests that you do what she calls "fast flicks": contract and relax those same pelvic muscles as rapidly as possible. Dr. Ladas recommends 100 of these a day.

Have sex as often as possible. Women who have sex two or more times a week have twice as much estrogen circulating in their blood as women who don't, Dr. Whipple says. By having more sex, you generate more estrogen, which lubricates the vagina, making sex easier for you.

Relax and Sleep Well

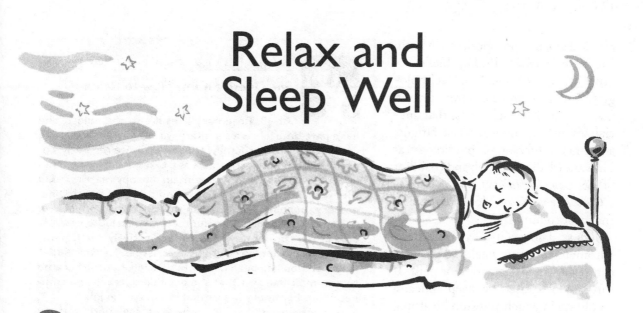

Sleeping Beauty. Remember her story? She pricked her finger on a spindle, then slept for a hundred years.

Getting some rest should be so easy! In fact, women make up the majority of the 84 million Americans who experience insomnia at least occasionally, insomnia being the inability to get enough sleep.

How much is enough? According to Peter Hauri, Ph.D., codirector of the Sleep Disorders Center at the Mayo Clinic in Rochester, Minnesota, it varies from person to person. For some, as little as 4 hours will do, while for others, 9 hours is a must. The average person functions just fine on 7 to 8.

If you're not getting the sleep you need, you won't need to check into a rest home, but you may feel like you belong in one. It's probably no surprise that, among other things, sleep deprivation cuts energy levels, reduces your ability to concentrate, and can make you moody—affecting everything from your work performance and your relationships to your driving skills. Not to mention causing those other, yet all-important, eye "problems"—unsightly bags and circles.

On the other hand, getting the right amount of sleep can—overnight—help you to think, look, and feel younger. Just think what a little shut-eye did for Sleeping Beauty. When that handsome prince fell for her peaceful, resting face and woke her with a kiss, she was well over a hundred years old! Talk about a youth enhancer.

The Mind-Body Connection

So why is it so hard for some of us to crawl under the covers—and stay there? For one thing, sleep difficulties may be one of the consequences of leading an extremely busy life, says Meir Kryger, M.D., professor of medicine at the University of Manitoba in Winnipeg, Canada, and past president of the American Sleep Disorders Foundation. "In our society, we have demanding careers that extend beyond 5:00 P.M., extracurricular activities after we leave the office. We can watch 24-hour television, and we can stay up all night surfing the Internet," he explains.

But there are a variety of other factors, both

physical and psychological, says Martin Moore-Ede, M.D., Ph.D., chief executive officer of Circadean Technologies, a research and consulting firm in Cambridge, Massachusetts, that specializes in reducing workplace fatigue; a former professor of physiology at Harvard Medical School; and coauthor of *The Complete Idiot's Guide to Getting a Good Night's Sleep*. Here are some of the most common.

Illness. The quality of your sleep is a barometer of your health. Insomnia can result from depression or pain. It can also be caused by sleep apnea, a condition in which you stop breathing for 10 to 60 seconds at a time, then wake up for a few moments, then fall back asleep—sometimes without even being aware that your sleep has been disturbed. Restless leg syndrome, which makes your legs feel jumpy so that you have to move them to get relief, can also keep you awake. And then there's periodic limb movement disorder, which causes you to kick while sleeping. (The bruises on your partner's legs will tell you if you have this problem.)

External factors. Some common lifestyle-related causes of sleep problems include drinking alcohol or caffeinated drinks late in the evening, eating foods that could cause heartburn before going to bed, arguing with your mate before bedtime, worrying about unfinished business from the workday, and engaging in vigorous exercise after 6:00 or 7:00 P.M. (Experts say that having sex is the exception to this rule; *that* type of exercise may actually help you release tension and relax.) An uncomfortable bed or a bed-

REAL-LIFE SCENARIO
She Doesn't Know How to Relax

At 40, Rosemary lives life to the fullest. She has a part-time job as a secretary with the local library. She cooks meals for her family, tries to exercise regularly, coordinates family activities, acts as a taxi service for her adolescent twins, and tries to maintain a happy marriage. On the weekends, she cleans house and does the laundry and grocery shopping. She's also on the building committee of her church, occasionally volunteers to distribute newspapers at the community hospital, and actively participates in an e-mail forum on environmental issues. Her one outlet for relaxation had been ballroom dancing, but she became so accomplished at it that she decided to teach and compete; thus her hobby has turned into a second job.

As engaged with her life as she feels, she's noticed lately that she's been experiencing headaches, and she's unable to sleep at night. In fact, sometimes she feels so old and tired and out of control of her life that she vacillates between losing interest in everything and frantically trying to keep up with it all, as if she's on the verge of a breakdown. What should she do?

Rosemary's life has become a merry-go-round, and she's at risk of falling off. She's an extrovert who has naturally gravitated toward people-oriented activities, but, unfortunately, she's overextended herself, and she's experiencing diminishing returns.

On the positive side, Rosemary has tried to create balance in her life by exercising, nurturing her family, and working no more than part-time. But she's a doer, and these types of people add more and more to their schedules until they wear themselves out, long before their time, both physically and psychologically. No wonder she's feeling old and tired.

room that's too light, too hot, or too cold are also likely to stand between you and dreamtime.

Mind games. If you've been having trouble sleeping, you're more likely to begin worrying the moment you hit the sheets about whether

The solution is for her to adopt certain lifestyle changes that will help her comfortably ease out of her stressful situation and return to the youthful enthusiasm and energy she has a right to.

She should begin by setting aside an hour each day dedicated to herself: taking a bath, listening to music, or doing relaxation exercises such as rhythmic breathing, progressive relaxation (in which she tenses, then relaxes, one body part at a time), or autogenic training (which consists of self-suggestion relaxation techniques such as "My arms are feeling warm and heavy.").

Once she begins to let go of stress, she'll notice that she's feeling more alert, refreshed, and focused. From this calmer, more centered frame of mind, Rosemary should reflect on her life and priorities. Now she's in a position to simplify her life by focusing on the projects that are most important to her and letting go of the low-priority ones.

Realistically, given her personality type, Rosemary is still likely to keep herself busier than most women. To stay healthy, she'll need to incorporate relaxation exercises into her daily routine. For example, she should learn to recognize certain early warning signs of tension—such as tightening of the muscles in her jaw, neck, and shoulders—and use these internal cues as reminders to stretch, breathe deeply, and consciously release the stress.

Expert consulted
Martha Davis, Ph.D.
Author of The Relaxation and Stress
    Reduction Workbook
Psychologist
Department of psychology at Kaiser Perma-
    nente Medical Center
Santa Clara, California

asleep. This creates anxiety, which actually *does* prevent them from relaxing and falling asleep."

Turning Out the Lights, Naturally

Rest easy. There are lots of things that you can do to ensure a blissful night's sleep. Here are the very basic ones from the experts.

Make time. Allow yourself at least 45 minutes to an hour to unwind before you lie down in bed. Let the leftover tension from your long day drift away. Avoid working on finances or watching the late news or stimulating your mind in any way too close to bedtime.

Don't be a clock watcher. Remove your clock from your bedside; in fact, remove it from the room, if possible. A watched pot never boils, and a watched clock won't let you sleep.

Work it off early. Exercise regularly during the day and find as many waking outlets for your stress as possible. The object is to be physically and mentally stress-free by bedtime.

Cozy up. Create a comfortable bed and bedroom. From room temperature to the crispness of the sheets, everything should be just the way you like it when you turn in for the night.

you're going to have trouble sleeping again. It's a cruel irony of insomnia. "People learn behavior that prevents them from falling asleep," explains Dr. Kryger. "It's a conditioned reflex called psychophysiologic insomnia, in which people associate going to bed with having a problem falling

Easing toward Dreamland

It's no accident that children, whom one rarely hears complaining about sleeplessness, have an elaborate set of bedtime rituals. "Rituals are sequences of behavior that help you wind

WOMEN ASK WHY

Why do older people get up early when they don't have to?

Various stages of life bring changes in our sleep patterns. Aging appears to involve a resetting of our biological clocks, which causes us to experience the internal signals that tell us both when to wake up and when to go to sleep earlier in the day. This is most likely the result of changes in our bodies' release of melatonin, a hormone secreted by the pineal gland deep within the brain, which regulates the wake/sleep cycle.

Also, as you age, you're likely to notice that both the timing and the quality of your sleep are undergoing changes. For example, the older you get, the less time you'll spend in the deep stage 3 and stage 4 sleep, and the more (proportionately) you'll spend in stages 1 and 2—the lighter stages.

As a result of getting less satisfying sleep, you might find yourself becoming groggy and going to bed earlier in the evening. Because your body only requires a certain number of hours of sleep per night, you're likely to wake up earlier the following morning. That, in turn, may lead you to go to bed early that evening, and before you know it, you've established a new sleep pattern.

If this is the case and your internal clock is out of whack, reset it by going to bed 10 minutes later each night for 6 consecutive nights. Continue this regimen for several weeks, if necessary, until you are able to go to bed as late as you like. As for getting up early, relax and enjoy the time.

Expert consulted
Dian Dincin Buchman, Ph.D.
New York City
Author of The Complete Guide to Natural Sleep

Whatever comforting things you do before bed—throwing on your favorite pajamas, tucking in your sheets, or brushing your teeth—do them in the same order every night and take as many of them on the road with you as you can when you travel. Establishing and following a relaxation ritual that works for you is a key factor in avoiding sleep problems.

Here are some relaxing steps from experts that you might want to add to your bedtime ritual.

Sip a natural relaxer. Tranquilizing herbal tea blends made with chamomile (such as Celestial Seasonings Sleepytime Tea), valerian, or passionflower are age-old sleep aids for their ability to induce drowsiness, while warm milk contains tryptophan, a chemical that also helps make you sleepy, says Dr. Moore-Ede.

Create the mood. While getting into your before-bed mode, turn down the lights and illuminate with candles to create a soft, warm glow. While you're at it, choose candles with scented lavender, a fragrance known for its calming properties. (Just make sure to put out those candles before you finally turn in.)

Soothe your senses. Off with the car chases, bad sitcoms, and general blare of the TV, and on with soft music, a traditional relaxation tool. Choose jazz, classical, R&B—whatever style you prefer as long as it's smooth and mellow. Tuning in should help you tune out your troubles.

down and get ready for bed; it's part of the relaxation process," explains Dr. Moore-Ede. Even if you factor teddy bears and bedtime stories out of the equation, adults need bedtime rituals, too.

Engage your imagination. Reading poetry, short stories, or other relaxing fare can help transport your thoughts away from your world for a short time. Those who have a really hard time falling asleep should probably avoid thrillers, scary science fiction, and any other pulse-quickening genres.

Get that warm, fuzzy feeling. Since studies show that petting an animal can lower your blood pressure, bedtime might also be a good time to gently brush your dog or cuddle your cat—in turn, treating yourself to a bit of furry relaxation therapy.

Immerse yourself. Slipping into a warm bath for 20 minutes can ease the transition from a stressful day to a quiet evening. As the heat helps open blood vessels and relaxes tired muscles, let your mind drift to pleasant thoughts, says Dr. Kryger.

Calm your mind. Prayer and meditation can also bring peace and allow you to shut off the cares of the day. They require some self-discipline and may take a little practice, but it's time well spent a few minutes before bed.

Tap the power of touch. If you're fortunate enough to have a partner with you, exchange light, not-too-stimulating massages. If you're alone, you can still gently run your hands over your own body, feeling yourself relax as you go along.

Get into a rhythm. Practicing rhythmic breathing can help take your focus off your mind and direct it toward your body. Simply breathe deeply—filling first your stomach and then your lungs with air—and exhale slowly, allowing yourself to become more drowsy and calm each time you exhale.

Stretch your limits. Stretching or tensing muscles one at a time for a few seconds and then relaxing them helps release tension. And a relaxed body is one that will drift off to sleep easily, says Dr. Kryger.

When All Else Fails

What if you still can't fall asleep? Should you take medication?

"Sleeping pills and tranquilizers can be helpful in the short term," says Dr. Hauri. "They allow you to get to sleep if you're in a different time zone and absolutely need to be well-rested and alert, or if there's been a death in the family, and the grief and stress have made it impossible for you to sleep. But if you're taking them more than once or twice a week, that may be a problem. Anytime your inability to sleep interferes seriously with your daytime functioning for more than a month or two, that's the time to seek professional help," he says.

Indeed, if your insomnia is chronic, says Dr. Moore-Ede, "you should try to work your way around medication; you're far better off dealing with the environmental and lifestyle issues that are likely to be keeping you awake."

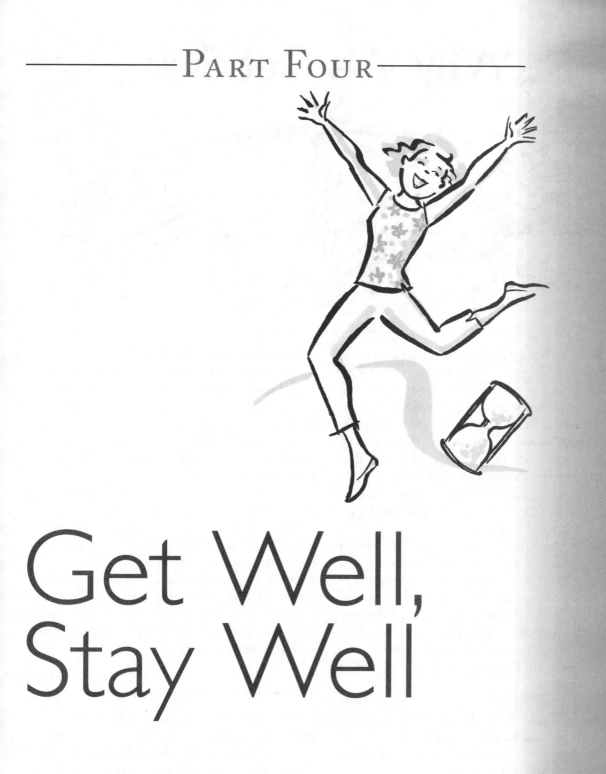

PART FOUR

Get Well, Stay Well

Why We Get Sick

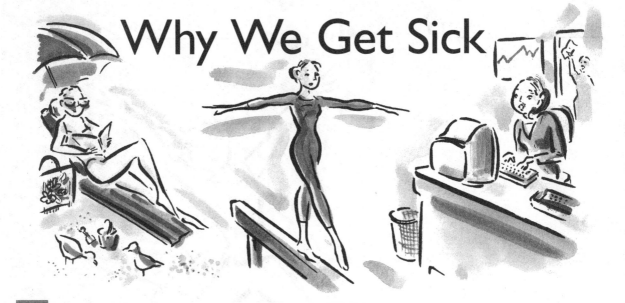

There's a word that describes a perfect state of balance: *equipoise*. It's a state we strive for in every aspect of our lives. We have families to care for, homes to maintain, careers to pursue, and personal needs to meet. We work, play, eat, and rest. And we try not to give any one part of our lives so much time, energy, or feeling that another part suffers. We're all aware of the pitfalls of putting career too much ahead of family or of all work and no play (it makes dull girls too). Balance is better.

Our health is the same way. The key to staying healthy is to keep all the aspects of our *selves*—the physical, emotional, and spiritual—in balance. When we do, we feel and function at our best. We're happy, creative, and productive. We have lots of energy, enjoy strong relationships, and are more able to handle the stressors in our lives. In short, we're healthy. Everything is in equipoise.

"Some people call it the zone," says Elaine Ferguson, M.D., a holistic physician practicing in Chicago and author of *Healing, Health, and Transformation*. "It's when you've reached the state where you're in harmony."

Illness, on the other hand, is a state of disharmony. We're functioning below our peak because some area of our health is out of balance, says Dr. Ferguson. Perhaps we have a serious illness such as cancer or a chronic disorder such as arthritis, or maybe we simply don't feel our best because of nagging headaches or fatigue.

"I see wellness and sickness as a continuum more than as distinct states," says Marcey Shapiro, M.D., a holistic physician practicing in Albany, California, who specializes in herbal medicine. At one end of the spectrum is optimal health, and at the other is serious illness. "Very few of us are at the extremes of having ideal health or being terribly ill," she says. "Most of us are somewhere in between."

Heeding the Signs

The symptoms we all get from time to time—stomachaches, insomnia, muscle tension—are warning signs that we're moving away from optimal health. We may not even be sick with a diagnosable illness, but our bodies are trying to tell us that something is out of balance, Dr. Ferguson says.

"We all have this intelligence within our bodies that speaks to us. The message could be a pain or a thought, but our bodies always tell us when something's wrong," Dr. Shapiro says.

It's our job to recognize these signs and pay attention to them. Heeding our bodies' signals will help us get back on the path to optimal health, but first we need to know what signals to watch out for. Here are the common physical, emotional, and mental symptoms that experts say can point to an imbalance in your health.

Muscle tension. Your muscles, especially in your neck, shoulder blades, and back, are full of tight knots.

Fatigue. Your energy level is so low that you just barely get through the day and then crash when you get home from work.

Loss of appetite. You don't feel hungry at mealtimes, and nothing seems appetizing to you.

Weight gain or weight loss. You've dropped or put on several pounds but haven't changed your eating or exercising habits.

Aches and pains. You have frequent, unexplained pain, such as headaches, stomachaches, or heartburn.

Difficulty sleeping. Several nights in a row, you have trouble falling or staying asleep.

MEDICINE THAT COMES IN PINK AND BLUE

"Sugar and spice, and everything nice, that's what little girls are made of. . . . Snips and snails, and puppy dog tails, that's what little boys are made of."

It's a nursery rhyme that speaks volumes. Scientists in the field of gender-based biology are now discovering that men and women actually are made of different stuff. "Women are not just small men," says Sherry Marts, Ph.D., scientific director of the Society for Women's Health Research, based in Washington, D.C. It turns out that men and women are different at the most basic level, the cellular level.

This discovery came about almost by accident. Researchers studying various drugs began noticing that some work better in women, while others are more effective in men. Take the over-the-counter drug ibuprofen, for example. When it comes to bringing down fevers and inflammation, ibuprofen works about the same in men and women. But it relieves pain much more effectively in men.

The differences don't end there. Diseases affect men and women in different ways as well. "Men tend to get diseases that are more urgent and tend to be more lethal. Women's diseases often start at a slower pace and cause disability long before death," explains Florence Haseltine, M.D., Ph.D., originator of the term *gender-based biology* and cofounder and former president of the Society for Women's Health Research.

By finding out why autoimmune diseases such as multiple sclerosis are much more common in women and why women develop heart disease decades later than men, we'll learn more about these diseases and develop better treatments for both women and men, Dr. Haseltine says.

As a result of these findings, someday doctors will treat the same disease differently, depending on the patient's sex, predicts Dr. Marts.

"It will translate itself almost immediately in the cardiac field," Dr. Haseltine says. "But I think the most exciting area of research is the study of structural differences in the brain and how brain disorders such as stroke are treated."

Hair loss. You notice more hair than usual in your brush or around the shower drain.

Dizziness or faintness. You feel weak and light-headed, especially when standing up. You may even have fainting spells.

Shortness of breath. You get winded when you walk to your car or up a flight of stairs.

Diarrhea or constipation. Your bowel movements are more frequent or less frequent than normal.

Anxiety. You feel tense and irritable and can't seem to escape your worries.

Disorganized thoughts. You have difficulty concentrating. You may lose things or forget appointments.

Depression. You are down in the dumps and feel hopeless.

Mood swings. Instead of being your typical pleasant self, you're moody and cranky much of the time.

"These are the signs that happen along the way when we move from optimal health toward illness," says Dr. Shapiro. "Usually, things start out as smaller signs that get louder and louder if people don't attend to them."

The problem is that it's easy to blame these symptoms on getting older or on the stresses of everyday life, so we end up dismissing them as quickly as they appear.

"We're so externally focused in terms of how we're taught to think and live that we don't pay attention to our bodies or our inner voices," Dr. Ferguson says. And the more we ignore our bodies, the further away we move from optimal health.

The good news is that we women have a built-in tool that helps keep us tuned in to our bodies. All we have to do is take advantage of it.

HAPPY TO BE HOSPITALIZED

We've all played hooky at least once in our lives—calling in sick when we barely had a sniffle. But some people practically make a career out of faking illness. They're sometimes called professional patients or hospital hobos by doctors because they travel from hospital to hospital claiming to be sick when, in fact, they don't have a physical illness at all. They have a mental disorder known as Munchausen syndrome.

The lives of people with this syndrome revolve around pretending to be sick. "They typically have poor relationships and spotty job histories," says Marc Feldman, M.D., an expert on Munchausen syndrome, an associate professor of psychiatry at the University of Alabama at Birmingham, and author of *Patient or Pretender*.

They lie about or exaggerate symptoms. Some even go so far as to make themselves sick. They may take poison, use their own feces to cause infections, and subject themselves to unnecessary surgery. If they're found out, they simply move on to another hospital in another city.

Often, they're seeking the attention, care, and concern that they lack in their lives, Dr. Feldman says. Or they may do it for the thrill of outsmarting highly trained, highly educated people. "Some patients describe it as an addiction, like gambling or alcoholism," he says.

How do they manage to dupe so many doctors? First of all, they play off doctors' expectations. "Physicians expect to

Women's Edge

Some women call it their intuition. Others say it's their sixth sense. Whatever you call it, women are more in touch with their bodies—and that gives them an edge over men when it comes to their health. "Men are taught from childhood to ignore pain rather than to stop and take care of it," says Royda Crose, Ph.D., associate director and associate professor of the Fisher Institute for Wellness and Gerontology at

see patients who are sick and want to be well—not patients who are well and want to be sick," Dr. Feldman says. Many of these people know a lot about the illnesses they fake. Some have worked in the medical field as receptionists or nurses. Others use the Internet to learn about the conditions they mimic. "The Internet has also given those with Munchausen syndrome a new forum," he says. They join on-line support groups and claim to suffer from chronic or incurable diseases, seeking warmth and support from the rest of the group.

Another form of this syndrome, called Munchausen by proxy, involves a parent faking or inducing illness in a child to gain "dutiful caregiver" status. Again, it's about getting attention as well as having some more complex needs met, says Judith Libow, Ph.D., coordinator of psychological services and training director in the department of psychology at Children's Hospital in Oakland, California. At least 95 percent of the time, the mother is the perpetrator, and it's estimated that 10 percent of these cases end in death, she says. A typical case involves a very young child who can't yet speak, a mother with an interest or training in health care, an uninvolved father, and a physician who becomes intensely involved in trying to solve the medical mystery.

"There are about three million reports of child abuse each year in this country. It would be wonderful to know how many of those involve Munchausen by proxy," Dr. Feldman says. "I receive an inquiry about Munchausen by proxy every day."

and that we feel physically and emotionally different throughout our cycles. Our periods are just the beginning. Our bodies make sure that we pay attention to them in many other ways as well.

When we get pregnant, for example, our bodies go through constant change for 9 months. During that time, we experience a part of being women that teaches us to be especially in tune with our physical well-being, Dr. Crose points out.

Even when we're not pregnant, most of us have annual gynecological exams and, after 40, mammograms. Eventually, of course, we also experience all the physical changes of menopause, such as hot flashes, mood swings, and the end of our monthly periods. "It's yet another time when our bodies go through changes and we become sensitive to everything that's going on inside of us," Dr. Crose says.

Call a Timeout

Because all of these physical changes and trips to the doctor make us more aware of what's going on within our bodies, we're in a better position to recognize symptoms of illness when they crop up. But recognizing them isn't enough. We need to act. "When we notice signs that we're not feeling our best, we need to stop and take stock of our lives," Dr. Ferguson says. "I tell my patients to get very quiet and still and to listen and let their bodies tell them what they need to do."

We also need to question ourselves and our habits and examine the things that we've been doing, adds Heather Morgan, M.D., a holistic physician practicing in Centerville, Ohio.

Ball State University in Muncie, Indiana, and author of *Why Women Live Longer Than Men*. Male professional athletes, for example, are notorious for playing while injured.

Women, on the other hand, are good at listening to their bodies. We're better listeners, in part, because the female body requires us to pay attention to its changes. "Our reproductive systems keep us tuned in to our bodies," Dr. Crose says. Because we menstruate, we learn at a young age that our bodies go through constant changes

REAL-LIFE SCENARIO

She's Running Herself Ragged and Getting Sick All the Time

Suzanna, 44, had it all: a beautiful home, an exciting job as a stockbroker, two daughters away at college, and a 25-year marriage. Then one night, her husband announced that he was divorcing her. Instead of caving in emotionally, Suzanna made him move out, then she threw herself into her work. She stayed at the office 12 hours a day, even on weekends. She didn't have time for breakfast or lunch—let alone time to think about the divorce. Soon, her body rebelled. She began feeling sluggish, then started getting frequent colds and headaches. She knows that she is wearing herself out but thinks that it's more important to get through this emotional crisis now and straighten out her health habits later. Is she right?

If Suzanna doesn't invest some time and effort into her physical and emotional health, she could be a stockbroker headed for a crash. Her headaches are no doubt a by-product of all this stress, and her weakened immune system is likely a result of stress and poor diet. She could be setting herself up for a serious illness, such as heart disease.

Suzanna is not taking care of herself emotionally either. It's perfectly normal for someone going through a divorce to be sad, angry, and scared. She should see a psychotherapist, who can help her face her feelings and teach her healthier ways to cope with stress.

Suzanna can also do some things on her own. She needs to make time for breakfast and lunch and start an exercise program. She'll relieve stress, increase her energy level, and improve her emotional well-being—all things that positively impact the immune system. Suzanna also needs to set aside some quiet time each day to connect with her feelings, perhaps through yoga or meditation. And above all, she has to get together with friends on the weekends instead of isolating herself at the office.

Expert consulted
Mary Claire Wise, M.D.
Holistic family physician
Rochester, New York

Any number of events can knock us off-kilter. Maybe we have picked up a virus, are grieving the loss of a loved one, or are questioning our spiritual beliefs, Dr. Ferguson says. Perhaps we are under a lot of stress, aren't getting enough sleep, or are routinely passing up nutritious food for high-fat fare. "Everything from our relationships and emotions to what we eat, breathe, and touch affects our health," she says. Our hormones, our expectations, and, of course, our genes all play a role.

So does the fact that we're women. "Scientists are just beginning to discover the enormous impact that our sex has on our health," says Sherry Marts, Ph.D., scientific director of the Society for Women's Health Research, based in Washington, D.C.

Beyond Having Babies

Our ability to bear children is not the only thing that makes us different from men. Being female has a great deal of influence over our health. "We're starting to see that there are definitely a lot of physiological differences between men and women," Dr. Marts says. Because our bodies are different than men's, various illnesses and treatments affect us differently as well, she says.

For example, women appear to be more susceptible than men to certain chemical substances, such as alcohol and the carcinogens in cigarettes. Research shows that women develop cirrhosis of the liver after a shorter period of heavy drinking than men do. Women also have a 20 to 70 percent higher risk of developing lung cancer than men at every level of exposure to cigarette smoke.

Women also suffer from certain diseases more often than men. About 75 percent of all people with autoimmune diseases, such as multiple sclerosis and lupus, are female.

When we do get sick, women experience symptoms that are different from men's for the same conditions. A man suffering a heart attack, for example, is likely to have gripping chest pain, while a woman is more likely to have subtle symptoms such as abdominal pain, nausea, and extreme fatigue.

Beyond symptoms, diseases may actually progress differently in men and women. Women with multiple sclerosis, for example, tend to experience periods of remission followed by relapses, while men with the disease tend to have continuously progressive symptoms. In addition, some research suggests that HIV-positive women progress to AIDS at a lower viral load than men, which means that women have less virus in their blood when they start to develop opportunistic infections and other symptoms of full-blown AIDS.

There are even differences between men and women where treatment is concerned. Drugs are processed and handled differently in a woman's body and affect its systems differently. Ibuprofen, for example, is less effective at providing pain relief for women. Women also wake up from anesthesia an average of 4 minutes faster than men.

It all comes down to something most of us intuitively know: To prevent and heal illness, we not only need to listen to our bodies and keep ourselves in balance, we also have to establish health habits that address our special needs as women.

MY MAMA TOLD ME

Can reading in dim light really ruin my eyes?

You may find reading in dim light hard to do, but it won't hurt your eyes. Moms probably tell their kids not to read in the dark because they have a tough time doing it themselves. It turns out that kids' eyes can gather more light, so children need less light to read than adults do.

If Susie likes reading with a flashlight under her blanket, there's no need for her to close the book. She can finish the story, and Mama can rest easy.

Expert consulted
Anne Sumers, M.D.
Ophthalmologist
Spokesperson for the American Academy of
    Ophthalmology
Ridgewood, New Jersey

How Healthy Women Stay Well

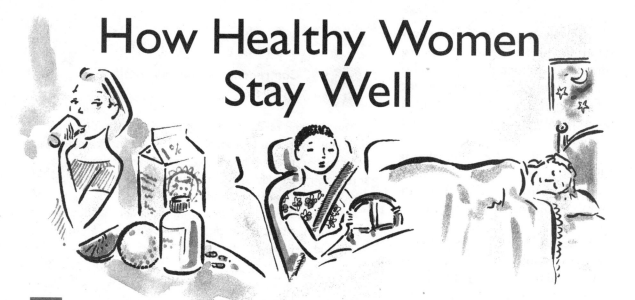

"There is no animal more invincible than a woman," said poet and playwright Aristophanes. And in one way, he may have been right. Although men clearly have physical advantages over women in strength, height, and muscle tone, when it comes to longevity, there's no contest. According to documented mortality data, women have been outliving men since at least the 1500s, and these days we outlive them by an average of 5 years—life expectancies are 79 years for women and 74 years for men.

Our predisposition to live longer does not, however, mean that we can sit back at our leisure and enjoy better health with no effort. To gain from our biological advantages, we have to work at taking good care of ourselves. Here's a top 10 list of health habits we all should strive for.

1. Move Your Body

Exercise improves cardiovascular health, which helps prevent heart disease, high blood pressure, and diabetes, explains Sherry Marts, Ph.D., scientific director of the Society for Women's Health Research, based in Wash-

ington, D.C. It also helps you look better, have more energy, and be less likely to get depressed. To get the most mileage for your sweat, exercise both aerobically and with weights. "There is also some data showing that weight-bearing exercise prevents osteoporosis, particularly when it's done in your twenties and thirties," she says.

Get your heart pumping. "Walk, and walk faster," says Trudy L. Bush, Ph.D., professor of epidemiology and preventive medicine at the University of Maryland School of Medicine at Baltimore. "All you need is a pair of athletic shoes." For both your heart and your waistline, the American College of Sports Medicine recommends that you exercise aerobically at a moderate pace for 20 to 60 minutes a day 3 to 5 days a week.

Pump yourself up. "Resistance training, such as lifting weights, increases and maintains muscle and bone, which improves body composition and appearance and increases your metabolism," says Jennifer Layne, a certified strength and conditioning specialist and exercise physiologist at the Jean Mayer USDA Human Nutrition Research Center on Aging at Tufts

University in Boston. And resistance training builds your strength, which makes daily life activities easier. The American College of Sports Medicine recommends doing a routine, 2 or 3 days a week, consisting of 8 to 10 exercises that work the major muscle groups. Strive for 8 to 12 repetitions of each exercise.

2. Eat a Healthful, Diverse Diet

Eating a nutritious, varied diet helps lessen your risk of heart disease and certain cancers, such as colon cancer. "Eat lots of fiber, fruits, and vegetables, and a reasonable amount of fat," advises I-Min Lee, M.D., assistant professor of epidemiology at Harvard School of Public Health and assistant professor of medicine at Harvard Medical School. The American Heart Association (AHA) considers no more than 30 percent of daily calories to be a reasonable amount of fat, with less than 10 percent coming from the saturated fats contained in animal products. "It's also important to watch your total calorie intake," she says.

Get your fruits and veggies. The AHA recommends that you eat five or more servings of vegetables, fruits, or fruit juices a day. Fruits and vegetables pack lots of vitamins, minerals, and fiber without adding many calories. If fruits and vegetables sound boring—and let's face it, sometimes they are—Ann Gentry, chef and owner of the organic, vegetarian Real Food Daily Restaurant in Los Angeles, recommends that you boost their appeal by

My Mama Told Me

Will going barefoot really give me flat feet?

Going barefoot may make your feet dirty, but it won't make them flat. Some people are born with the collapsed arches that give a person flat feet. Your arches can also collapse if you spend a lot of time on your feet but don't have adequate arch support in your shoes.

Your mom probably told you not to go barefoot outdoors because she knew of all the dangers. You could hurt your feet by stepping on glass or a rusty object. Hard surfaces like asphalt are hot and may be hard on your feet. If you have any heel pain or foot problems, walking on concrete or asphalt can aggravate the condition. What's more, if you go barefoot on wet surfaces, such as at a public pool or in community showers, you could pick up the microbial organisms that cause athlete's foot or painful plantar warts.

Expert consulted
Pamela Colman, D.P.M.
Director of health affairs
American Podiatric Medical Association
Bethesda, Maryland

buying them fresh (preferably from a farmers' market) and by putting more thought into the way you arrange and serve them. "Think color and texture," says Gentry. Put three to five different-colored vegetables on a plate, and use bigger pieces, smaller pieces, and different cuts. A variety of colors also indicates a variety of nutrients.

Control your appetite for critters. The AHA recommends that you keep your daily intake of poultry, fish, or lean meat to no more than 6 ounces. If greasy ribs are your only passion at mealtimes, try using different meats, such as lean cuts of wild game, buffalo, or ostrich, and add flavor with some spices.

WOMAN TO WOMAN

She Made Kicking the Habit a Family Affair

Longtime smoker Agatha Johnson-Page, 57, had tried to quit before, but hypnosis and stopping cold turkey didn't do the trick. Now, thanks to a popular drug and the support of her family, she has kicked the habit for good. Here's her story.

I had my first cigarette at age 16. My friends smoked, so I tried it—and before long, I was hooked. At that time, no one knew it was a health hazard.

I smoked half a pack a day for about 20 years. Then I quit cold turkey but started smoking again 6 months later when I needed a way to relieve stress.

Since then, I've tried to quit a number of times. I even went to a group hypnosis session where we all tossed our cigarettes in the trash as we left.

Finally, two of my kids and I quit together, and none of us has had a cigarette since June 1998. The support system we created really helped. We shared our success stories, encouraged each other, and called each other if we thought we might slip. Quitting with my kids also gave me an extra incentive: I didn't want to falter, because I didn't want them to falter.

My daughter used nicotine patches, and my son and I took the prescription drug Zyban. After the first week, I didn't get much pleasure out of smoking anymore. And now I can't stand being around cigarette smoke. I find it offensive.

I figured that at my age, after smoking for some 40 years, quitting wouldn't really improve my health. Boy, was I wrong. I always used to cough and blow my nose in the morning, but since I've quit smoking, I don't wake up congested anymore. I'm also able to hold my notes longer when I sing in my car. And I'm a much cleaner, healthier person.

I did gain a few pounds, but I didn't let that discourage me. I figure that's the next thing I'll work on.

Several of my friends still smoke, and at first I was worried I'd slip back into the habit when I was around them. But I just went on a 4-day trip with two of my friends, and I didn't have a single craving. That was my big test, and I aced it.

Expand your food horizons. You can find an endless number of tasty and healthful foods if you open up your mind along with your mouth. "To add more variety to your diet, add exotic vegetables like yams and winter squash, and experiment with spices," says Dr. Bush.

Basic spices can give food great flavor. "Use basil, oregano, thyme, rosemary, and cilantro," Gentry suggests. "And definitely put them on during the cooking." She also suggests cooking with miso, which is a soybean paste. "Whether you're making soups, pastes, sauces, or spreads, miso can really go a long way."

3. Bone Up on Calcium

Before the onset of the agricultural age 10,000 years ago, humans appear to have been high consumers of calcium. Nowadays, we probably eat only one-fourth to one-third the calcium that our ancestors did, and that's not enough. Osteoporosis affects 20 million American women, and one of the best ways to prevent the disease is with calcium. Here's how to boost your intake.

Dine on some dairy. "Eat yogurt and other calcium-rich foods," says Dr. Bush. The National Institutes of Health suggests that you get 1,000 to 1,500 milligrams of calcium daily. Try to choose nonfat or low-fat dairy products such as fat-free milk or low-fat cheese.

Supplement it. "Most Americans don't get enough calcium in their diets," says Dr. Lee. To up your intake, you can take supplements.

But keep your total daily intake from diet and supplements below 2,500 milligrams, says Lila A. Wallis, M.D., clinical professor of medicine at Weill Medical College of Cornell University in New York City and coauthor of *The Whole Woman*. Higher doses must be taken under medical supervision.

4. Get Enough Sleep

The quality of your Zzzs may determine not only your well-being the next day but also your physical health for years down the road. "Sleep deprivation may reduce your body's defenses and increase your risk of disease," says Dr. Lee. It's believed that when you fall asleep, infection-fighting blood cells move from your bloodstream into your tissues, attacking viruses and bacteria as you snooze.

Sleep deprivation can also affect your emotional well-being. You may be more testy, and your attention span may suffer, says Rosalind Cartwright, Ph.D., director of the Sleep Disorder Service and Research Center at Rush–Presbyterian–St. Luke's Medical Center in Chicago. Here are suggestions to help you improve your sleep patterns.

Replace lost hormones if you are postmenopausal. "Since the hormones we lose at menopause are implicated in the breathing disorders of sleep, supplementation is a

---

TOP 10 KILLERS OF WOMEN

Young Women (Ages 25 to 44)
1. Cancer
2. Accidents
3. Heart disease
4. AIDS
5. Suicide
6. Homicide
7. Stroke
8. Chronic liver disease and cirrhosis
9. Diabetes
10. Pneumonia and influenza

Middle-Aged Women (Ages 45 to 64)
1. Cancer
2. Heart disease
3. Stroke
4. Chronic obstructive pulmonary disease
5. Diabetes
6. Accidents
7. Chronic liver disease and cirrhosis
8. Pneumonia and influenza
9. Suicide
10. Blood infection

Senior Women (Ages 65 and Up)
1. Heart disease
2. Cancer
3. Stroke
4. Chronic obstructive pulmonary disease
5. Pneumonia and influenza
6. Diabetes
7. Accidents
8. Alzheimer's disease
9. Kidney disease
10. Blood infection

THE WORST HEALTH HABITS
A WOMAN CAN HAVE

Unfortunately, not all of the choices we make regarding our health are good ones. In fact, when it comes to bad habits, these top the list.

Lighting up. Unless you've been in hiding for the last 30 years, you know that smoking is bad for you. In addition to being a major factor in heart disease, lung cancer, and stroke, smoking causes emphysema, skin wrinkling, and bone loss. But despite the repeated warnings, about 23 percent of all women still smoke.

Basking in the sun. About 80 percent of skin cancers are caused by sun exposure—a big price for a good tan. "Sunbathing also promotes wrinkling and dry skin," says Trudy L. Bush, Ph.D., professor of epidemiology and preventive medicine at the University of Maryland School of Medicine at Baltimore.

Hitting the sauce too hard. "Drinking large amounts of alcohol is definitely a no-no," says I-Min Lee, M.D., assistant professor of epidemiology at Harvard School of Public Health and assistant professor of medicine at Harvard Medical School. Overconsumption of alcohol has been linked to an increased risk of breast cancer and possibly to an increased risk of certain types of stroke. Small amounts are okay since alcohol lowers the risk of heart disease, she says. For optimum health, limit yourself to three to four drinks a week and no more than one drink in a day, says Dr. Bush.

Being a couch potato. A sedentary lifestyle puts you at risk for a long list of problems, such as heart disease, osteoporosis, obesity, and depression, says Lila A. Wallis, M.D., clinical professor of medicine at Weill Medical College of Cornell University in New York City and coauthor of The Whole Woman. Any type of motion that separates you from the sofa is better than none. For best results, Dr. Wallis suggests that you regularly engage in a repetitive activity that increases your breathing and heart rate.

Having bad eating habits. A diet high in saturated fat, sugar, and meat, and too low in vegetables and whole foods is likely to take a negative toll on your body, possibly leading to heart disease, cancer, and chronic gastrointestinal problems.

good idea," says Dr. Cartwright. "Hormone supplements also reduce sleep disturbances caused by hot flashes."

Stick to a regular schedule. "If you don't sleep long enough one night, don't go to bed earlier the next night," says Dr. Cartwright. Going to sleep and getting up at the same time every day will help establish a regular sleep/wake cycle.

Behave yourself before bedtime. Your activities immediately before you hit the sack can interfere with your sleep. "Avoid heavy meals or booze before bedtime," says Dr. Cartwright. Heavy meals could cause heartburn, and alcohol, although it makes you drowsy, will wake you up about 3 hours later. And although walking has been shown to promote good sleep, don't work out less than 4 hours before hitting the sack, because exercise's stimulating effects may up your sheep count.

If you must nap, keep it short. "If you need to extend your waking hours, a 15- to 20-minute nap midday will help," says Dr. Cartwright. "Longer naps make you wake up with a 'sleep hangover' and may interfere with your sleep that night."

5. Stop Stressing

"Stress results from the perception that you are ill-equipped to meet the demands on your mind and body," says Margaret Caudill, M.D., Ph.D., codirector of the department of pain medicine at Dartmouth-Hitchcock Medical Center in Manchester, New Hampshire. Stress can also result from an overload of positive activities, such as when planning a wedding. "Unchecked stress can cause decreased sleep, muscle tension, heart palpitations, shortness of breath, and irritable bowel symptoms," she says. Long-term stress may lead to the development of chronic health problems such as high blood pressure and decreased immune function. To help destress yourself, consider this advice.

Listen to your body. "It's important for people to identify their stress symptoms," says Dr. Caudill. Most of us know how we react to stress—your neck tenses up, your stomach hurts, you can't sleep, you suddenly have a headache, or you feel irritable. The key is to home in on the symptoms early so you can quickly take steps to deal with the stressful situation that's causing them.

Do something for yourself. If you're like many women, you nurture everyone else at the expense of satisfying your own needs. It helps to make a commitment to yourself, says Dr. Caudill. "Do something on a regular basis to relieve tension," she says. It doesn't take much—get some exercise or just take a few deep breaths.

Meditate. "Repeatedly focusing on a word, phrase, breath, or motion can cause the relaxation response during and after meditation, which can reduce stress-related changes in your body," says Dr. Caudill. Meditate once a day for 10 to 20 minutes to rejuvenate both your body and your mind.

6. Pay Your Doctor a Visit

Yearly exams can prevent a number of conditions, including breast and cervical cancers and osteoporosis, says Dr. Wallis. Have your body screened with these tests.

Get a mammogram. "The mortality rate from breast cancer is decreasing, which is prob-ably related to the detection of early lesions by mammogram," says Paula Szypko, M.D., a pathologist at North State Pathology Associates in High Point, North Carolina, and spokesperson for the College of American Pathologists. Premalignant and early noninvasive tumors can be detected by a mammogram before they can be felt. Dr. Szypko suggests going for an annual mammogram every year after age 40. "In addition, do monthly self-examinations and have an annual examination by your health-care practitioner," she says.

Prevent cancer with a Pap test. "The death rate from uterine cervical cancers has dropped significantly since the Pap test became available almost 50 years ago. It went from being number one to not even being in the top 10," says Dr. Szypko. The preventive effects of the test are tremendous. Eighty percent of women who die of cervical cancer have not had a Pap test in 5 years. She recommends that you have an annual Pap test starting at age 18. "A lot of women believe that they don't need to have Pap tests if they're beyond their childbearing years, but 60 percent of cervical cancers occur in women over age 55," she says.

Give the rest of your body a once-over. In addition to a Pap test and mammogram, you should have an annual flu shot and cholesterol and blood pressure checks, says Dr. Bush. Women over 45 should have a dual-energy x-ray absorptiometry (DEXA) bone scan to check for osteoporosis. If you're over 50, you should also undergo a screening for rectal and colon cancers every 5 to 10 years.

7. Buckle Up

"I'm only going a few blocks." "I don't want to wrinkle my dress." The list of excuses goes on. But every hour, somebody dies as a result of failure to wear a seat belt. And if the threat to

WHY WOMEN LIVE LONGER THAN MEN

It's been documented for hundreds of years and known for thousands: Women live longer than men. But why? Here are some possibilities suggested by Royda Crose, Ph.D., associate director and associate professor of the Fisher Institute for Wellness and Gerontology at Ball State University in Muncie, Indiana, and author of *Why Women Live Longer Than Men.*

Testosterone is troublesome. "Testosterone seems to be related to increased activity, impulsiveness, and aggressiveness, which can lead to risky behavior," says Dr. Crose. In their younger years, men are more likely than women to die from accidents, suicide, and homicide. Later in life, testosterone increases bad low-density lipoprotein cholesterol and decreases good high-density lipoproteins, putting men at a greater risk for heart disease.

Estrogen protects. "Medical scientists believe that premenopausal women enjoy a buffering effect from illness, because of estrogen," says Dr. Crose. Estrogen is believed to protect women against heart disease, osteoporosis, and possibly brain disorders such as Alzheimer's disease.

Illness gets crossed out. "Scientists believe that females have an advantage in having two X chromosomes, because the second X chromosome provides a backup if something goes wrong with a gene on the first one," says Dr. Crose.

Pears are healthier than apples. Women typically gain weight in their lower bodies—their hips, buttocks, and legs—giving them more of a pear shape, while men are more apple-shaped. "The apple-shaped pattern of obesity is believed to be a strong predictor of increased high blood pressure, diabetes, heart disease, and stroke," says Dr. Crose.

If you still absolutely refuse to buckle up when you're driving alone, at least buckle up in front of your children. If you don't, you send a message that it's okay to go without a seat belt. The American College of Emergency Physicians (ACEP) reports that when a driver is not wearing a seat belt, young passengers will be buckled only 30 percent of the time, versus 94 percent for buckled drivers' young passengers.

And remember that *all* passengers should buckle up. The ACEP states that in a 55-mile-per-hour crash, an unrestrained backseat passenger could fly forward at a force strong enough to seriously injure or even kill a person in the front. So for your own safety and that of your fellow passengers, make sure that everyone is belted.

Finally, make sure that you're buckled properly. According to the AAA, a seat belt worn incorrectly could do more harm than good. The belt should be over your hips and pelvis, in front of your chest, and over your shoulder. A belt worn behind your body could cause your head to hit the dashboard, and a belt worn under your arm could break your ribs and lead to serious internal injuries.

your life won't convince you, maybe the threat to your wallet will. A primary seat-belt law in 16 states and the District of Columbia allows a police officer to pull you over and cite you specifically for not buckling up. There's really no excuse for not spending the 3 to 7 seconds it takes to fasten your seat belt.

8. Renew Your Relationships

"People who are emotionally connected to other people do better in terms of disease risk than people who are not connected," says Dr. Lee. The effects of isolation are even worse for people with chronic illness. People with coronary artery disease who have spouses or confidantes, for example, are 30 percent more likely to survive than patients who are isolated. "Whether it's church, your partner, or your friend, just having support helps," she says. Here are a few ways you can stay connected.

Build a support network. "People with good social health have relationships that are interdependent and complementary, where each person helps the other," says Royda Crose, Ph.D., associate director and associate professor of the Fisher Institute for Wellness and Gerontology at Ball State University in Muncie, Indiana, and author of *Why Women Live Longer Than Men*. "Such interdependent relationships provide a safety net that's important for survival throughout life but is especially crucial in old age."

Keep your love alive. To remain zestful, love relationships need a constant supply of fresh energy. Be spontaneous with your partner, whether you make a last-minute decision to walk in the park or to fly to the Bahamas. And remember to laugh—it boosts the joyful spirit that connected you in the first place, says Dr. Crose.

Explore your spirituality. Religious activities can give meaning to your life and provide personal satisfaction outside your family. "Spiritual and religious connections provide motivation and hope—outlooks that can promote longevity," says Dr. Crose.

9. Laugh Out Loud

Laughter is the physiological response to humor. Research suggests that laughter produces physiological benefits, including increased antibodies, decreased stress hormones, and a higher pain threshold. "Laughter is also good for your emotional health," says Dr. Bush.

According to a study done at Loma Linda University in California, when heart attack patients added a 30-minute humorous video to their cardiac rehabilitation, they had lower blood pressure, fewer stress hormones, and lower medication requirements.

10. Have a Hobby

"Women spend too much time doing things for others," says Dr. Bush. Doing an activity for your own sake provides a source of enjoyment that can reduce stress and improve well-being, she says. To incorporate a new activity into your life, try the following.

Look back to your youth. "Renew a hobby you had earlier in life," suggests Dr. Bush. Whether it's painting, playing cards, or even mall walking, if you enjoyed it before, take it up again.

Dig in the dirt. Gardening is an excellent hobby, says Dr. Bush. Garden work has been shown to spark creativity and optimism, and physically, it burns calories and can lower blood pressure.

Volunteer. "I think that volunteering, the idea of altruism, is important," says Dr. Caudill. "It's been demonstrated that people who make connections with people and do things for others are healthier."

By volunteering, you can enhance your own life as you learn new skills and form new relationships, says Dr. Crose.

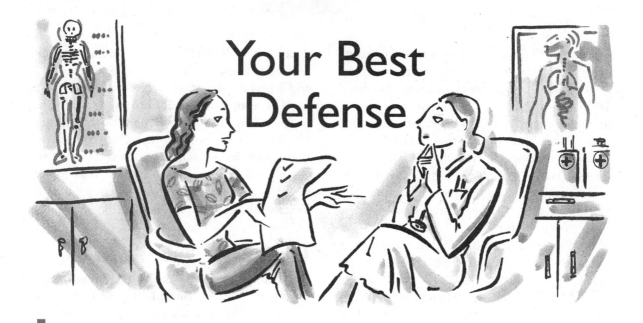

Your Best Defense

If it's true that an apple a day keeps the doctor away, we must be eating an awful lot of apples, because our doctors aren't spending much time with us at all. In fact, a typical primary-care physician spends less than 13 minutes with each patient every 6 months.

That doesn't leave much time for the kind of basic preventive medicine that can help to keep us healthy. In a 1998 survey conducted by the Commonwealth Fund, only 55 percent of women reported that their blood cholesterol had been tested in the previous year. Nearly 40 percent said that they had not had physical exams or Pap tests. One in three had not undergone clinical breast exams. And one in six had not received any preventive care during that time.

But time is not the only problem. A lack of incentives—doctors aren't compensated by insurers for most types of preventive care—also tends to discourage physicians from suggesting precautionary measures that would have long-term impact on women's health, points out Linda Hyder Ferry, M.D., associate professor of preventive medicine and family medicine at Loma Linda University School of Medicine in California. In addition, many doctors simply haven't been adequately trained in preventive care.

"Physicians traditionally are not taught how to be good prevention counselors," Dr. Ferry says. "I did my own survey of every medical school in the United States. The survey asked about the training available concerning tobacco. The results were discouraging. Tobacco use is the leading preventable cause of death in the United States, yet most medical schools do not require clinical training in helping patients to stop smoking. Nutritional training is even worse."

So, like it or not, the burden of responsibility for preventive care rests primarily on our own shoulders.

"Women must become consumer advocates for themselves. They need to read everything they can about preventive care because most physicians, unless they have taken time on their own to learn about these issues, aren't likely to provide the best prevention strategies," Dr. Ferry says.

Eat Good Food to Sidetrack Ailments

The USDA Food Guide Pyramid is an excellent foundation for helping people prevent many illnesses, says Jennifer Brett, N.D., a naturopathic physician in Stratford, Connecticut. The pyramid says that women should eat 6 to 11 servings daily of bread, cereal, rice, and pasta; 2 to 4 servings of fruits, such as apples, strawberries, and bananas; 3 to 5 servings of vegetables, such as broccoli, tomatoes, and lettuce; 2 to 3 servings of milk, yogurt, cheese, and other dairy products; and 2 to 3 servings of meat, poultry, fish, dried beans, eggs, or nuts. Fats should be used sparingly. But the pyramid is just one of many tools that women should use to maintain their health.

"Your entire health derives from what you do every day. All the pills in the world aren't going to make up for a bad foundation. So you have to start off with balanced nutrition," Dr. Brett says. "Of course, there are specific needs for individuals that must also be accounted for. A woman with recurring yeast infections, for instance, might help herself prevent those infections if she eats foods that contain less sugar, starch, and other refined carbohydrates."

Although every woman's dietary needs differ slightly, here are a few general guidelines that, in addition to the food pyramid, can help keep you in peak nutritional condition.

BETTER FOODS FOR BETTER HEALTH

Eating more organic, natural products can help you maintain your health, says Jennifer Brett, N.D., a naturopathic physician in Stratford, Connecticut. Many commercial products on a typical grocery shelf these days contain chemicals, hormones, and other unnatural additives that can trigger food allergies and compromise your overall health. Naturally grown staples and other organic products are available at most health food stores. For starters, consider adding the following natural foods to your shopping list.

- **Amaranth.** It is a near-complete protein, loaded with calcium and other vital nutrients. It's available as a seed, as flour, or puffed.
- **Arrowroot.** Instead of cornstarch, which may cause constipation, diarrhea, and vitamin loss, use arrowroot as a thickening agent in recipes. Arrowroot also has less of an aftertaste than cornstarch. For people who are allergic to corn, it is a perfect substitute.
- **Cayenne.** A good food seasoning, this red pepper helps break up mucus and cholesterol. It also may improve circulation. An excellent substitute for black pepper, it is available in mild, medium, or hot varieties.
- **Eggs.** Purchase free-range or organic for better taste and no hormones.
- **Foods for liver health.** Beets, carrots, artichokes, lemons, parsnips, dandelion greens, and watercress all help keep your liver healthy.
- **Millet.** This tasty gluten-free whole grain is very nutritious and easy to digest.
- **Nutritional yeast.** Yeasts, such as brewer's, are stocked with nutrients, including B vitamins. Sprinkle these yeasts on popcorn, breads, or cereals.
- **Spelt.** A member of the wheat family, spelt can often be tolerated by people with gluten or wheat allergies and by people with celiac disease. It contains more protein and fiber than wheat.
- **Stevia.** Also known as honey leaf, stevia is a mighty herbal sweetener without the unwholesome side effects of artificial sweeteners. Just 1 to 3 drops is plenty to sweeten a cup of tea.

WOMAN TO WOMAN

She Had to Force Her Doctors to Diagnose Her

Since she was 17, Dede Wilson of Cincinnati had suffered from gastrointestinal problems that left her doctors perplexed. Specialist after specialist and years of testing failed to find the root of the problem. So Dede diagnosed herself. Her doctors scoffed at first, but they soon found out that her instinct was dead-on. Here's her story.

In the beginning, I had no clue what the problem was. I would eat lunch and then feel sick to my stomach. Nausea, vomiting, diarrhea, pain. My family doctor had no clue. He just wrote it off as nerves and prescribed Valium.

Eventually, I was referred to a gastroenterologist. Again, the tests were negative. So I received a one-size-fits-all diagnosis: irritable bowel syndrome. I endured months of useless medication.

Then, I began having irregular bleeding, which seemed odd since I was taking birth control pills to help regulate my periods. That's what pushed me over the edge. All my aunts had been telling me that I had endometriosis. They were right. In fact, it runs in our family—seven of us have it. But getting my doctors to believe it was a tremendous struggle. Every time I mentioned endometriosis, they shot it down. They said that there was no way I could have it because I was just in my early twenties. Finally, I was in so much pain I called my gynecologist and demanded treatment. He did a laparoscopy and at last diagnosed the disease correctly. I was grateful that he had found it, but I didn't feel comfortable with his treatment or bedside manner. So once again, I sought another doctor. And another. It took 4 years, but now I am seeing a physician who actually listens to my concerns.

My advice to others: Don't take a backseat to your doctor. Treating endometriosis is a partnership. If I see an article about endometriosis that I think may help my doctor understand the disease better, I mail it to him. I don't want to be just someone lying there in his office with a cloth over her naked body. I want him to know who I am and how this disease affects my life.

Peel me a grape. Bite into the fresh fruits and vegetables that you enjoy, experiment with new ones, and eat a variety of all of them, Dr. Brett urges. The phytochemicals (plant chemicals) that they contain may help ward off such catastrophic diseases as cancer, heart disease, and stroke. No one is certain how phytochemicals work, but researchers suspect that various mixtures of compounds neutralize free radicals, those unstable molecules that damage or destroy healthy cells. Since phytochemicals work as groups, you need a lot of them to make a difference. No single fruit or vegetable contains all of the phytochemicals that you need. The greater the variety of fruits and vegetables you consume, the better off you will be.

Snap up beans. Navy, pinto, lima, and other dried beans are virtually fat-free and are tremendous sources of protein that can slash or even eliminate the need for fat-laden meats in chili, stews, and salads.

To cut down on gas, soak your beans overnight in a bowl of water, then use fresh water for cooking them. Over-the-counter products such as Beano, which contains the enzyme alpha-galactosidase, also can help prevent gas by breaking down sugars in your digestive system.

Don't let meat hog your plate. Avoid letting meat crowd the fruits and vegetables off your plate. Instead, limit yourself to no more than 6 ounces of cooked meat a day. Use a small portion of meat (2 to 3 ounces after cooking) to complement, not dominate, each meal. Or, think of it this way: For every bite of meat, take four bites of fruits, vegetables, beans, and grains.

Sneak in soy. Soy contains isoflavones, which are substances that block the formation of blood vessels around new tumors, stop cancer cells from multiplying, and prevent the absorption of tumor-promoting estrogen. So instead of beef, chicken, and other meats, use soy products such as tofu, available at most grocery stores, as a main course in your meals.

Wear a milk mustache. Milk is fortified with vitamin D, which your body needs to absorb calcium. Calcium helps prevent osteoporosis, a degenerative bone disease that affects women four times more often than men. Drinking 2½ to 3 glasses of fat-free milk a day can help you reach a goal of 1,000 milligrams through your diet. Other good sources of calcium include yogurt, Cheddar cheese, sardines (with bones), tofu, and calcium-fortified orange juice.

Take your breath away. Eating one-half of an onion or a clove of garlic a day helps regulate bacteria and other organisms in both your intestines and reproductive tract. Both onion and garlic also contain a great number of cancer- and heart disease–fighting antioxidant compounds.

Heave hydrogenated foods. Foods such as commercially baked goods and margarines are often loaded with hydrogenated or partially hydrogenated oils. This means that hydrogen has been added to unsaturated fat to make it solidify. This process creates saturated fat and trans fatty acids—a gruesome pairing that raises blood levels of low-density lipoproteins (LDL), the bad cholesterol that clogs arteries. So if you read

---

THE WARNING SIGNS OF CANCER

Caught early, many cancers can be subdued. Here are the signals to look for, according to the American Cancer Society.

- Any change in bowel or bladder habits
- A sore that does not heal
- A lump or thickening in the breast or elsewhere
- Unusual bleeding or discharge
- Chronic indigestion or swallowing problems
- An obvious change in a wart or a mole
- A nagging cough or hoarseness

In most cases, these signs are symptoms of some disease other than cancer. But to be on the safe side, if you notice any of them, notify your doctor immediately. If it does turn out that you have cancer, the sooner you get started on treatment, the better your chances will be for a complete recovery and a long, healthy life.

---

the word *hydrogenated* on a food label, put the package back on the grocery shelf.

Reach for a supplement. Getting adequate amounts of all the nutrients that you need to stay healthy can be a challenge, even if you eat a well-balanced diet, so take a once-a-day multivitamin. It should include 100 percent of the Daily Values for calcium, magnesium, niacin, iron, folic acid, chromium, and vitamins A, C, D, E, and B$_{12}$. In particular, the antioxidant vitamins in these preparations will help prevent heart disease and other tissue damage.

Jump-Start Your Exercise Routine

Regular exercise has long been known to reduce the risk of heart disease and stroke among women, but that's not all.

(continued on page 200)

YOUR TREE OF KNOWLEDGE

Research your family history of ailments by talking to your parents, grandparents, aunts, uncles, and siblings. If a blood relative has a disease or condition, you need not panic, but you should be aware that you are at an increased risk.

The more relatives you talk to, the better. You should also know something about their lifestyles. For example, did they drink or smoke?

Serious but potentially preventable conditions are the ones you should pay the most attention to, including cancer, high blood pressure, diabetes, alcoholism, heart disease, and depression.

The sample family tree below depicts ways that you can chart your family's medical history. (Deceased members are crossed out, with ages of death in circles next to them.)

Sample Family Tree

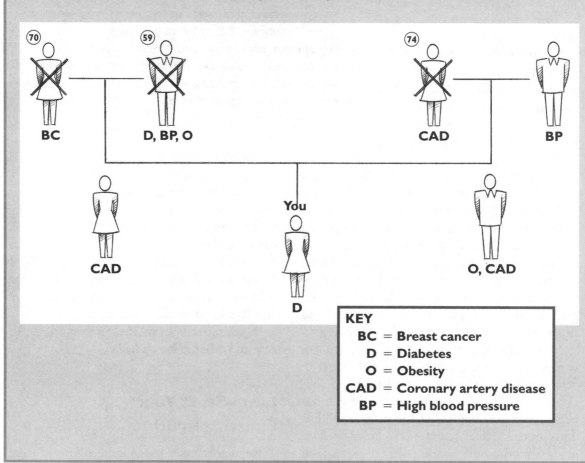

KEY
BC = Breast cancer
D = Diabetes
O = Obesity
CAD = Coronary artery disease
BP = High blood pressure

Organize your findings into a chart as shown in the sample. This will allow you to view the medical histories of several of your relatives all at once. You'll need to assign a letter to each medical condition or disease that occurs in your family and place that letter under each affected relative. Use the key to note which conditions the letters represent. Also note the age of death if the relative is deceased.

When your medical family tree is as complete as you can make it, review it with your physician to get a clearer understanding of your risks.

Your Family Tree

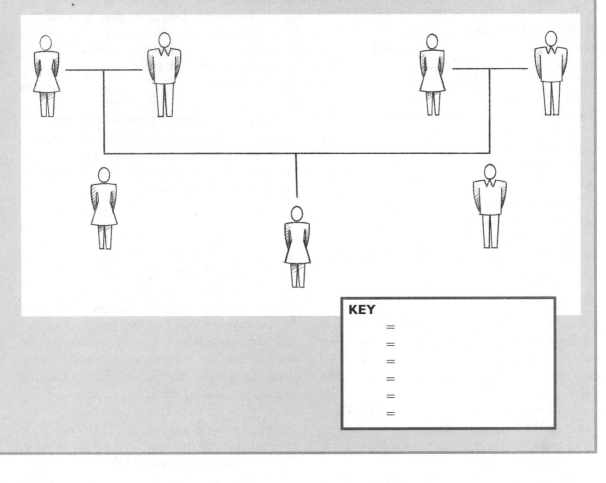

KEY

=
=
=
=
=
=

Women who exercise an hour a day may also reduce their risk of breast cancer by 20 percent, according to findings from the Nurses' Health Study, one of the largest studies (involving 121,701 women) ever done on women's health. Other researchers who have evaluated data from the Nurses' Health Study found that women who did the most weekly exercise had significantly lower risks of developing type 2 diabetes than did women who exercised the least.

Weight-bearing exercise, such as walking, jogging, and running, can also help women maintain bone mass and derail osteoporosis—the thinning and wearing away of bone that occurs as we get older, says Marianne Legato, M.D., founder and director of the Partnership for Women's Health at Columbia University College of Physicians and Surgeons in New York City and author of *What Women Need to Know*.

Simply walking 40 minutes a day, four times a week, can make an enormous difference in your body's ability to defend itself against a multitude of ailments.

Rest Easy

Sleep helps your body rebuild muscle tissue and replenish chemicals in your brain. Without adequate sleep—typically, 7 to 9 hours a night—you may be less energetic and more irritable, have greater difficulty concentrating, and be more prone to accidents, Dr. Brett says. Taking 200 to 300 milligrams of calcium and of magnesium every evening can help you get more restful sleep, she adds.

Valerian, an herbal remedy, has been shown to

HOW TO BE A HEALTH DETECTIVE

Resources abound, both in bookstores and on the Internet, for getting information about your health or a particular illness that may be challenging you. Here a few book titles you can find at the public library.

➤ *Mayo Clinic Family Health Book* and *The American Medical Association Family Medical Guide*, used together, provide basic health information in easy-to-understand language. *Mayo Clinic Family Health Book* provides information on more than 1,000 ailments and disorders. *The American Medical Association Family Medical Guide* includes illustrations and diagnoses for common symptoms.

➤ *Health Care Almanac: Every Person's Guide to the Thoughtful and Practical Sides of Medicine*, by the American Medical Association, is arranged in alphabetical order with addresses of medical associations and a variety of health-related information.

➤ *The Female Body: An Owner's Manual*, by the editors of *Prevention* Magazine Health Books, is designed to answer many concerns that women have about their health.

➤ *Our Bodies, Ourselves for the New Century*, by the Boston Women's Health Book Collective staff, continues to be considered the best in providing women with comprehensive coverage of health care.

---

have tranquilizing and sedative properties similar to the prescription drug diazepam (Valium), but without the side effects. Plus, valerian is nonaddictive. Dr. Brett suggests taking two 400-milligram capsules 30 minutes before bedtime. Valerian is also sold as a tea, but Dr. Brett says that it stinks like dirty, old socks and can be difficult to drink. Do not use valerian with sleep-enhancing or mood-regulating medications, because it may intensify their effects. It may cause heart palpitations and nervousness in sensitive individuals. If it stimulates you that way, discontinue using it. Valerian is available at most health food stores.

In addition, according to Dr. Brett, heeding

For information that's constantly brought up-to-date, both medical and public libraries are equipped with collections of electronic databases and Internet connections. Here are some Internet sites to look for.

➤ Healthfinder (www.healthfinder.gov), a government Web site, offers a searchable topic interface with additional links to professional organizations, academic institutions, and libraries.

➤ The American College of Obstetricians and Gynecologists Web site (www.acog.org) addresses a variety of women's health issues.

➤ CancerNet (http://cancernet.nci.nih.gov) from the National Cancer Institute provides current cancer information covering diagnosis, treatment, and cancer physicians and facilities.

➤ The National Women's Health Information Center (www.4woman.org) is maintained by the U.S. Department of Health and Human Services. Updated health-related news stories, consumer information, and links to medical dictionaries and glossaries are features of this Web site.

➤ The North American Menopause Society Web site (www.menopause.org) discusses scientific studies related to menopause.

the following advice also can help you sleep better.

Stick to a schedule. Try to go to bed and wake up at approximately the same times each day.

Kick back and unwind. Take a few moments before you turn in for the night to unload the stresses of the day through meditation or deep breathing. And avoid doing strenuous exercise an hour or two before you go to bed. The physical and psychological stimulation may wire you up.

Drink milk or herbal tea. Milk is loaded with L-tryptophan, which helps some people sleep. Drinking a cup of herbal tea before bed is a soothing ritual that can help you relax.

Avoid alcohol and caffeine. Either one of these substances, taken up to 8 hours before bed, will disrupt your natural sleep patterns.

Eat light. A large dinner or late-night snack might keep you tossing and turning as your digestive tract works overtime.

Strangle Stress

Women, particularly mothers, are more likely than men to feel stressed, according to a survey by Roper Starch Worldwide, a marketing research and consulting firm based in New York City.

While 21 percent of women in 30 countries report feeling an immense amount of stress, only 15 percent of men share those feelings. Among the most stressed women in the world are full-time working mothers with children under the age of 13, with nearly one in four feeling stress almost every day. More single women than single men around the world feel intense daily stress, and the number of stressed separated or divorced women exceeds that of stressed separated or divorced men by a 3-to-2 margin.

Of course, excessive stress is more than just a nuisance. It can make women more susceptible to infections and hormonal imbalances, Dr. Brett says. Meditation, yoga, and other techniques can go a long way toward reducing the stress that you feel and, in turn, reduce your risk of disease.

Listening to music is the number one stress-buster for more than half of the world's women, according to Roper Starch Worldwide. Reading,

WOMEN ASK WHY

How do I get a mammogram if I'm a AA-cup kinda woman?

Although smaller-breasted women may be concerned about whether an adequate mammogram can be done on them, they should be assured that the size of their breasts doesn't matter, even if they are A or AA cups. Technicians seldom have to treat small-breasted women differently from women who have larger breasts. The compression is the same. It doesn't hurt any more or less if you have smaller breasts.

But the truly important message here is for small-breasted women to get annual mammograms after age 40 like everyone else. Some women with smaller breasts may think that they are at lower risk for cancer because they have less breast tissue. But that's not true. Breast cancer is no more common among large-breasted women than among smaller-breasted women. No matter how much breast tissue she has, every woman has the same percentage of risk as any other woman in her age group.

Expert consulted
Deborah Capko, M.D.
Breast surgeon and associate medical director
Institute for Breast Care at Hackensack
University Medical Center
New Jersey

than 40 should undergo, according to Dr. Legato. Some of them may be familiar and a regular part of life. Others may not be, and in those cases, you should ask your doctor about adding them to your schedule of routine medical care.

- A blood pressure reading by a doctor or nurse at least once a year. High blood pressure (readings consistently above 140/90) is a known risk factor for stroke and heart disease.
- A mammogram at least every other year after age 40 can help detect breast cancer.
- A manual breast exam by a knowledgeable physician once a year, in addition to a mammogram.
- A complete head-to-toe skin exam by a knowledgeable physician once a year.
- A cholesterol screening once a year. Since heart disease is the number one killer of women, Dr. Legato believes that monitoring total cholesterol, LDL, high-density lipoproteins (HDL), and triglycerides is an essential component of preventive care.
- A thyroid-function test every year after age 50. For this test, your blood sample is analyzed at a laboratory.
- A bone-density screening to help determine your risk of developing osteoporosis. You only have to have this test done once.
- A serum estradiol test every 2 years after age 45. Low blood levels of estradiol (less than 50 picograms/deciliter) may mean that you need hormone-replacement therapy.

walking, or taking a bath or shower are other popular ways to unwind.

Make an Annual Pilgrimage

Regular physical exams and medical tests can help detect small problems in your body before they get big. The type and number of tests you'll need each year will depend on many factors, including your age and previous medical history. But here are a few critical tests that women older

- An electrocardiogram (EKG) every year. More than one in three heart attacks that occur in women are silent, without any outward warning signals. An EKG can help determine if you've had any heart damage in the previous year.
- A fecal occult blood test every year after age 50. This test can disclose any hidden blood in your stool that may be a warning sign of colon cancer and other diseases.
- A digital rectal exam once a year. In this test, which Dr. Legato highly recommends, a physician inserts a gloved finger into your rectum and feels for growths, abnormalities, and signs of bleeding.

   "I use it all of the time," Dr. Legato says, "and I think many more women's lives would be saved, in terms of death from colon cancer, by an early detection of polyps in the colon. It can take years for those polyps to become cancerous, but all become malignant eventually. Some of the cardinal ways to detect them are with a simple digital examination and by testing the stool for blood."

In between these tests, always be sure to do monthly skin and breast self-examinations at home, Dr. Ferry urges.

Manage Your Meds

Medicines can heal, but they also can harm. In fact, in ancient Greece, *pharmakos*, the root word of pharmacy, meant both remedy and poison. So be careful whenever you take medicines. In particular, be wary of drug interactions.

Dr. Ferry urges that your primary-care physician should know all of the medications, both prescription and over-the-counter, that you're taking. And don't forget about herbal remedies and other alternative treatments that you may be ingesting. Like any drugs, these remedies can cause side effects or interact with other drugs. Some herbs, such as chaparral, can trigger hepatitis and other liver damage. Before you leave your doctor's office, pharmacy, or alternative health-care provider's office with a new drug, make certain that you fully understand how to take the drug properly. Be sure to ask the following questions.

- What is the name of the drug and what will it do?
- How often should I take it?
- When should I take it?
- If I forget to take it, what should I do?
- What side effects might I expect, and should I report them?
- Will I need periodic blood or urine tests to monitor adverse effects?
- Is there any information about this drug that I can take home with me?

In addition, keep in an easy-to-find place in your purse or wallet a list of all medications that you are taking—again, including over-the-counter drugs and complementary treatments—and their dosages, Dr. Ferry says. That could be extremely helpful in an emergency, if you're incapacitated and can't communicate with the health-care professionals trying to save your life.

Take Charge of
Your Health Care

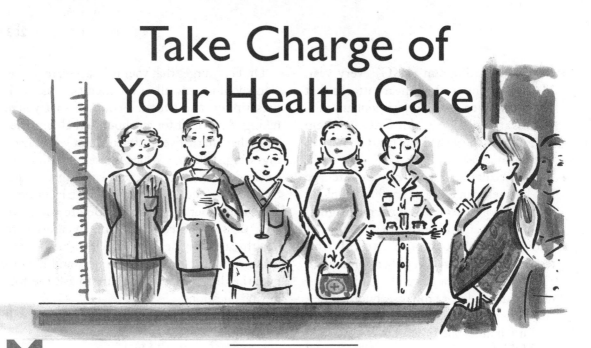

Many of us spend more time and effort on locating a good hairdresser than on finding a good doctor. Who can blame us? Shopping for doctors is intimidating. They all hang diplomas—written in Latin, which no one understands—on every wall of their offices, so we presume they're extremely well-educated. And most are not exactly fond of being interviewed about their competency by people who know nothing about medicine. But finding the right doctor is something we all need to do—and we need to do it now, when we're well, not when we're on the way to the hospital.

To complicate matters even more, as women, we have special health issues that our doctors should be familiar with. Can your doctor, for instance, give female-specific advice about preventing heart disease? Can she answer your questions about hormone-replacement therapy? Does she know enough about alternative medicine—herbs, supplements, and the like—to have an intelligent conversation with you about any alternative treatments you are using? Maybe you have both a regular and an alternative doctor. Wouldn't it be wonderful if the two of them

could talk together about your care once in a while? Wouldn't it be nice if your health-care team were as good a match for you as your hairdresser is? Here's how to make that happen.

Finding Dr. Right

Nowadays, two types of doctors perform the role formerly played by the general practitioner: the family practitioner and the internist. While doctors in both of these specialties receive similar training, there are some significant differences between them.

Family practitioners study general adult medicine as well as pediatrics, gynecology, obstetrics, and in-office surgical procedures. So their training is broad. Internists, on the other hand, receive more in-depth training in the diagnosis and treatment of adult illnesses, such as diabetes and heart disease.

Gynecologists also sometimes act as primary-care doctors for women. They can offer some preventive care, monitor your blood pressure and cholesterol, and do screening tests for thyroid function and colon cancer. But gynecology is actually a medical-surgical specialty, and a gynecologist's skills are best used to treat illness of your reproductive organs.

One of the best ways to find a competent doctor is to ask around, but don't ask just anyone. If you can, question people who work in the medical field. Emergency room physicians and nurses are often in a good position to judge the abilities of local doctors. If it's a gynecologist you're after, ask midwives and nurse practitioners, says Karla Morales, vice president of communications for People's Medical Society, a nonprofit organization devoted to consumer health issues, in Allentown, Pennsylvania.

Doctor-referral services can also be somewhat helpful, but you need to be aware of their limitations. Listed in the yellow pages, these services are usually run either by a local hospital, which lists only doctors employed there, or by a county medical society, which is a paid-membership organization.

At the least-sophisticated level, these services simply give callers the names of doctors from a rotating list of members. The better services, on the other hand, list basic information concerning board-certification and specialties of their doctors. And most of them weed out doctors who are trouble or who have been the subject of numerous complaints. "But these services do not give true comparisons or negative information about doctors," says Morales. For that information, contact the American Board of Medical Specialties at 1007 Church Street, Suite 404, Evanston, IL 60201.

WOMEN ASK WHY

Is it better for me to see a doctor who's a woman rather than one who's a man?

It's true that female doctors are more likely than male doctors to offer advice on preventing illness. They also tend to be better listeners and are less likely to interrupt their patients. But, on average, they rate only slightly better—10 percent—at these skills than male doctors. In fact, differences among female doctors are often greater than the average difference between male and female doctors.

So making female gender your number one priority when you're doctor shopping isn't necessarily going to find you the best doctor in your area. It's probably better to look for a doctor, male or female, who encourages you to ask questions, listens to you, explains things clearly, and treats you with respect.

However, when it comes to intimate personal examinations, women and men tend to be more comfortable and more frank with someone of their own gender and ethnicity. A woman who is uncomfortable with a pelvic or breast examination usually prefers seeing a female gynecologist for her care. Maybe that's one reason that female doctors now make up the majority of gynecologists.

Expert consulted
Erica Frank, M.D.
Associate professor in the department of
*   family and preventive medicine*
Emory University School of Medicine
Atlanta

Taking the Alternate Route

If you're looking for a doctor practicing alternative medicine, consider a naturopathic doctor, or N.D. An N.D. is trained in all forms of alternative medicine, including nutrition and herbal remedies. Look for one who is a member of the American Association of Naturopathic Physicians (AANP). These doctors have all graduated from one of the four U.S. or Canadian colleges recognized by the Council on Naturopathic Medical Education.

To find an N.D. in your area, you can check the AANP's Web site at www.naturopathic.org. Or for a small fee, you can receive a national membership list and a brochure describing naturopathic physicians and their services from the AANP, 601 Valley Street, Suite 105, Seattle, WA 98109-4229.

Eleven states license N.D.'s., and four states (Connecticut, Montana, Washington, and Alaska) require that health insurance providers cover N.D. care. In states where N.D.'s are not licensed, anyone can claim to be a naturopathic doctor, so checking credentials and education is important.

What about Dentists?

If you're looking for a dentist, experts again suggest that you ask for help from people you know and trust, including health-care professionals such as your doctor. You can also call to ask faculty members of the nearest dental school, which is often associated with a medical school. About three out of four dentists also belong to the American Dental Association (ADA), which means that they have some interest in continuing education and maintaining a professional practice, says Kimberly Harms, D.D.S., a dentist from Farmington, Minnesota, and consumer advisor for the ADA. The ADA can give you a list of its members in your area. Contact it at the ADA, 211 East Chicago Avenue, Chicago, IL 60611. You can also request information via e-mail on its Web site at www.ada.org.

The staff of the dentist's office should allow you to come in to look around or to have a get-acquainted visit with the dentist, where you

---

WHAT TO LOOK FOR IN A FIRST-RATE HOSPITAL

Generally, your doctor, not you, chooses the hospital you will go into for surgery. So if you want to go to a particular hospital, you'll have to become the patient of a doctor who has operating or attending privileges there. Good doctors are more likely to be affiliated with good hospitals, but how can you be certain that your doctor is sending you to the best hospital for *your* problem? According to Karla Morales, vice president of communications for People's Medical Society, here are some things to consider.

➤ Is the hospital accredited? About 80 percent of U.S. hospitals are accredited by either the Joint Commission on Accreditation of Healthcare Organizations or the American Osteopathic Association. This means the facility is inspected every 3 years for a long list of items.

➤ Is the staff top-quality? The doctors who will be treating you in the hospital should be board-certified by their specialties' professional societies. Find out, too, how the hospital is equipped to treat your particular illness or to perform your type of surgery. How often do they treat your kind of illness? What success rates do they have? You can start with a phone call to the hospital administration office for answers to these questions. Studies show that hospitals get better at procedures they often perform, and the results are better, too.

---

simply discuss your concerns and get to know each other, Dr. Harms says. A good dentist will have a clean, organized office and friendly staff; will use proper sterilization techniques, including wearing a face mask and gloves; will take a comprehensive dental and medical history before working on you; and will openly discuss treatment options and fees, she says. Many dentists these days work with a dental hygienist, who cleans your teeth, so you'll want to meet the dental hygienist as well.

By the way, D.D.S. and D.M.D. degrees are basically the same thing.

- Is there an all-R.N. staff? The best hospitals have moved in this direction, replacing practical nurses and others with more highly trained R.N.'s.

- What's the staffing level? Make sure that the hospital is not understaffed. One nurse for every three to eight patients can help assure good care. You can obtain information about a hospital's nursing staff from the hospital itself, your state affiliate to the American Nurses Association, or the American Hospital Association.

- What is the hospital's infection rate? The national average for infections acquired in hospitals is growing, but most infections are avoidable. In fact, the Harvard Medical Practice Study in 1991 found that 70 percent of all wound infections could be prevented when proper procedures are followed.

- What are the hospital's morbidity (nonfatal complications) and mortality statistics for your procedure? While this does not tell you everything, it gives you a measure for comparison of one hospital with another.

Get information from your doctor and local hospitals, but also ask other health-care professionals, clergy, and business leaders. If there is a major quality difference among hospitals, your sources are likely to tell you. If there is a doctor in your region who is well-regarded for her work, find out at which hospital she works.

All about Counselors and Therapists

As anyone who has ever tangled with depression will tell you, emotional well-being plays an important role in overall good health—but finding the right therapist can be tricky. If you've never used one before, you may not even know what to look for.

The following guidelines can help you identify a therapist who is both professionally qualified and the best personal match for you.

You should feel comfortable. You need to trust this person enough to openly talk about your thoughts, feelings, and behavior, says Faith Tanney, Ph.D., a psychologist practicing in Washington, D.C. "You may feel challenged or disagree with things, but you should have a basic trust in the therapist and feel as though she is listening and interested in you and understands who you are."

It may take about two sessions to decide if you feel comfortable working with a particular therapist, Dr. Tanney says.

The therapist should act like a professional. Psychologists and other mental health professionals are expected to adhere to a code of ethics that includes confidentiality and certain boundaries. Those boundaries involve not having an outside relationship with a client while she's in treatment; not counseling someone with whom there is a preexisting relationship, such as friend, employee, or student; not having any kind of sexual contact with the client; and structuring financial arrangements clearly and honestly.

Warning signs of a lack of professionalism manifest themselves when the therapist is often late beginning or ending sessions, takes phone calls during sessions, confuses you with other clients, forgets what you've said in past sessions, or talks about herself instead of keeping the primary focus on you, advises Dr. Tanney.

The therapist should work with you to establish treatment goals. In these days of managed care, you're lucky if your insurance company pays for six treatment sessions. Focusing on your central issues and setting goals to help resolve those issues is the best use of your

Women Ask Why

Why do people sometimes go into the hospital well and come out sick?

Hospitals are full of sick people, and sick people are sometimes contagious. Organisms can be transmitted in the air, by direct human contact, on towels and sheets, via the housekeeping crew, by contact with surgical wounds, and through the use of urinary catheters, drainage tubes, and ventilator tubes. Studies show that most people don't develop a hospital-acquired infection until at least 72 hours after admission, so some infections may not become apparent until after you've been discharged from the hospital.

How can you protect yourself? Ask your doctor about the hospital's track record for infections. (People at the hospital itself may paint too rosy a picture.) Make sure all hospital personnel who come in contact with you wash their hands. Ask them to do so in your room, in your presence.

Nurses who wear fake fingernails are more likely to harbor harmful organisms than those who don't. In a recent study, 68 percent of nurses wearing fake nails were carrying harmful bacteria on their hands even after washing, so ask nurses who wear fake nails to put on gloves before treating you.

If you're concerned that a sick roommate has something you could catch, ask your doctor or nurse about your risk. Change your room at once if there is any chance that you could become infected.

If you're undergoing a procedure that requires the removal of hair, refuse to be shaven the night before surgery. A low rate of infection is achieved by using a chemical depilatory or barber clippers to remove hair on the morning of the surgery.

If you have a urinary catheter, a nurse should check it regularly to make sure that it is draining correctly. This may help you avoid a urinary tract infection.

Expert consulted
Karla Morales
Vice president of communications
People's Medical Society

time, Dr. Tanney says. For this, a therapist needs to be focused.

The therapist should empower you. A good therapist doesn't attempt to solve problems for you. At best, she provides helpful insights and offers new ways of looking at your situation, serving more as a catalyst to help you develop the ability to problem-solve for yourself, Dr. Tanney says.

The therapist should have good credentials. Many different types of professionals, including the following, practice psychotherapy. Psychiatrists are, essentially, physicians, and with a few exceptions, they are the only mental health professionals licensed to prescribe drugs. Clinical or counseling psychologists (Ph.D., Psy.D., or Ed.D.) spend an average of 7 years in postgraduate school developing expertise in human behavior, diagnosis, and treatment. Clinical social workers (M.S.W.) have earned master's degrees in social work and are trained in individual, family, and group counseling with an emphasis on tapping community resources. Psychiatric advanced nurse practitioners (R.N.) are registered nurses with advanced training in the prevention and treatment of mental health problems. And marriage and family therapists have earned, at minimum, master's degrees and are specialists in their respective fields.

Licensure is an important credential. Through licensure you can be certain that an independent review of the professional's training and experience has been conducted. All physicians, psychologists, nurses, and social workers are licensed in every state. Marriage and family therapists are licensed in most states. Most insurance companies require licensure for payment for mental health services, and licensure also assures that you'll have legal recourse if inappropriate care is provided.

When Should You Fire Your Doctor?

What if you're seeing a doctor you just don't care for? No doctor is perfect—you have to balance her strengths and weaknesses. You may want to discuss your dissatisfactions with her before you start shopping for a new doctor. There may be room for reconciliation.

Still, most experts say that it's time to end the relationship if your doctor puts you down or judges you, fails to exercise good medical judgment, orders the same test several times when once would do, does not perform thorough physical exams, or minimizes serious side effects or risks of a treatment. Likewise, think about going elsewhere if your doctor blocks your attempts at communication or makes you feel so intimidated that you don't speak up, isn't interested in your worries and concerns, ignores psychological and social causes of illness as well as job-related health problems, or is disrespectful or verbally abusive to you or others.

DOES YOUR DOCTOR HAVE THE RIGHT STUFF?

Whether the doctor you're considering is traditional or alternative, you need to check her credentials and other more subjective aspects of her practice, says Karla Morales, vice president of communications for People's Medical Society. Call the doctor's office for this information. It's a good way to find out if her staff is consumer-friendly and willing to answer your questions. Here are some of the questions you should ask.

- Is the doctor accepting new patients?
- Is the doctor board-certified? Board certification means that the doctor has taken extra training and passed the vigorous examination given by a national board of professionals in that specialty field. Board certification is an important way by which doctors judge their colleagues' credentials. Keep in mind that alternative physicians are not likely to be board-certified.
- Does the doctor have get-acquainted visits? How long are they? (Expect 10 to 15 minutes.) How much do they cost?
- At what hospitals does the doctor have privileges to admit, treat, or operate on her patients? Privileges are rights granted to a doctor by a hospital review board, depending on the hospital's need for doctors and on a doctor's qualifications.
- Does the doctor accept phone calls from patients? At what hours? Does she have e-mail? The doctor's staff can frequently answer questions over the phone, but you should have access to the doctor herself if you feel that's necessary.
- Does she have any evening or weekend hours?
- How far in advance is the doctor booked for routine appointments? How quickly can you get in for an emergency?
- Does the doctor work in a group? How many doctors are in the group? Are they all board-certified? Who backs up the doctor when she's on vacation?
- Does she work in conjunction with alternative practitioners or make referrals to them?

Disease-Proof Your Lifestyle

Heart disease runs in my family. I'm either going to get it or I'm not. There's nothing I can really do about it."

Sound familiar?

Maybe heart disease isn't your worry. Maybe it's some other disease of "aging," like diabetes, cancer, or osteoporosis. Whatever the illness, it's easy to imagine it waiting like an unavoidable chasm in the road ahead. Genetics, as we know, is the blueprint of our lives. We believe it holds our fate, in the same way the ancients believed that fate was written in the stars.

Well, here's a news flash: Your fate isn't in the stars, and it isn't in your genes. You hold it in your very own hands.

"Certainly some diseases might have a genetic component, but the evidence clearly shows that other environmental issues—like lifestyle—play a key role," says Julie Buring, Sc.D., professor of ambulatory care and prevention at Harvard Medical School and Brigham and Women's Hospital in Boston. "Whether we develop a condition like cancer or heart disease, for example, is not something that's totally out of our control. There are many things we can do to reduce our risk."

What's more, it's never too late to make positive changes in your lifestyle—even if you're a fifty-something smoker who's overweight. "You may think that you should have made healthier choices when you were a teenager—and it's true that the earlier you do it the better—but we've found that even when elderly people quit smoking or start exercising it greatly benefits their overall health," Dr. Buring says.

The average 40-year-old woman still has another 40 years of life to look forward to. So start making healthy changes now, and you'll feel as good—or even better—throughout the second half of your life as you felt through the first.

Gene-Proof Your Health

Thanks to the men and women in white lab coats who've done countless hours of research, we now know that there are specific preventive measures we can take to lower our risk for many diseases as we age. Here are 10 key things you can start doing right away to help keep you healthy and feeling young.

210

Toss the smokes. Lung cancer, heart disease, stroke, high blood pressure, osteoporosis. The list of age-related diseases that smokers are at higher risk for goes on and on. Not to mention the wrinkles and stained teeth that make you look far older than your years. If you don't smoke, raise your right hand and swear you never will. Then give yourself a pat on the back. If you do smoke—stop. "Without a doubt, it's one of the best things you can do for your health," says Elizabeth Ross, M.D., a cardiologist at Washington Hospital Center in Washington, D.C.; spokesperson for the American Heart Association; and author of *Healing the Female Heart*. Within minutes of puffing your final cigarette, your blood pressure and pulse rate drop to normal. And after just 24 hours, your risk of having a heart attack decreases.

Add activity. Close to five million American adults say they don't do anything physically active in their leisure time. Now that's a lot of couch potatoes. And it turns out that more women are inactive than men. Everyone knows exercise is good for you—so why are so many women still stuck on the sofa? Perhaps you haven't found a fun activity that keeps you coming back for more. Or maybe you think you don't have the time. But it takes a lot less time than you probably realize.

"You don't have to go to a gym every day or become a marathon runner to get the benefits of exercise," Dr. Buring says. "The current recommendation for physical activity is something that virtually all of us can do." That's 30 minutes of accumulated moderate physical activity most days of the week. Walking the dog, gardening, housework—they all count.

Need another reason to trade in your recliner for a treadmill? How about 250,000 reasons? That's how many deaths per year in this country can be attributed to a lack of regular physical activity. In fact, regular exercise helps prevent everything from heart disease and diabetes to breast cancer and osteoporosis.

Control your weight. It's no secret that we tend to put on pounds as we grow older. A growing middle may seem like a harmless, natural part of aging, but it's not. "In this country, we gain an average of 7 pounds a decade," Dr. Buring says.

That adds up fast. If you weighed 125 at age 20, that means you'll tip the scale at 160 by the time you're 70. That rate of weight gain puts you at risk for a number of diseases including diabetes, heart disease, arthritis, and even gallstones.

Losing weight isn't easy. So your best bet is not to gain it in the first place. "Focus on maintaining your weight rather than trying to lose the extra pounds after you've already gained them," Dr. Buring says.

If you've already put on some pounds, try losing just 10. Even small reductions can go a long way in helping improve your condition if you have a problem like arthritis or high blood pressure, Dr. Buring says.

Pile your plate with fruits and veggies. That's right. One key to living a long, disease-free life can be found in the produce section of any grocery store. In fact, a study of 52 Italians aged 70 and older found that the healthy one-hundred-and-somethings ate more than twice as many vegetables as the younger folks.

That's not surprising since eating five servings of fruits and vegetables a day is associated with lower risks of several diseases, including cancer and stroke. And researchers have identified all sorts of healthy components in our produce. Not only are fruits and vegetables a natural source of antioxidants, vitamins, minerals, and fiber—they also contain phytonutrients like quercetin, lycopene, flavonoids, and ellagic acid, which are potential heart protectors and cancer fighters.

Eat a low-fat diet. Too much fat does a lot of nasty things to our bodies. First, it can clog up the arteries in our hearts and block blood vessels in our brains, putting us at risk for heart disease and stroke. Excess fat can also overstimulate our gallbladders and create the right conditions for painful gallstones. And of course, too much fat can make us, well, fat, which increases our risk for other diseases like cancer and diabetes.

Most experts agree that a low-fat diet should get no more than 25 percent (and preferably less) of its calories from fat. But not all fats are bad. The main one to limit in your diet is saturated fat, found in foods like meat, butter, and dairy products. Researchers say that the best way to cut down on saturated fat is to limit meat servings to 3 or 4 ounces a day, use little or no butter, switch to low-fat dairy foods, and cook with corn, canola, or olive oil.

Other fats to be wary of include the trans fatty acids found mostly in margarine and prepackaged snacks. They may be just as unhealthy for our hearts as saturated fat. You can cut your trans fatty acids by using trans-free margarine (partially hydrogenated oils are not listed as an ingredient) instead of regular margarine and by limiting the amount of snack foods you eat that contain partially hydrogenated oil.

Fill up on fiber. Eating a high-fiber diet may lower your risk for several diseases, including heart disease, diabetes, high blood pressure, obesity, and diverticulosis. And several small studies suggest that filling up on fiber can lower your risk of colon cancer. How does fiber protect against such a variety of diseases? For one thing,

WOMAN TO WOMAN

She Turned Her Health Around with a Simple Strategy

Sky-high blood pressure, the aches of arthritis, and 15 extra pounds gave 71-year-old Jennie Cargill of Cleveland Heights, Ohio, a powerful incentive to change her diet and beef up her exercise program. But as she peeled off the pounds, she got a bonus—it's as if she turned back the clock. Here's her story.

I was about 15 pounds overweight when I went in for my stress test. I had been dealing with a lot of family problems, and my blood pressure was already high. But I was about to find out just how high. The doctors put all these wires on me before I got on the treadmill.

"Well, let's get her reading," the technician said.

"It's 220 over 110," the nurse told him.

The technician hesitated. He said, "Excuse me, is that a blood pressure reading you're giving me?"

"Yes it is."

Well, after that, they wouldn't even let me take the stress test; my blood pressure was way too high. A little later, my doctor took me aside and said, "You know, we really have to do something about this." He knows that when he gets serious or acts concerned, I'll respond.

He immediately put me on a medication that would reduce my high blood pressure, and I was already taking a diuretic and another drug for heart problems. But I didn't want to rely on drugs.

Now, I've always exercised—we have lots of parks here—and I would try to walk at least 2 to 3 miles a day. But I de-

it acts like a sponge as it passes through our bodies, soaking up potentially harmful substances like cholesterol and binding to extra estrogen in the digestive tract, then removing them in our stool. Fiber also fills us up so we eat less.

The problem is that most people get only 11 to 13 grams of fiber a day—that's about half of the 25 to 35 grams experts recommend. To give

cided I wanted to do more. So I started walking even faster. Before long, I could do a mile in 15 minutes. In addition, I signed up for a seniors' exercise class and toned and stretched my muscles for 1½ hours 4 days a week.

I also read somewhere that fiber helps fill you up. So I started eating a cereal called Fiber One and later switched to Post Shredded Wheat, which has less sodium. When I wanted to snack, instead of grabbing potato chips or something, I'd eat a handful of cereal and drink a cup of tea. Or I'd have cottage cheese and fruit, which I knew were low in fat and calories. And then for dinner, I would eat beans or something that would be filling along with chicken or fish.

To me, it's easier to eat this way. People would say, "Well, you should just go on a diet . . ." But I didn't want to go on a diet. I wanted a new way of eating. If you decide that you're not going to eat any pie or cake, then you just say, "I won't eat any cake at all." It's easier than saying, "Well, I won't eat chocolate cake, or I won't eat vanilla cake." Very simple.

In 4 to 6 weeks, I started feeling better. My clothes fit more loosely, and it seemed to help my arthritis. Suddenly, I could fly up and down the stairs. I'm not sure what helped me the most, but it was probably a combination of things. Losing the weight, the fish in my diet—these may help keep me limber.

My blood pressure came way down, too. The last time I was in my doctor's office, it was 134 over 82. And he was really pleased. He said to keep up the good work.

I told my daughter I'm going to live to be 100. I'm even reading a book now on how to do it. But that's not my only goal—I want to feel as great as I do now for the next 29 years.

your plate a fiber face-lift, add more foods like fruits, vegetables, beans, and whole-grain breads, cereals, rice, and pasta.

Supplement your diet. Our bodies need vitamins, minerals, and other important nutrients to function at their best. And if we all ate a low-fat diet high in fruits and vegetables every day, we'd probably get enough of these vital nutrients,

Dr. Buring says. But many of us don't. That's why it's important to take a multivitamin/mineral supplement that provides the Daily Value for most nutrients. Think of it as an insurance policy for those days when our diet isn't up to snuff. But don't think because you're taking a vitamin that you don't have to eat a healthy diet, exercise, or quit smoking, Dr. Buring adds.

Another good reason to take a multi is the mounting evidence that supplementing your diet in this way may help you ward off disease. "People who take a multivitamin a day are less likely to have heart attacks," says Kathryn Rexrode, M.D., instructor at Harvard Medical School and associate physician in the division of preventive medicine at Brigham and Women's Hospital in Boston.

That may be because nutrients like folate, vitamin B_6, vitamin E, and beta-carotene have all been found to promote heart health. Folate may also help prevent colon cancer, cervical cancer, and strokes. Vitamin D lowers your risk for colon cancer and osteoporosis. Calcium may reduce rectal cancer risk along with preventing osteoporosis. Vitamin C and magnesium can help strengthen your bones and keep your blood pressure in check. The trace element selenium can protect a man's prostate from cancer. And beta-carotene has been shown to prevent cancer in lab animals.

With all that protection in a single pill, it's no wonder that one out of every two M.D.'s takes supplements or vitamins. "The benefits of taking a multivitamin are not absolutely proven," Dr. Rexrode says. "On the other hand, it's pretty cheap and safe."

Limit yourself to one drink.
While having one alcoholic drink a
day may lower your risk of death, especially from heart disease, more than
one may put you at risk for a whole
host of other diseases including breast
cancer, stroke, and osteoporosis, explains Marianne J. Legato, M.D.,
professor of medicine at Columbia
University College of Physicians and
Surgeons and founder/director of the
Partnership for Women's Health at
Columbia, both in New York City, and
coauthor of *The Female Heart*. What's
more, many heart specialists don't even
recommend a drink a day to their patients.

"If they don't drink or they drink in-
frequently, I don't advise them to start,"
Dr. Legato says. "If they do imbibe, I
tell them to keep it to one drink a day."
So if you enjoy a good bottle of Lam-
brusco on occasion, pour yourself just
one glass and recork the rest for later.

Get screened. Most women get a
Pap smear once a year as part of their
annual gynecological exam. But that's
not the only potentially lifesaving test
a woman should regularly have done.
After age 40, a mammogram (earlier if
there's a family history of breast cancer) and
skin-cancer screening, for example, should also
be included in every woman's yearly checkup.
Later in this chapter, we discuss other health
screenings that women shouldn't skip.

Know your risk factors. Many diseases run
in families. So it's wise to know what that means
for you. If a parent or sibling has had a condition
like colon or breast cancer, for example, you
should get the recommended screenings even at
a younger age, Dr. Buring says. The same goes
for diabetes.

WOMEN ASK WHY

*Why are men encouraged to take an
aspirin a day to keep their hearts
healthy, but women aren't?*

In fact, some women with heart dis-
ease could very well enjoy the mild, blood-thinning benefits
taking an aspirin a day provides. The problem is, we don't
know enough about heart problems in women to make that
kind of recommendation—yet.

Why? For years, most medical experts assumed that heart
disease was exclusively a male problem. In fact, surveys
showed that one out of three doctors wasn't aware that
heart disease was the leading cause of death in women. Two
out of three believed that women had the same heart disease symptoms as men. And an even higher percentage believed that if women do get heart disease, they do "better"
than men.

As a result, relatively few female heart disease studies were
conducted. But more information is slowly emerging. For one
thing, we now know that women develop heart disease a
little bit later than men. While the vast majority of guys are
affected between the ages of 45 and 55, research shows that
most women don't develop heart disease until after 55—a
phenomenon attributed in part to estrogen levels.

It seems that estrogen helps keep your good high-density

No matter what your family history, you
should have your blood pressure and cholesterol
checked regularly. For cholesterol, that means
every 5 years if your levels are normal. "Normal"
is defined as having a total cholesterol of 150 or
lower, with a total/high-density lipoprotein
(HDL) ratio of 4.0 or lower. That ratio, which
tells you how much of your total cholesterol is
HDL, or "good" cholesterol, is a better predictor
of heart disease risk for women than total cholesterol, HDL, low-density lipoprotein (LDL),
or triglycerides, say doctors. If your cholesterol

lipoprotein (HDL) cholesterol high and bad low-density lipoprotein (LDL) cholesterol in check. As you go through menopause and lose estrogen, however, your total cholesterol can begin to look more like a man's, raising your risk for heart disease. So much so, in fact, that by the time you're 65, your cholesterol levels could actually exceed those of a man.

For these and other reasons, some experts do recommend that women at greater risk for heart disease, such as those who have had a relative die from a heart attack, consider taking an aspirin a day. But if that's you, don't rush to your medicine cabinet just yet. There's evidence it may raise your risk for stroke or boost your blood pressure—obviously a problem for someone already suffering from hypertension. And aspirin has been known to cause stomach upset—as well as provoke asthma and allergies.

The best advice until we know more: If you're at risk for heart disease, get 30 minutes of exercise a day, eat less fat, find a way to relieve stress, and talk to your doctor about whether aspirin is right for you.

Expert consulted
Elizabeth Ross, M.D.
Cardiologist and spokesperson for the American Heart Association
Washington Hospital Center
Washington, D.C.

numbers are high, you should have them taken again in 4 months.

When it comes to your blood pressure, the American Heart Association suggests that you have it checked at least once every 2 years. An optimal reading is less than 120 over 80, and normal is less than 130 over 85. If you've had a higher reading, decide with your doctor how often you should have it checked.

"High blood pressure, which significantly raises your risk for stroke, is a silent disease. You could have it for years and not even know it," Dr.

Buring says. "And you could be eating a healthy diet but still have high cholesterol, if it runs in your family. That's why you should have both your blood pressure and cholesterol checked regularly."

They are important to know because high levels are associated with increased risk of serious conditions such as heart disease and stroke, Dr. Buring says. If your levels are high, there are things you can do to lower them—like exercising and switching to a low-fat diet. In some cases, your doctor may want to put you on medication to help lower your levels.

Stop Disease before It Starts

As we grow older we start to feel, well, old. We may slow down a bit, and as a result, our bodies may slow down, too. Our joints ache a little more and our food is harder to digest. That's when disease prevention often becomes a priority in our lives, because we want to be as healthy and live as long as possible—aching joints and all. And it's true that the older we are, the higher our risk of developing certain diseases. But almost all of the life-shortening or slow-you-down diseases can be prevented. From dietary measures to early detection, here are the best prevention strategies for the most common diseases that affect women.

Arthritis

Arthritis. It's the nation's leading cause of disability among adults, and it's more likely to

BREATHE DEEPLY TO FIGHT DISEASE

Take a deep breath. Notice how your belly feels as if it's filling with air? Chances are you don't breathe that way most of the time, but instead take short shallow breaths that inflate your chest rather than your abdomen.

Some doctors believe shallow breathing so deprives our bodies of much-needed oxygen that it can lead to disease, so they teach their patients how to breathe properly. As silly as that may seem, they claim it significantly improves your health and may even help you live longer—much like aerobic exercise can. Here, three doctors explain the connection between breathing and health.

➧ "The human body is designed to discharge 70 percent of its toxins through breathing. Only a small percentage of toxins are discharged through sweat, defecation, and urination. If your breathing is not operating at peak efficiency, you are not ridding yourself of toxins properly. If less than 70 percent of your toxins are being released through breathing, other systems of your body, such as your kidneys, must work overtime. This overwork can set the stage for a number of illnesses," writes Gay Hendricks, Ph.D., a psychologist, in his book *Conscious Breathing*.

➧ "Breathing is unquestionably the single most important thing you do in your life. And breathing *right* is unquestionably the single most important thing you can do to *improve* your life. If you're interested in preventing illness, proper breathing may help you protect against angina, heart disease, respiratory infections, and fibromyalgia. It will also help you live a longer, more energetic, and stress-free life," writes Sheldon Saul Hendler, M.D., Ph.D., a doctor specializing in internal medicine, in his book *The Oxygen Breakthrough*.

➧ "Proper oxygen delivery to all parts of your body is crucial to health and well-being. . . . Breathing is the process by which oxygen enters the bloodstream, via the lungs. Thus, proper breathing, and correcting common breathing disorders, is the ultimate form of aerobics," writes Robert Fried, Ph.D., a psychology professor, in his book *The Breath Connection*.

So if you want to breathe easy about your health, try breathing deeply. It just might work.

strike women than men. At least 26 million women in the United States have some type of arthritis. The most common type—osteoarthritis—tends to occur more often in older people, usually striking between the ages of 45 and 65. That's because the cartilage around our joints can get worn down from years of wear and tear. Without cartilage to cushion them, bones rub together and cause pain, stiffness, and swelling. Several areas are particularly vulnerable, including the knees, hips, wrists, fingers, toes, neck, and lower back.

Many people may have osteoarthritis and not realize it because they have no symptoms, says Yvonne Sherrer, M.D., director of clinical research at the Center for Rheumatology, Immunology, and Arthritis in Fort Lauderdale, Florida. That's probably because certain lifestyle factors, which are described below, can prevent symptoms from ever occurring. Here are the key actions experts recommend to keep osteoarthritis—or at least its symptoms—from bothering your bones.

Shed a few pounds. The more you weigh, the more stress certain joints have to bear. And the more stress you place on your joints, the more wear and tear that occurs. It just makes sense. "We know that if you keep your weight down to ideal body weight, then you're less likely to have problems with osteoarthritis of the knees," Dr. Sherrer says. If you are overweight, just losing 10 to 20 pounds can substantially reduce your risk of developing osteoarthritis symptoms, she says.

Get some exercise. Strong muscles equal healthier joints. That's because weak muscles cannot effectively protect the joint they surround and may eventually cause it to slip out of alignment, explains Dr. Sherrer. As a result, certain areas of the joint may sustain a lot of pressure. But regular exercise increases your muscle strength, which helps to adequately protect the joints and also makes them more flexible. Activities that don't put a lot of stress on the joints, such as walking and swimming, are best.

Don't overexercise. Serious athletes are more likely to get osteoarthritis because they tend to overuse their joints, and overuse speeds up the wear-and-tear process, Dr. Sherrer says. "If you abuse your joints, then you pay a price," she says. "And athletes are the most notorious group when it comes to overstressing the joints."

Cancer

Cancer is the second leading cause of death in this country, after heart disease. More than half of cancer deaths in women are from lung, breast, and colorectal cancers.

Our risk for cancer increases as we grow older. Take colorectal cancer, for example. One in 150 women ages 40 to 59 developed this type of cancer from 1993 to 1995. Raise the age to 60 to 79 years, and the ratio jumps to 1 in 32.

"There's a very dramatic increase with age for most adult cancers," says Demetrius Albanes, M.D., senior investigator in the Cancer Prevention Studies Branch at the National Cancer Institute in Bethesda, Maryland. Scientists are not sure why cancer is largely an older person's disease, he says, but they theorize that it takes many

years of exposure to a variety of carcinogens to eventually cause the genetic damage that results in cancer. And they think that the weakening of our internal defenses as we grow older may also play a part in the disease.

There's at least one common type of cancer that is an exception to the aging rule and that's melanoma, a potentially deadly type of skin cancer. "Melanoma is actually a disease of young people," says Jessica Fewkes, M.D., assistant professor of dermatology at Harvard Medical School. "If you look at the largest group, the median age is around 40."

Whether you're 30, 40, or 60, you can take steps to lower your risk for any type of cancer. The most important thing you can do is obvious—don't smoke. Lighting up is to blame for up to 90 percent of all lung cancer cases—and lung cancer kills about 25,000 more women a year than breast cancer does. If you do smoke, quitting now can dramatically lower your risk. Five years after kicking the habit, an ex-smoker's risk of dying from lung cancer decreases by about half. And after 10 smoke-free years, the risk is similar to that of a nonsmoker.

Keeping your weight within a healthy range and eating a diet that's low in dietary fat can also help lower your risk for lung, breast, and colon cancer, Dr. Albanes says. So can exercising regularly, he adds. In fact, a study of more than 1,800 women found that those who were moderately active had a 50 percent lower risk of breast cancer. Women who did more vigorous activity like swimming or running at least once a week were 80 percent less likely to develop breast cancer than inactive women.

Whether or not cancer runs in your family, you can further cut your cancer risk with these preventive measures.

Follow the five-a-day rule. When you sit down at your next meal, remember this catchy phrase: The food on your plate determines your fate. It may sound like a bit of a cliché, but research backs it up.

An analysis of more than 200 studies shows that a diet high in agricultural produce cuts your cancer risk in half. Consuming lots of fruits and vegetables can help prevent all three of the top cancer killers—lung, breast, and colon cancer, Dr. Albanes says. Researchers don't think there's just one component in produce that protects against cancer, but rather a bunch of components—such as the beta-carotene found in sweet potatoes and carrots, the vitamin C in green peppers and citrus fruit, and phytonutrients like the isothiocyanates found in broccoli. To improve your chances of staying cancer-free, aim for at least five fruits and vegetables a day.

Go for fiber. Perhaps you've heard that fiber may not be as beneficial in warding off colon cancer as was once thought. That's based on the findings from a study of nearly 89,000 nurses who got most of their fiber from fruits and vegetables but ate very little of the wheat bran fiber that many other studies have found prevents colon cancer. More research is being done to confirm the benefits of fiber, but until then, keep in mind that even the authors of the study involving the nurses say it's very important to stick with a high-fiber diet.

How might fiber help prevent colon cancer? By causing stool to move more quickly through the body. That's important because the less time harmful compounds in the stool stay in the colon, the less likely they are to do damage.

Eating a high-fiber diet may also help cut your risk for breast cancer. That's because fiber routinely binds to estrogen in the digestive tract and removes it from the body, Dr. Albanes explains. The less estrogen women are exposed to over their lifetimes, the lower their risk of breast cancer.

Pass up charred food. A survey of more than 900 women found that those who often ate well-cooked meat such as hamburger, beefsteak, and bacon were nearly five times more likely to develop breast cancer than women who preferred their meat rare to medium. Researchers say that may have been a result of exposure to cancer-causing compounds called heterocyclic amines, which form when meat and fish are cooked at high temperatures. You may be able to lower your risk of breast cancer by taking that steak off the grill before the black, crispy edges form.

Take a multi. There's some evidence that higher intakes of the trace mineral selenium and several vitamins such as A and E, along with some carotenoids, like beta-carotene, may lower your risk for cancer, Dr. Albanes says. "We're also looking closely at dietary folate," he adds. And at least one study of 930 people suggests that taking extra calcium may help prevent colon cancer. While there isn't really strong evidence yet, it wouldn't hurt to take a multivitamin/mineral supplement every day.

Wear sunscreen. Unless you work on a submarine, you're bound to spend some time in the sun. The best thing that you can do to protect your skin from the sun's harmful rays is to wear sunscreen. "I recommend sunscreen with an SPF (sun protection factor) of at least 15 and full UVB/UVA protection," Dr. Fewkes says. And if you're going to be outside for a while, you should reapply the sunscreen every 2 to 3 hours, she adds.

Get tested. Cancer's a mysterious disease. You can do everything right from not smoking to eating a healthy diet and still find a lump that turns out to be malignant. Perhaps that's because the disease often has a genetic component—especially when it comes to melanoma, breast cancer, and colon cancer. Since you can't lower your cancer risk 100 percent, it's important to undergo screenings that can detect a tumor before you even have symptoms—when the cancer is most curable.

To help detect breast cancer in its earliest stages, women should have a yearly mammogram starting in their forties and should do self-exams every month, according to the National Cancer Institute. They should also have a clinical breast exam as part of their annual gynecological checkup. Some doctors suggest women begin getting yearly mammograms at age 50, but research shows that women under age 50 whose breast cancer was found through mammography had a 90 percent chance of survival. That's compared to the 77 percent survival rate of women whose cancer was found during a clinical breast exam.

To catch colorectal cancer—which is highly curable when found early—women over age 50 should have a fecal occult blood test at least every 2 years. An 18-year study by researchers at the University of Minnesota found that this simple test can lead to a 33 percent reduction in deaths when done every year. When the test was done every 2 years, the drop in deaths was 21 percent.

To head off skin cancer, you should see a dermatologist for a full-body screening every year if you're 41 or older and every 3 years if you're between the ages of 20 and 40. And you should also be on the lookout for any changes in your freckles and moles—it turns out that about half of all melanomas are found by the patient.

ALZHEIMER'S DISEASE: PIECING TOGETHER THE PUZZLE

Alzheimer's disease. Those two words strike fear in the hearts of many women. That's partly because until the 1980s we didn't know much about the disease. Now we do.

Many complex processes slowly occur in the brains of Alzheimer's patients. For starters, a protein fragment called beta amyloid builds up around nerve cells, forming dense deposits called plaques. Inside these nerve cells are twisted strands or tangles of fiber. In the regions attacked by Alzheimer's, some nerve cells die. Others lose their connections or *synapses* with nearby nerve cells. "Basically the brain is dying," says Claudia Kawas, M.D., associate professor of neurology and clinical director of Johns Hopkins Alzheimer's Disease Research Center in Baltimore.

More women than men develop Alzheimer's, most likely because women tend to live longer, Dr. Kawas says. The only known risk factors for the disease are age and genetics. "The risk of developing Alzheimer's doubles with every 5 years of life starting at age 65." And those with a family history of the disease have nearly double the risk.

There is currently no cure for Alzheimer's, but researchers are now focusing on three potential treatments.

The first is estrogen. A 14-year study of more than 8,000 women found that those on hormone-replacement therapy were 35 percent less likely to develop Alzheimer's.

The second uses nonsteroidal anti-inflammatory drugs like ibuprofen. In one study, people who took ibuprofen frequently had half the risk of developing Alzheimer's.

The third uses antioxidants such as vitamin E. In a study of 341 people with midstage Alzheimer's disease, those taking high doses of vitamin E were able to perform daily activities 25 percent longer. Supplementation of vitamin E also delayed entrance to nursing homes by an average of 7 months.

We probably haven't found a single cause or treatment yet because one may not exist, Dr. Kawas says. "Instead, what I think we're going to find is that Alzheimer's is like cancer in that there are several types of the same disease, each responding to different therapies."

Diabetes

Diabetes affects more than 15 million people in the United States—about 8 million of them women. And the majority of people with diabetes are age 65 and older. The disease becomes more common as we age for a couple of reasons. We tend to gain weight gradually over the years, and that puts us at greater risk for diabetes. And diabetes often goes undiagnosed for many years, making it appear that older people are more prone to the disease, but in reality, it's probably far more common among the middle-aged population than we realize, says Judith Gore Gearhart, M.D., associate professor of family medicine at the University of Mississippi Medical Center in Jackson.

People with type 2, or adult-onset, diabetes have elevated levels of the sugar glucose in their blood. This sugar buildup has two causes: either the body isn't producing enough insulin, which it uses to break down and utilize glucose, or the insulin is no longer doing its job properly. Oftentimes it's a combination of the two. Elevated glucose levels can lead to a whole host of complications, including blindness, kidney disease, and nervous system disease. People with diabetes also are two to four times more likely to have heart disease or a stroke than adults without diabetes.

There *are* key lifestyle factors that can significantly lower your risk for diabetes. The following suggestions from our experts can help you prevent the disease and the many complications that come with it.

Watch your weight. People who are overweight are much more likely to develop diabetes. "As a person gains more and more weight, they become insulin resistant," Dr. Gearhart says. That means the receptors in the cells that help insulin work are not sensitive to the insulin. The receptors are like a lock and insulin is the key—but when you're insulin resistant, the two don't fit. "Losing weight improves insulin sensitivity and helps tremendously with glucose control," she says. "In fact, many people are able to control their diabetes without medication when they lose enough weight."

Get moving. Regular exercise can also improve insulin sensitivity and can help you lose weight, Dr. Gearhart says. In fact, aerobic exercise almost immediately improves your blood sugar level and your insulin response—at least temporarily. And if you do it every day, it becomes a long-term effect, explains John Duncan, Ph.D., an exercise physiologist at Texas Woman's University Center for Research on Women's Health in Denton. That's why we recommend that people with diabetes exercise 5 days a week, he says.

Request the test. Diabetes tends to run in families. If you have a family history—or if you're overweight, have high blood pressure, high cholesterol, or any symptoms like intense thirst or frequent urination—ask your doctor about getting a fasting plasma glucose test, which measures the amount of glucose in your blood after an 8-hour fast. The earlier you catch diabetes, the earlier you can control it. "Many people have the disease for several years before being diagnosed," Dr. Gearhart says. "And as a result, they may already have organ damage."

Everyone age 45 or older should be tested, whether you have a family history or not. If the results of the test are normal, it should be repeated every third year after that.

Digestive Problems

A number of digestive problems tend to creep up as we age. One is diverticulosis, a condition especially common in people over 50, where the lining of the intestine bulges outward, forming tiny pouches called diverticula. These pouches are created by pressure that builds up from waste in the colon. The condition is usually painless, but if the pouches become infected, it can lead to a painful and more serious condition called diverticulitis.

Older people are also five times more likely to be constipated, and chronic constipation can lead to diverticulosis as well as hemorrhoids. And the over-60 crowd tends to have lower amounts of acid in their stomachs, which makes them more prone to gastritis (inflammation of the stomach lining).

Plus, painful gallstones affect about one in five people over age 65—most of them women—partly because the gallbladder may not contract as well when we're older, explains Melissa Palmer, M.D., a gastroenterologist and hepatologist in Plainview, New York. As a result, the stuff in the gallbladder that helps your body digest fat may form into hard stones, and they can clog up the ducts in the gallbladder or those that lead into the small intestine.

All of these digestive complaints can be treated, but there are steps you can take that may help prevent them as well. With these dietary and other preventive measures, you and your gut can be problem-free well into your seventies and beyond.

Get your fill of fiber. Eating a high-fiber diet can help prevent a number of digestive problems, including constipation, hemorrhoids, diverticulosis, and perhaps even gallstones. That's mainly because diets that are high in fiber lower the pressure generated in the bowel, says Susan Gordon, M.D., professor of medicine at MCP–Hahnemann University in Philadelphia. Experts recommend getting between 25 and 35

LIFE EXTENDER
Slow Heart—Long Life

The express aisle. Fast food. Speed dial. In today's frantically paced world, quick often equals quality. But when it comes to longevity, it turns out slower is better. Research shows women who have slower hearts live longer.

A study of more than 7,000 French women found that those with lower resting heart rates were less likely to die of almost any cause than those with higher heart rates. What's the best way to slow down a fast heart? With regular aerobic exercise, experts say. Just make sure to see a doctor before starting any exercise program.

grams of fiber a day. Try spreading out your fiber intake by eating foods like raisin bran, oatmeal, a sandwich on whole-wheat bread, broccoli, or an apple at every meal. Or you can take psyllium, which is a natural fiber supplement such as Metamucil, she says.

Flush out your pipes. Another way to lower pressure in the bowel is to drink enough fluids. "You need adequate fluids for proper bowel function in general," Dr. Gordon says. "And for fiber to work properly, you need adequate fluid in the bowel." A good rule of thumb is to drink at least eight 8-ounce glasses of fluids like water and juices every day. But beverages that contain caffeine or alcohol actually make you lose more fluids than you take in because of their diuretic effect. So don't count them toward your eight a day.

Lose weight slowly. Women who are overweight are more prone to getting gallstones, Dr. Gordon says. But losing weight too quickly can also put you at risk for developing the painful stones. So can yo-yo dieting, which is when you frequently lose weight and gain it back. That's one reason doctors recommend losing no more than 1 to 2 pounds a week.

Get off the couch. Physical activity can help keep you regular. Exercise gives your metabolism a boost, increases blood flow to the bowel, and helps the wastes move through your body faster, Dr. Gordon says.

Check your meds. If you frequently take aspirin or nonsteroidal anti-inflammatory drugs like Advil for arthritis or another condition, you may be putting yourself at risk for digestive problems. These drugs—when taken every day—can sometimes injure the stomach, which can lead to chronic conditions like gastritis and ulcers, Dr. Gordon says. If cutting back on the drugs isn't an option, taking enteric-coated pills can help, but it won't eliminate the risk, Dr. Palmer says.

Heart Disease and Stroke

Ask most people what the leading cause of death is for women, and they'll probably say breast cancer. Good guess, but it's wrong. Heart disease is the number one killer of both men *and* women in this country. In fact, a woman's risk of dying from a heart attack is five times greater than that of dying from breast cancer.

Most women are unaware of their heart disease risk because they think it's a man's disease—as did many doctors for a long time, Dr. Ross says. The focus has probably been on men because they tend to develop heart disease a decade earlier than women, she says. "We think that estrogen may be what protects women before they hit menopause," she adds.

Stroke—which is like a heart attack that occurs in the brain—is the third leading cause of death in this country. A stroke usually occurs when a blood vessel in the brain is blocked, either by a blood clot or by the same plaque buildup that can cause a heart attack. As a result, part of the brain is starved of blood and oxygen, and the cells in that area die.

Heart attacks and strokes both occur suddenly, but the conditions that cause them take years to develop. For starters, artery-clogging cholesterol builds up slowly over time. We tend to gain weight gradually as we grow older. And most people with diabetes—which is a major risk factor for heart disease and stroke—are age 65 or older. High blood pressure, another major risk factor for both diseases, is more common in women age 55 and older. "Heart disease and stroke have a lot of contributing risk factors," Dr. Ross says. "And many of those risk factors become more common as we age."

Since the two diseases have many similar causes and risk factors, most of the measures you can take to prevent one disease prevent the other as well. Take diet, for example. Eating low-fat, high-fiber fare prevents both heart disease and stroke by keeping your weight and blood pressure down and your arteries clear. Controlling your weight—especially the pounds that tend to stick to your middle—lowers your risk for both diseases. And so does reducing stress. When you're under stress, your body produces chemicals that over time can cause your arteries and blood vessels to stiffen—and that sets the stage for cholesterol buildup, Dr. Ross explains. So find ways to destress. Exercise, take a hot bath, read a romance novel—whatever works for you.

There are plenty of other ways to head off heart disease and stroke. Here are more strategies to help disease-proof both your heart and brain.

Kick the habit. The experts we talked to said the most important thing women can do to cut their risk for heart disease is to quit smoking—or better yet—never to start in the first place. "You quit smoking today, and your risk of heart disease goes down by tomorrow," Dr. Ross says. "Patients always say the damage has already been done, so it won't matter if they quit. It absolutely matters." Within 3 months of quitting, your circulation improves. After a year, your heart disease risk is half that of a smoker. And by 15 years, your risk is the same as that of a nonsmoker.

Smoking is a risk factor for stroke as well. In fact, it's probably the second highest risk factor after high blood pressure, Dr. Rexrode says. That's because smoking constricts blood vessels, speeds up the formation of plaque deposits, and makes it easier for blood clots to form. So putting out that cigarette for good will benefit both your heart *and* your head.

Find time to get physical. Regular exercise prevents heart disease and stroke in a number of ways. For starters, physical activity lowers blood pressure and stress levels and improves cholesterol by raising HDL levels. It also helps you to stay slim. Aerobic exercises, such as brisk walking, cycling, and swimming, help keep your cardiovascular system in great shape. "Exercise tackles all those things that put us at risk for heart disease and stroke," Dr. Ross says.

Mind your peas and cantaloupes. Fruits and vegetables contain all sorts of heart- and brain-friendly compounds from antioxidants to minerals like potassium, which helps by lowering blood pressure, Dr. Ross says. In fact, a study of more than 87,000 nurses found that women who ate the most fruits and vegetables were 40 percent less likely to have a stroke than those who ate the least. And experts say that munching on at least five servings of produce a day is good for your heart, too.

Call in a replacement. Women who have used hormone-replacement therapy have a 40 to 50 percent lower incidence of heart disease, Dr. Legato says. Estrogen's protective effect helps explain why the heart disease rate in women greatly increases after menopause. Estrogen protects the heart in several ways. First, the hormone has a positive effect on cholesterol. It

keeps the levels of HDL—that's the "good" cholesterol—up. It can also lower blood pressure by keeping blood vessels relaxed and wide open.

"I think every woman should consider hormone-replacement therapy," Dr. Ross says. "One of the newest estrogen therapies may actually be protective against breast cancer as well."

Hormone-replacement therapy may help prevent strokes, too. In one study that compared long-term users of postmenopausal estrogen to nonusers, the women who took estrogen had a 73 percent reduction in risk of death from vascular problems—including stroke. With all of estrogen's possible benefits, women really should talk to their doctors about whether hormone-replacement therapy is right for them, Dr. Ross says.

Take some extra E. Antioxidants such as vitamin E can help protect your heart from the ravages of free radicals—harmful oxygen molecules your body produces that damage tissues throughout the body. Inside your body, rogue free-radical molecules cause cholesterol to cling to artery walls and clog them up. Vitamin E can help prevent the cholesterol buildup by getting rid of free radicals before they do any damage.

The evidence is so convincing that some doctors even recommend vitamin E to their patients. "I recommend that my patients take supplemental vitamin E, because it can be hard to get enough of in a low-fat diet," says Dr. Ross, who suggests women take between 200 and 400 international units (IU) a day.

As for stroke, the research hasn't clearly shown that vitamin E can prevent stroke, Dr. Rexrode says. "There are much more convincing data for heart disease," she adds.

Go nuts. Research shows that nuts such as almonds, walnuts, and peanuts can be an important part of a heart-healthy diet. A 10-year study of more than 86,000 women by researchers at the Harvard School of Public Health found that

LIFE EXTENDER

Get the Benefits of Wine without Imbibing

We've all heard the news about booze: One glass of red wine a day can lower your risk of heart disease. But for those of us who don't make a habit of uncorking the Chianti, there are still ways to enjoy the health benefits of wine—such as guzzling a glass of grape juice.

The flavonoids found in both red wine and purple grape juice help prevent blood platelets from clumping, so they're less likely to form clots that can trigger a heart attack. One study by researchers at the University of Wisconsin found that folks who drank two 5-ounce glasses of purple grape juice a day for a week reduced the tendency for blood clots to form by 60 percent. Just make sure you choose purple grape juice made from Concord grapes. Red and white grape juices don't have the same effect.

women who ate more than 5 ounces of nuts a week were about a third less likely to develop heart disease than those eating less than an ounce a month. The unsaturated fats found in nuts help to lower cholesterol and may be what gives the nuts their protective effect, suggest researchers. Nuts are also high in other heart-healthy substances: vitamin E, potassium, magnesium, protein, and fiber. So if you're a frequent flier, don't pass on the cashews.

Take care of your teeth. What's the connection between your teeth, your heart, and your brain? It turns out that the bacteria that cause gum disease can travel through the bloodstream to your heart, where it can damage the heart walls or valves, explains Dr. Ross. The bacteria may also cause the release of clotting factors that can trigger a heart attack or stroke, she adds. Common signs of gum disease are red, swollen gums and bleeding after brushing. To keep your gums—and your heart and brain—healthy, brush your teeth at least twice a day, floss once a day, and see your dentist regularly, she suggests.

Osteoporosis

Ten million people in the United States have osteoporosis—and 80 percent of them are women. The problem is, you may not even know you have the disease until your bones become so weak that a bump or minor fall causes a fracture. In fact, one out of every two women will have an osteoporosis-related fracture in their lifetime, according to the National Osteoporosis Foundation. Women are more prone to developing osteoporosis because the steep drop in estrogen at menopause speeds up bone loss.

Even so, doctors are sending the message to women that this is not really an illness of aging. "It has been said that osteoporosis is not a geriatric disease, but a pediatric disease—and that's largely the truth," says Stanley Wallach, M.D., clinical professor of medicine at New York University School of Medicine, codirector of the Osteoporosis Center at the Hospital for Joint Diseases, and director of the American College of Nutrition, all in New York City. That's because behaviors that lead to osteoporosis—such as not getting enough calcium—often begin in childhood. Still, doctors agree it's never too late to bone up on bone. Just be aware that the older you are, the lower your baseline bone mass will be when you start.

Even if you're no teenager, experts say these five strategies can help strengthen your skeleton.

Nibble the right nutrients. Eating a calcium-rich diet from the time you're a little girl is the best way to build and maintain strong bones, says Dr. Sherrer, who is also author of *A Woman Doctor's Guide to Osteoporosis.* But for many teens and young women, milk, cheese, and other sources of calcium are off-limits. That's because these foods are typically high in fat, and girls in our culture are concerned about their weight at a very young age, Dr. Sherrer says. As a result, they're not building adequate bone during their peak developmental years and end up putting themselves at risk for osteoporosis later in life.

Even women way past their teen years can benefit from getting enough calcium. You may not be able to *add* bone, but you can maintain what you have, Dr. Wallach says. The bottom line is that premenopausal women need 1,000 milligrams of calcium a day through diet and supplements plus 400 IU of vitamin D, which helps your body absorb calcium. Postmenopausal women need even more: 1,500 milligrams of calcium and between 600 and 800 IU of vitamin D.

Get active. Physical activity is another key preventive measure that should be started at an early age and continued throughout life. Regular exercise—both aerobic, like fast walking, and lifting light weights—not only strengthens and maintains the bone you have but can also increase your bone mass. As you build and strengthen muscle—which is attached to your bones—you build bone as well, Dr. Sherrer explains. Try to work in at least 30 minutes of weight-bearing activity like brisk walking at least three times a week. Other weight-bearing activities, which simply means that they require you to bear your own body weight, include running, dancing, tennis, even bowling. Swimming and cycling, on the other hand, are not weight-bearing.

Measure your bone mass. Women should get a baseline bone-density test somewhere around the onset of menopause followed by a screening about one year after the start of menopause, says Dr. Wallach. Doctors can compare the numbers then to see if you've lost (or have failed to acquire enough) bone. If you have a family history of osteoporosis, you should be tested even earlier. The typical test is called the DEXA, which is a quick and painless x-ray that measures the density of the hip and spine.

Consider using hormone-replacement therapy. Giving women synthetic estrogen once their bodies have stopped producing their own can greatly reduce the risk of osteoporosis. That's because women who aren't taking estrogen can lose up to 20 percent of their bone mass in the 5 to 7 years following menopause, making them more susceptible to osteoporosis. Hormone-replacement therapy helps by preserving the bone you have, and in some cases it can add bone, Dr. Sherrer says. As with taking any prescription drug, hormone-replacement therapy is not without risks—certain kinds of estrogen, if taken inappropriately, may cause a small increase in your risk for breast cancer. So talk to your doctor about whether hormone-replacement therapy is right for you.

Avoid the big three. Another way to prevent further bone loss is to participate in the social graces as little as possible, Dr. Wallach says. "What I mean by that is smoking, alcohol use, and excessive caffeine use," he says. "All of these promote bone loss at any age."

How much is too much? Any amount of smoking is detrimental—not only to your bones but to your cardiovascular system as well, Dr. Wallach says. One alcoholic drink a day is okay, but drinking more than one a day may weaken your bones. And when it comes to caffeine, more than three cups of coffee a day or the equivalent in cola drinks can cause bone loss. So stick to decaf.

PART FIVE

Doctors'
Best Disease
Fighters

Colds, Sore Throats, and Flu

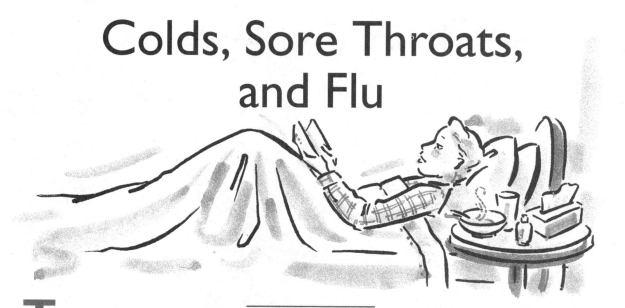

The common cold costs the American economy 15 million days in lost work every year. Influenza drives the number even higher. So what? If you have a cold or the flu right now, you want relief, not statistics.

Unfortunately, as everyone knows, there is no way to cure a cold or influenza once you're infected. But there are steps that you can take to help your body cope and heal as quickly as possible. Better yet, there are strategies that you can use to avoid coming down with these illnesses altogether.

Risk Factors

The most obvious risk factor for catching the cold or flu is exposure to the germs that cause it, but that doesn't necessarily mean standing in the direct line of fire of a sneeze or cough, says Carlene Muto, M.D., director of infection control and epidemiology in the division of infectious diseases at the University of Pittsburgh Medical Center. Although both diseases can be transmitted through the air, colds are actually more likely to be spread by touch. "All you need to do is touch something that someone sick touched or coughed on or sneezed on, then touch your own face, nose, or mouth," she says.

Time of year is also a risk factor. Colds and flu have a season, and it's fall/winter, says Dr. Muto. That's because in cold weather you spend more time indoors, in close quarters, and have more opportunity to be infected with germs and to infect others.

The rhinovirus (a virus that can cause the common cold) has a season that actually peaks in September and early October. The start of a new school year may be another contributing factor, as respiratory illness is more easily spread in the classroom and then is brought home to the other members of the family.

Some researchers also believe that your menstrual cycle, allergies that affect your nose and throat, and emotional stress can all make you more liable to catch a cold.

People with weakened immunity due to some other illness, poor nutrition, stress, or smoking are not at an increased risk of viral exposure; however, once exposed to a cold or flu virus, their bodies may be less capable of fighting off the infection, Dr. Muto says. Some types of respiratory allergies can also alter the mucous membranes in the nose and throat, making you more vulnerable to viral infections.

On the other hand, it's also true that if you've just had a cold, you're less likely to pick up another one right away. We're exposed to more than 100 types of cold viruses, and each type is distinct. Once you've had one of them, you develop an immunity to that particular virus that lasts about 2 years. You also develop a generalized immunity that protects you against the other 99 cold viruses for about a month.

Prevention

The steps to prevent colds and flu are simple and effective, but they require that you be vigilant, break old habits, and create new ones.

Flee from sneezers. Stay away from people who are coughing and sneezing. If you can't avoid them altogether, try not to get too close, and make your visits as brief as possible.

Wash up. Often, that rids your hands of any nasty viruses that may be waiting for a ride up to your nose or mouth.

Put your hands down. To make doubly sure that no cold or flu germs find their way into your body, keep your hands away from your face even after you have washed.

WOMEN ASK WHY

Why can't you get Lyme disease from a regular tick—and what's a deer tick, anyway?

*B*orrelia burgdorferi, the spiral-shaped organism that transmits Lyme disease, can move from a tick's midgut to its salivary glands in only two species: the deer tick in the Northeast and Midwest and the Pacific tick in the Northwest. Once the organism is in the tick's salivary glands, it can be injected into the bloodstream of whatever the tick snacks on—animals and humans. In general, the tick has to be attached for 36 to 48 hours before the Lyme disease organism is transmitted. So you have some time to remove the tick while your risk of getting Lyme disease remains low.

A deer tick is smaller than the common dog tick, the kind you're most likely to recognize. In its nymph stage, the deer tick is the size of a poppy seed. When it is engorged with blood, however, it can blow up to five times this size. An adult deer tick is about the size of a sesame seed and can get as big as a Raisinet after sucking your blood for a few days.

It can be difficult to tell an engorged deer tick from a regular tick. If you've been bitten, you may want to save the tick and ask someone from your local health department to identify the species. Most doctors do not prescribe antibiotics for a deer tick bite unless you develop symptoms of Lyme disease—skin rash around the site, headache, fever, stiff neck, aches and pains, and fatigue. If you are pregnant when you are bitten, however, prophylactic antibiotics are prescribed. A vaccine is recommended for people living in areas with a high prevalence of Lyme disease. It requires three shots: two given a month apart, usually in April and May, and one given a year after the first shot.

Expert consulted
Clarita E. Herrera, M.D.
Clinical instructor in primary care
New York Medical College
Valhalla

Disinfect. Three hours—that's how long rhinoviruses can live on surfaces outside a human body. Scrubbing those surfaces down with a virus-killing disinfectant may help stop the spread of disease.

Take a shot. Getting your annual flu vaccination shot is one of the nicest things that you can do for yourself. So do it.

Take a good multivitamin. So many vitamins and minerals are involved in proper immunity that it's a mistake to zero in on some and neglect the others, says Rachel Wissner, M.D., a family practitioner in Baton Rouge, Louisiana. A good multi will cover your bases.

Chew less fat. Fats, especially polyunsaturated fats, tend to suppress the immune system. Cut your total fat intake to 25 percent or less of your daily calories, says Dr. Wissner.

Destress—or else. Long-term psychological stress can inhibit many aspects of the immune response, including natural killer cell activity, T cell response, and antibody production. If you're getting lots of colds, you may need to consider stress as a factor, experts say.

There are lots of ways to reduce stress—exercise, meditation, breathing exercises. The trick is to find a balance that works well for you. It's not so surprising that the same nutrients that help ward off colds and flu, such as vitamins C and E and zinc, play a role in the body's production of stress hormones and in the hormones that help keep you relaxed.

HOW TO USE A THERMOMETER

What is a normal temperature for one person may not be quite the same for another, says Clarita E. Herrera, M.D., clinical instructor in primary care at New York Medical College in Valhalla. Generally speaking, a normal oral reading would be about 98.6°F. Rectal readings usually run a degree higher, at 99.6°; and axillary (or armpit) readings run 0.5 to 1 degree lower than oral.

Mercury thermometers used to be considered the gold standard, the most accurate, for taking a temperature, but digital thermometers now work just as well and are safer since they don't break.

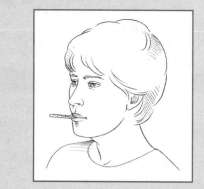

To use a mercury thermometer, shake it down, using quick flicks of your wrist, until it reads less than 96°F. Place the bulb under your tongue, just to one side of the center. Keep your lips closed; breathe through your nose. (If you have a stuffy nose, you can take a rectal or underarm temperature instead.) Leave the thermometer in place for 4 minutes.

Digital thermometers are safe, accurate, and fast. Look for one that claims to be accurate to within at least 0.2 degree. Some are accurate within 0.02 degree, but these may be a little more expensive. With most digital types, readings are obtained within a minute. The temperature is displayed much like the numbers on digital wristwatches.

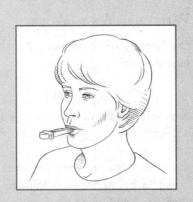

The digital thermometer can be used under the tongue, in the rectum, or in the armpit. Since turning the thermometer off clears the display, you do not need to shake it down beforehand. Usually, a beep or series of beeps indicates that the reading is done.

Ear (infrared) thermometers are accurate, quick, and relatively comfortable, but using one correctly requires some training. Follow package instructions carefully. The temperature is taken by placing the small cone-shaped end of the thermometer in the ear canal. The thermometer usually gives a reading within seconds.

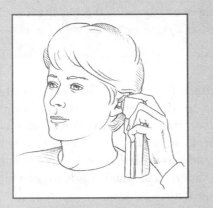

Heat given off by the eardrum and surrounding tissue is used to calculate body temperature. The thermometer converts the temperature to an oral or rectal reading and displays it on a digital screen.

Signs and Symptoms

Cold symptoms usually start 2 to 3 days after you have been infected, and include a sore throat, cough, headache, sneezing, and a clogged, runny nose. You may also have a slight fever of less than 100°F.

Flu symptoms usually appear within 2 to 4 days of your being infected. You're likely to have a headache, chills, and a dry cough, followed by body aches, fever, nasal congestion, and sore throat. The flu is highly contagious, and you can spread the virus for another 3 to 4 days after your symptoms appear.

Who Do I See?

Colds are a leading cause of visits to the family doctor, and people frequently receive antibiotics for colds when they do not need them. Colds are caused by viruses, not bacteria, and antibiotics won't faze them. "Sometimes, though, a cold can lead to a secondary bacterial infection of the middle ear or sinuses, in which case antibiotics may be in order," says Dr. Muto. "A high fever, shortness of breath, significantly swollen glands, severe facial pain in the sinuses, or a persistent cough that produces mucus all suggest you may have more than a simple cold and should see a doctor soon."

What Can I Expect?

Cold symptoms can last from 2 to 14 days, but two-thirds of all people infected recover in a week.

Flu viruses, on the other hand, have a whole-body effect that can leave you feeling tired for weeks. Give yourself up to 2 weeks to ease back into your normal routine. You will bounce back faster than if you push yourself, Dr. Muto says.

Conventional Wisdom

Many conventional doctors will tell you that there's not much they can do for you when you have a cold except advise you to get lots of rest and drink plenty of fluids. As for chicken soup, it actually may help. Sipping hot broth helps keep protective mucous layers in your nose and throat flowing, which in turn flushes away cold virus particles.

Here's what else traditional doctors suggest.

Take your pharmaceuticals. If you are coming down with the flu, you can take prescription antiviral drugs such as amantadine (Symmetrel) or rimantadine (Flumadine). If started within 2 days of symptoms, antiviral drugs can decrease the severity of symptoms and the duration of a bout of the flu. These drugs, however, work for only one kind of flu, called Type A.

Instead, your doctor may recommend a prescription powder inhaled through the mouth, called zanamivir (Relenza). In a study, this drug reduced the duration of a bout of the flu by a day or two. It also cut the chance of catching the flu by 72 percent. This drug works for two types of flu, A and B. A pill form of the flu antiviral drug oseltamivir (Tamiflu) is also available by prescription.

Use a humidifier. Dry air dries out your nasal membranes, making them less resistant to

WOMEN ASK WHY

Do I really have to get a flu shot every year?

Getting a flu shot is one of the best bargains in medicine. It really can protect you from getting the flu, and in a worst-case scenario, it might just save your life.

The influenza vaccine is actually a killed virus or a mix of viruses, and it works by making your immune system develop antibodies. So if and when your body becomes exposed to the virus, those antibodies are set to attack. Additionally, the antibody-producing part of your immune system actually has a memory. So if it has made antibodies against a particular virus once and is exposed to the same virus again, it can crank up production much faster the second time. It's almost as though it had the template already made.

Each year, a vaccine is made for whatever strains are most likely to strike, based on analyses of flu outbreaks around the world.

Vaccination is recommended for all people age 65 or older and people of any age with chronic diseases of the heart, lung, or kidneys; diabetes; compromised immune systems; or

attack from viruses. Keep your air humidity at 35 to 45 percent, Dr. Muto recommends. Indoor air-conditioning can be just as drying as heat, so you'll want to adjust your cooling system as well. If you're congested at night, keep a vaporizer at your bedside to get a direct shot of moist air.

Great Alternatives

There are hundreds of self-care herbal and nutritional remedies that can minimize the symptoms of a cold or flu, help you recover energy faster, and ward off future infections. "The

severe forms of anemia or asthma. It is also recommended for people who live in nursing homes or other places where people with chronic medical conditions live, for health-care workers, and for people who live in a household with a person who fits into any of these categories. Also, children or teenagers receiving long-term aspirin therapy, who therefore may be at risk for developing Reye's syndrome after a flu infection, should get vaccinated, as should women who will be in the second or third trimester of pregnancy during the flu season (which is November to April, making September through mid-November the best time to get the vaccine).

Most people don't have any side effects from a flu shot, but some feel soreness at the shot spot or develop a headache and slight fever for about a day after the vaccination.

A flu vaccine in the form of a nasal spray rather than a shot is expected to be available for the 2001–2002 flu season. The preventive whiff may eventually prove more protective than a shot.

Expert consulted
Clarita E. Herrera, M.D.
Clinical instructor in primary care
New York Medical College
Valhalla

trick is to pick the ones that work best for you, given your symptoms," says Jasmine Carino, N.D., a naturopathic physician with the Canadian College of Naturopathic Medicine in Toronto. Here are the details.

Don't skimp on the vitamin C. You need to take 1,000 to 3,000 milligrams a day of vitamin C to reduce your cold symptoms, Dr. Carino says. "You want to increase your dosage until you begin to have loose stools, then back off a bit." In studies that used this range of dosages, cold symptoms and durations were reduced by about 30 percent. Doses under 1,000 milligrams were ineffective.

Take 250 to 500 milligrams every few hours as soon as you are aware that a cold is coming on, and continue taking it for a few days more, even if your symptoms start to wane.

If you've had kidney stones or gallstones, take a smaller dose, up to 1,000 milligrams a day.

Add echinacea. "Of dozens of herbs used to treat colds and flu, echinacea, or purple coneflower, is one of the best," says Dr. Carino. Echinacea contains a diverse array of active components that stimulate different functions of the immune system to mount a response to a virus or bacteria.

Here again, it's best to start taking echinacea at the first signs of a cold or flu. How much you take depends on the severity of your symptoms. For the worst colds, take 1/2 to 1 teaspoon of a liquid form (tincture or extract) every 2 hours. As symptoms improve, gradually decrease the dosage and frequency to 1/4 teaspoon three times a day, Dr. Carino says.

Don't use echinacea if you're allergic to closely related plants, such as ragweed, asters, and chrysanthemums. Don't use it if you have tuberculosis or an autoimmune condition, such as lupus or multiple sclerosis.

Suck on zinc. You may be able to cut your symptoms of sore throat, coughing, and nasal congestion from 8 to 4 days if you use zinc gluconate tablets or lozenges, according to a study done at the Cleveland Clinic. How much do you need to do the trick? In the Cleveland study, participants took a daily average of 4 to 8 lozenges containing 13.3 milligrams of zinc. This dose was effective. Possible side effects are nausea and a bad residual taste. Zinc's effectiveness in relieving cold symptoms is controversial.

STREP THROAT

Streptococci bacteria are nothing to fool around with. Strep throat infections range from mild to severe. In severe cases, fever, chills, headache, and abdominal pain may occur. Strep can simply invade your throat, causing severe pain, or it can become deadly, moving into your bloodstream where the poisons it produces can cause toxic shock syndrome or lead to heart or kidney damage.

Strep throat is spread just like colds and flu, through contact with someone infected with the bug. Children often bring it home and sometimes infect other family members. Symptoms usually appear 1 to 3 days after exposure and include painful, red tonsils or throat; a fever; swollen lymph glands in your neck; and, sometimes, white dots of pus on your tonsils or the back of your throat.

It's hard to tell just by looking at your throat whether you have strep or some other throat infection. "Even doctors can diagnose accurately with visual inspection only about 60 percent of the time," says Berrylin Ferguson, M.D., associate professor of otolaryngology at the University of Pittsburgh Medical Center. That's why they vigorously swab the back of the throat to do a culture for bacteria to confirm a diagnosis of strep throat. Sometimes, however, if strep is a suspect, your doctor will simply give you antibiotics. A 10-day course of penicillin is the usual treatment, and it's important to take the drug all 10 days, even if your sore throat is soon gone.

Zinc is thought to help stop viral replication or to prevent viruses from entering cells in this application.

Take zinc lozenges as you feel a sore throat or cold coming on and for up to 2 days after you have recuperated, Dr. Carino says. You can find zinc gluconate lozenges at drugstores.

Hold the sugar. Sugar inhibits phagocytosis, the process by which viruses and bacteria are engulfed and then destroyed by white blood cells, says Dr. Carino.

Inhale herbal vapors. Throw a teaspoon of dried basil, thyme, or oregano into a pot of steaming hot water and inhale the steam for a few minutes to unplug your sinuses and soothe your mucous membranes, Dr. Carino says. "It's great. Both have menthol properties that aid decongestion." For safe steaming, remove the pot from the stove and place it on a stable, heat-resistant surface. Drape a towel over your head and shoulders to enclose steam. Keep your face at least 12 inches from the water to avoid burns.

Get your body moving. Moderate exercise is an immune booster. It takes about a half-hour of aerobic exercise to sweep back into circulation white blood cells—key immune system components—that are stuck in your blood vessel walls. Studies also show that the number of certain immune system cells increases, at least temporarily, following exercise. Ideally, you should get a half-hour of aerobic exercise 5 days a week.

If you are actually coming down with something, listen to your body and pay attention to your symptoms, Dr. Carino says. Some people find that exercise makes them feel better, especially if it makes them sweat; others feel they need to rest.

Allow yourself to run a bit of a fever. Your fever is there for a purpose—to help your immune system destroy the enemy. An adult can safely run a fever of up to 102°F for a day or two while fighting a cold, Dr. Carino says. Support your body during this time by drinking lots of fluids and by resting.

Cold Sores, Chapped Lips, and Gum Problems

A passionate kiss between lovers. A hearty laugh between friends. A tender smile between mother and child. For some of life's simplest pleasures, we have our mouths to thank. So let's give them the respect they deserve.

"The best thing a woman can do to keep the inside of her mouth healthy is brush and floss regularly," says Esther Rubin, D.D.S., a dentist in New York City. "Proper self-care can prevent most, if not all, teeth and gum problems."

Poor dental hygiene can lead to trouble down the line, starting with gingivitis and ending with periodontitis, serious gum deterioration that can lead to tooth loss if it is not treated in time. To nip tooth problems in the bud, here's what to do.

Gingivitis

Gingivitis is a form of gum disease caused when dental plaque (a gluelike film of bacteria, food, and saliva) invades the warm and inviting crevasses at and below the gum line. There it hardens into tartar (sometimes called calculus), triggering inflammation and infection.

Left untreated, gingivitis can lead to periodontitis, a condition characterized by severely receding gums and, ultimately, destruction of the jawbone, which anchors your teeth in place. But gingivitis doesn't have to get nearly that far. Combine the following strategies with regular brushing and flossing to combat gingivitis and keep your gums in the pink. If your gums continue to bleed each time you brush, make an appointment to see your dentist.

Make your own herbal toothpaste. Mix one tablespoon of the herb goldenseal in dried form with enough water to form a paste. Then brush your teeth as you normally would. Goldenseal, which is available in health food stores, can help heal inflamed, diseased gums. (If you are allergic to plants in the daisy family, goldenseal may cause an allergic reaction.)

Brush with baking soda. Mix baking soda with enough hydrogen peroxide to form a paste. With your toothbrush, gently rub the mixture onto your gums. Leave it on for a few minutes, then rinse.

Sip a soothing tea. Add two tablespoons of the dried herb anise and two tablespoons of

WOMAN TO WOMAN

She Cured Her Gingivitis and Kept Her Smile

Henrietta Johnson, 43, the owner of a pet service in New York City, was in danger of losing her teeth before she used natural remedies to turn the situation around. Here's her story.

When I was a kid, I had great teeth—not a cavity in my mouth. Then, when I was around 19 or 20, I started getting a barrage of cavities. My gums were in trouble, too. I'd eat an apple and they'd bleed—a classic sign of gingivitis. At that time, I was brushing my teeth once a day and I wasn't flossing at all.

Then a few years ago during a routine dental visit, my dentist found a 10-millimeter pocket between my back lower molar and the surrounding gum. Smaller pockets were forming around other teeth as well. Basically, I was in danger of my gums eventually loosening their hold on my teeth.

My dentist suggested gum surgery to repair the largest pocket. I said, "There has to be something else I can do." I was determined to heal my gums on my own.

I started brushing my teeth twice a day with Weleda Salt Toothpaste. I still do. It doesn't contain saccharin, and the salt helps tighten the gums. At night, I add two drops of tea tree oil to my toothpaste. (Essential oils can be toxic if swallowed, so don't use this on children.) It's a natural—and powerful—antiseptic, and it kills the bacteria that damage the gums. I floss twice a day as well. I take coenzyme Q_{10} every day. It boosts the body's immunity and is an excellent treatment for gum disease. Finally, I get my teeth cleaned four times a year instead of the recommended two times.

After following this regimen for a year, my gums improved dramatically. They don't hurt, they don't bleed, they don't itch, and they're not swollen. And that 10-millimeter pocket? According to my dentist, it actually shrank to 8 millimeters. Those other pockets got smaller, too. If I keep up the routine—keep those pockets clean—I believe that my gums will be okay. And best of all, I avoided surgery.

dried sage (both sold in health food stores) to one cup of freshly boiled water. Allow the herbs to steep for 10 minutes, then strain the tea and drink up. Repeat as needed to relieve sore gums.

Be generous with garlic. Garlic is nature's antibiotic. It helps to fight plaque-forming bacteria, which means that they are less likely to set up shop in your mouth. You can increase your intake of fresh garlic simply by adding it to most of your meals. Worried about garlic breath? Then take supplements instead—250 milligrams a day.

Take your Q. Coenzyme Q_{10} is a natural compound that may help treat gingivitis and can promote healthy gum tissue by increasing the flow of oxygen to cells. You will find coenzyme Q_{10} supplements in health food stores.

Sing for high C. Vitamin C can help gum tissue resist the bacterial onslaught that leads to gingivitis. Take 500 milligrams three times a day.

Note: Some people develop diarrhea when taking high doses of vitamin C. If this happens, cut back your dosage to a tolerable level.

Tooth Discoloration

Beginning in their late thirties, many women notice that their once pearly whites are taking on a different hue. Teeth naturally lose some of their outermost layer—the enamel—over the years. And because the material beneath the enamel is darker, your bright smile will begin to fade.

Unless you have a calcium deficiency, which will require a doctor's intervention, tooth discoloration is essentially a cosmetic problem. The following tips will discourage stains and spiff up your smile.

Whiten wisely. As a natural alternative to home bleaching kits, which can irritate gums, look in your health food store for a product called Peelu. It's a whitener made from tree root extract and sold as a toothpaste and a powder.

Chew gum as a chaser. After drinking coffee or tea, chew a stick of sugarless gum. This stimulates the production of saliva to help wash away the beverage's residues before they stain.

Sip water to stop stains. Out of gum? Then take a swig of water and swish it around your mouth. Water is enough to clean your teeth and prevent stains from building up.

Tooth Grinding

Most women who grind their teeth don't even know until someone else tells them about it. That's because tooth grinding (also called bruxism) often occurs during sleep.

Tooth grinding can lead to a variety of problems, including headaches, jaw pain, tooth sensitivity, and temporomandibular disorder, in which the hinges of the jaw malfunction. If you routinely have tooth or face pain when you wake up, see a dentist.

RAGING HORMONES, BLEEDING GUMS?

You brush. You floss. And still, your gums bleed. What's the deal?

You're a woman.

Menstruation, pregnancy, menopause, and birth control pills all cause hormonal changes that reduce the ability of a woman's gum tissues to fight the bacteria that cause gingivitis, says Barbara A. Rich, D.D.S., a dentist in Cherry Hill, New Jersey.

This hormonal roller coaster can decrease your gums' ability to become tough or less penetrable (what dentists call keratinization), one of the barriers that prevent bacteria from invading and damaging gum tissue, says Dr. Rich.

Bleeding gums can also signal that a woman's physical and emotional health is out of balance, says Andrea Brockman, D.D.S., board member of the Holistic Dental Association in practice at the Valley Green Center for Holistic Dentistry in Philadelphia. Chronic stress, poor diet, and inadequate sleep can weaken the immune system, allowing gum-damaging bacteria to thrive.

To avoid bleeding gums, you should cut back on red meat, sugar, processed foods, caffeine, and alcohol, says Dr. Brockman. "They can make saliva extremely acidic, and bacteria thrive in an acidic environment." Avoid smoking and eat more fish, whole grains, and raw fruits and vegetables. Also, get sufficient refreshing sleep, aerobic exercise, and fresh air and practice some form of stress-reduction technique.

For already sore gums, turn to tea tree, lavender, eucalyptus, or peppermint essential oils to inhibit the growth of bacteria and speed away infection, says Dr. Brockman. If you use a pulsating irrigation device such as a Water Pik or Hydro Floss, add up to five drops of one of these oils in five ounces of distilled water to the reservoir. "The oils will penetrate and stay in the gingival tissues," says Dr. Brockman.

Or, mix up to five drops of one of the oils with a few ounces of distilled water and swish it around in your mouth two or three times a day. (Essential oils can be toxic if swallowed, so don't use this on children.)

Fortunately, you can do things while you're awake to soothe a painful jaw and break the tooth-grinding habit. Here's what dentists recommend.

Get immediate relief with heat. Soak a towel in warm water, wring it out, and wrap it around a hot-water bottle. Apply this compress to your face for 15 to 20 minutes, frequently checking your skin to make sure that it's not getting burned.

Sip herbal tea before snoozing. Considering a nightcap to help you relax? Some research suggests that drinking alcohol before going to bed can exacerbate tooth grinding. Have a cup of herbal tea instead.

Follow the dots. Go to your nearest office supply store and buy a sheet or two of orange dot stickers. Paste them everywhere: on your mirror, your dashboard, and your refrigerator door. Every time you see one, take it as your cue to separate your teeth. This simple trick discourages tooth grinding.

Tooth Sensitivity

Its lightning bolt of pain can turn a sweet experience, like sipping an ice-cold glass of lemonade, sour real fast.

If you have a sensitive tooth, you may decide to deal with it by avoiding whatever triggers your pain. That's fine for a temporary fix. You really need to have the tooth checked out by your dentist to determine what's wrong. In the meantime, these self-care measures can minimize your discomfort.

Pass the jelly. Petroleum jelly doesn't feel or taste very good inside

BRUSHING AND FLOSSING: DO THEM RIGHT

You've been brushing your teeth all your life, so why would you need instructions on something so elementary? Because you probably aren't doing it right.

"A lot of women think that they're doing a great job of cleaning their teeth, but they've never had instruction and they're not using proper technique," observes Esther Rubin, D.D.S., a dentist in New York City.

Thoroughly brushing your teeth takes at least three minutes—not the 51 seconds that most women allow. Brushing *and* flossing are important because they prevent the formation of plaque, a sticky film of bacteria, mucus, and food particles that coats teeth and eventually causes cavities and gingivitis (swollen, bleeding gums).

Dentists agree that the easiest, most effective way to keep your teeth and gums healthy is to practice good oral hygiene. To do it right, follow these three steps, then finish by brushing the surface of your tongue, which can harbor bacteria and contribute to bad breath.

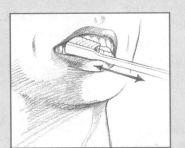

1. Position the brush at a 45-degree angle to your gum line. Use short back-and-forth strokes to clean the outside of your teeth and then the inside.

2. Brush the chewing surfaces of your teeth.

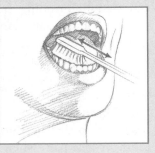

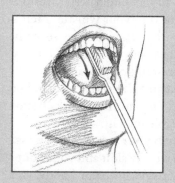

3. Clean the inside of your front teeth by holding the brush perpendicular to your gums. Move the brush from the gum toward the biting edge—up on your lower teeth, down on your upper teeth.

Ideally, your teeth should be brushed five times a day: in the morning, at bedtime, and after each meal. At least one of those sessions should be followed by flossing. "Personally, I think that flossing is the best investment a person can make in terms of dental health," Dr. Rubin says. "Proper flossing can save your teeth."

Be sure to pick the right floss for you. If you have rough fillings or if your teeth are close together, waxed floss works best. Unwaxed floss is thinner than waxed, but it also frays more readily. If your teeth are widely spaced or if you have a hard time flossing, dental tape is a good choice.

To practice proper flossing, follow these five steps.

1. Tear off a strand of floss about 18 inches long. Wrap the ends around the middle fingers of both hands until just 6 to 8 inches of floss is exposed.
2. Pinch the floss between the thumb and index finger of one hand. With the index finger of your other hand, guide about one inch of floss between your teeth.
3. Use a back-and-forth motion as you gently slide the floss up and down between your teeth.
4. Curve the floss around the base of each tooth. Gently move the floss back and forth beneath the gum line.
5. To remove the floss, use the same back-and-forth motion to bring it up and away from your teeth. Never snap or force the floss, or you might bruise delicate gum tissue.

your mouth, but it will quiet a sensitive tooth on a short-term basis. Simply apply petroleum jelly to the tooth.

Extend an olive branch. If tooth sensitivity results from an abrasion or erosion along the gum line, olive oil can help. Warm the oil by pouring a small amount into a saucepan and heating it until it starts to smoke. Dampen a cotton swab in the oil, then wave the swab in the air briefly to cool it off. Dry the affected tooth with a tissue or cotton ball and then dab the warm oil on your gum line a couple of times. Repeat as needed. (One treatment may last for months.)

Take a hard look at soft drinks. If you're drinking enough colas and root beers to float an armada, cut back. The darker sodas have high levels of phosphoric acid, which pulls calcium out of your body—and your teeth—like crazy.

Switch to a softer brush. A tooth can become sensitive because of overly aggressive brushing, especially with a brush that has hard bristles. This combination can push back the gum and expose the root surface. Use a toothbrush with softer bristles and adopt a gentler brushing technique.

Chapped Lips

Your lips do a remarkable job of keeping your teeth protected, and in doing so, they take their own form of abuse. For all the wear and tear that they endure, lips are remarkably unprotected. They lack the natural oils that keep the rest of your skin supple. They also lack melanin, the pigment that

Wisdom teeth, or third molars, are the last teeth to develop and appear in the mouth. They are so named because they usually appear during our late teens or early twenties—what has been dubbed the age of wisdom.

Dentists usually yank them because most of us don't have room for them in our mouths. And many dentists believe that if we get those big guys pulled before they're fully formed, we're much wiser for it. Saving a set of wisdom teeth "just in case" there's room could set you up for problems later in life. Here's why.

A wisdom tooth left to its own devices may become partially trapped, or impacted, under your 12-year molars (so called because that's the age at which they usually appear), where it can grow any which way. Food can easily get packed around partially impacted (partially grown in) wisdom teeth and the molar next to them, possibly causing an abscess or gum disease.

So why did nature give us a set of teeth too big to accommodate? Apparently, they served a purpose long ago. Evolution tells us that in the past, humans had bigger jaws, which were needed to gnaw at food before proper utensils were invented.

Expert consulted
Heidi Hausauer, D.D.S.
Spokesperson for the Academy of General
*   Dentistry*
University of the Pacific
Castro Valley, California

A few days of TLC—tender lip care—is all you should need to restore the wetness to your whistle. Here's what to do. (If you have severely cracked lips, see your doctor. You may need a prescription preparation.)

Smear on the old standby. For chapped lips, nothing works better than petroleum jelly.

Thumb your nose at dryness. If you have oily skin and you're outdoors with no lip balm handy, run your finger along the side of your nose to pick up some skin oil. Wipe the oil on your lips for short-term relief.

Fight yeast with yogurt. If the corners of your mouth appear red and cracked, you may have an overgrowth of yeast (a fungus), caused perhaps by antibiotics or stress. Go to the supermarket and pick up some yogurt containing live active cultures (check the label). Then, swish the yogurt around in your mouth several times a day. The live active cultures include *Lactobacillus acidophilus*, beneficial bacteria that control yeast.

Cover up your kisser. Always apply a lip balm with a sun protection factor (SPF) of 15 or higher before heading outside.

Lick your problem, not your lips. Licking your lips to moisturize them is only natural. Unfortunately, air evaporates the moisture, leaving your lips even drier than before.

provides some protection against sun damage. Combine these factors with exposure to blazing sun, strong winds, or moisture-sapping indoor heat, and you can understand why your lips sometimes become chapped.

Cold Sores

Nothing can ruin a beautiful smile like a nasty-looking cold sore. And if you get one once, you're likely to get them again and again.

You can credit their persistence to herpes simplex type 1, the virus that causes cold sores. Ninety percent of the people who carry the virus picked it up during childhood. It lurks in your system forever, lying dormant among the nerve ganglia beneath your skin's surface, just waiting for something to activate it.

For women, that something is usually stress. When you're under stress, your resistance to disease drops. The virus seizes the opportunity to instigate an outbreak.

If you have ever had a cold sore before, you are probably familiar with what doctors call the prodrome—a sort of introductory itching around the area where a sore is about to erupt.

A cold sore usually sticks around for one to two weeks. You can use these natural remedies to minimize any discomfort and shorten the duration of an outbreak.

Give it the cold shoulder. The minute you feel a cold sore coming on, wrap an ice cube in a handkerchief and hold it directly on the sore for about five minutes. Repeat every two to three hours. No virus, including herpes simplex type 1, can survive in a cold environment.

Try a little tenderizer. Mix meat tenderizer with a few drops of water to make a paste. Apply the paste to the cold sore and hold it in place with a dry washcloth for 5 to 10 minutes. Repeat every two to three hours for the first day of an outbreak, then cut back the treatments to three times a day. Continue until the sore heals.

Line up lysine. Before the advent of the prescription drug acyclovir (Zovirax) for cold sores, people swore by the preventive and healing properties of lysine. This amino acid counteracts arginine, a substance in various foods that seems to trigger cold sores in some people. Lysine tablets are available in drugstores and health food stores.

Shrink the sore with zinc. An essential trace mineral, zinc is essential for proper wound healing—especially cell production—and helps get rid of cold sores more quickly. During an outbreak, take 30 milligrams of zinc a day with food or water. Once the sore heals, cut back to 15 milligrams a day.

Note: If you're taking more than 20 milligrams daily, it's a good idea to inform your doctor.

Dab on some sun protection. If you have had a cold sore in the past, wearing lip balm with an SPF of 30 at all times can help prevent another outbreak. You can find lip balms with high SPFs in sporting goods stores and drugstores. (During an outbreak, use a cotton swab to apply the balm to your lips and the outside border of the cold sore. That way, you won't transfer the virus to the balm stick.)

Leave it alone. If you have a cold sore, don't pull it, stretch it, or otherwise touch it. You could get very painful cold sores on your hand, especially if the fluid from the blister gets under a hangnail.

Asthma and Emphysema

Breathe in, breathe out. Breathe in, breathe out.

For most of us, this basic bodily function doesn't take any conscious thought. But some 17 million Americans with asthma *do* have to think about it because a sudden asthma attack can cause wheezing, coughing, chest tightness . . . and on occasion, an inability to breathe at all. The disease kills more than 5,400 Americans each year.

It works like this: A trigger in the environment—often an allergen such as pollen, dust mites, or a viral infection—invades your bronchial tubes, which move air in and out of your body, and causes inflammation. The surrounding muscles then tighten, and your tubes fill with mucus, making breathing more difficult.

Asthma is another one of those diseases that seems to have a gender bias. It sends women to the emergency room nearly twice as often as men. But we don't have to become its victims. This chronic threat to our air force can be held off, stopped in its tracks, and even pushed back with today's arsenal of therapies.

Risk Factors

Even though environmental factors and allergens appear to affect the course of asthma, we're still not sure exactly what their role is. "We know that viruses and allergen exposure can exacerbate the disease, but we don't really know if they cause it," says Rebecca S. Gruchalla, M.D., Ph.D., chief of the allergy and immunology division at the University of Texas Southwestern Medical Center at Dallas.

For the time being, however, the generally accepted list of risk factors for asthma attacks comprises genetic, environmental, hormonal, allergenic, infectious, climatic, and physiological triggers. Marianne Frieri, M.D., Ph.D., director of allergy immunology training at Nassau County Medical Center/North Shore University Hospital in East Meadow, New York, and associate professor of medicine at the State University of New York in Stony Brook, details them in this way.

Hormones. Our regular hormonal shifts that occur around menstruation and pregnancy, and possibly hormone-replacement therapy for postmenopausal women, can trigger asthma.

Occupations. Nurses, teachers, day care–center workers—these largely female workforces report significant problems in their workplaces. These include latex allergies among nurses and, among all of these workers, viral infections from patients and students and reactions to animal dander on clothes and to dust.

Irritants. Plant pollens, mold, fungi, tobacco smoke, wood smoke, air pollution, chemical fumes, strong odors (including perfume), and sprays all can stimulate airways to tighten and clog. Parental smoking is especially harmful to children with asthma, according to one Canadian study. After following a group of children for 6 years, researchers found that those who still had asthma were almost four times as likely to have mothers who smoked heavily as were kids whose symptoms had disappeared.

Animal dander. The dander (not fur) and saliva of cats and the dander of dogs can trigger an asthma attack.

Cockroaches. Allergies to cockroaches pose risks for inner-city residents, especially.

Dust mites. In pillows, mattresses, carpets, and stuffed toys, our airways—not our eyes—detect the droppings of these tiny visitors.

Respiratory infections. Colds and the flu may bring on asthma troubles.

Exercise. Exercise-induced asthma is very common and controllable with medication. Research suggests that drinking water before,

---

EMPHYSEMA

Would you rather (a) die prematurely, (b) spend the rest of your life tethered to an oxygen tank, (c) develop a barrel chest, or (d) grunt every time you let out a breath? This multiple choice comes with a bleak bonus: If you have emphysema, you can pick all four.

As the most common cause of respiratory disease death in the United States, emphysema is tragic because it's almost entirely preventable. Up to 90 percent of cases can be blamed on smoking. (The rest are due to inherited gene deficiency.) It takes its time, too: "Emphysema can be a long, slow decline," says Monica Kraft, M.D., a pulmonologist and assistant professor of medicine at the National Jewish Medical and Research Center in Denver.

The word itself describes the disease. Its Greek root means "to inflate," and that's the problem: Lungs overinflate because of inefficient breathing. With emphysema, the air sacs in the lungs become overstretched or break. This makes your lungs less elastic, so air is trapped in your chest and you have to work harder to breathe (hence, the barrel chest and grunting on exhale).

In most of the two-million-plus Americans with emphysema, the disease has been doing its dirty work for years before it's diagnosed. The first symptom is often shortness of breath. Eventually, supplementary oxygen or even a lung transplant may be needed.

While emphysema prefers men by a margin of more than 50 percent, women are catching up.

There's some silver lining to this cloud of smoking disease. "It's never too late to quit smoking," assures Dr. Kraft. "We know that patients who smoke have an accelerated decline in lung function," she reports, but shortly after becoming smoke-free, an ex-smoker's rate of decline reaches that of a person who never smoked.

---

during, and after workouts is important for women with asthma. Women with the disease may start out with a hydration deficit that could make their asthma worse.

Cold, dry air. As some runners and skiers will tell you, breathing cold, dry air can launch an asthma attack.

Drugs. Aspirin, ibuprofen, and other nonsteroidal anti-inflammatory drugs (NSAIDs) are also offenders.

Anxiety. Stress and worry alone may not provoke an attack but may contribute to one.

Foods. Children in particular can be sensitive to milk, eggs, peanuts, nuts, soy, wheat, and fish. Sensitivity to shellfish is more common in adults.

Allergic rhinitis. Also known as hay fever, this condition is a red flag, too. It afflicts more than three-quarters of all people with asthma.

Prevention

Avoiding trouble in the first place is a big part of asthma prevention. Stay away from triggers and allergens that can spark an attack. If that isn't practical, allergy shots, or "immunotherapy," can make you less sensitive.

The next line of defense is early detection. "When it starts out, asthma is completely reversible," says Martha V. White, M.D., research director of the Institute for Asthma and Allergy at Washington Hospital Center in Washington, D.C. But once inflammation of the airways takes hold, the damage can be permanent. The lungs develop scar tissue that sometimes can't be reversed. Still, even at that point, proper monitoring can help keep attacks under control.

"What most people don't know about asthma is that it's really, really controllable," says Dr. White. But asthma can range from mild to life-threatening, so it's important to know where

---

REAL-LIFE SCENARIO

Her Bronchitis Just Won't Go Away

Anna, 43, has been running a day care center out of her home for years, and she's had great luck not only in her business but also with her health. Unlike the assistant providers she has hired, she has never fallen prey to the many cold and flu viruses that the kids bring with them to the center. But this year has been different. Although she has never smoked, gets plenty of rest and exercise, and takes lots of vitamin C, she has come down with a cold that just won't go away. It started as a scratchy throat, then quickly went to her chest. Now, 8 weeks later, she sometimes coughs hard, brings up mucus, and is short of breath. Her doctor had her lungs x-rayed, but there is no sign of disease. What should she do?

Anna may not have bronchitis at all. This word gets used very broadly to describe a number of respiratory ailments, but the coughing and mucus could be caused by something else.

As a day care worker, she's certainly exposed to lots of different viruses from the children at her center. She has probably developed an upper respiratory infection from one such virus, and the result is what we call twitchy, or reactive, airways. This means that the bronchial tubes that supply her lungs with air have become more responsive to various stimuli, including allergens, irritants, and viruses. As a result, the airways may have narrowed and become inflamed, leading to her coughing and shortness of breath.

---

your symptoms fall. That's where a device called a peak flow meter comes in.

Basically, it's a little tube you blow into twice daily that tells you how open or closed your large airways are. Because asthma rarely flares up without warning signs that appear hours beforehand, the meter works like an "asthma thermometer," Dr. White says, to detect trouble before it escalates.

Medications are a regular part of life for many women with asthma. Those with the mildest

Another strong possibility is that Anna has an underlying element of asthma brought on only by viral infection. We know that, like cold air, smoke, strong odors, or allergens such as ragweed, viral infection is one of the triggers that can bring on an asthma attack. Note that she's coughing and not wheezing: There is a syndrome called cough-variant asthma where people exhibit only coughing, as opposed to the classic wheezing of asthma.

The mucus that Anna is coughing up needs examining: If it's clear, that points to a viral infection that's producing twitchy airways. If it's green, she may have a bacterial infection on top of a possible allergy, and I'd probably put her on an antibiotic. If she has asthma and is coughing up yellow mucus, the problem may be an allergy rather than infection. The only way to tell is with a microscope, so I'd get a sample and examine the cells.

Anna should consult with either an asthma or allergy specialist to pinpoint just what's causing her symptoms, and then take appropriate action. If it turns out that she does have asthma, she may be able to stop it from becoming worse and to reverse her breathing problems.

Expert consulted
Rebecca S. Gruchalla, M.D., Ph.D.
Chief of the allergy and immunology division
University of Texas Southwestern Medical
Center
Dallas

form of the disease often are prescribed quick-relief, or "rescue," medications alone. These are bronchodilators taken with inhalers as needed. They work within about 10 minutes to open the airways. For more severe asthma, anti-inflammatory medicines called controller medications are used regularly to keep symptoms reined in. Most of these drugs, which include steroids, are also delivered to the lungs via inhalers.

Except for those with very mild asthma, most people require treatment with both types of medications, according to Dr. White. Taking medicine as prescribed is key to managing this disease, but not everyone follows that advice.

"People often think that controller medications should work right away, but these anti-inflammatories take awhile," relates Dr. White. "It's like taking an antibiotic: It takes a day or two before it kicks in." Those who think that their medication doesn't work fast enough tend to rely on rescue medication alone, leaving them more vulnerable to attacks.

Here are Dr. White's tips for breathing easier with (and without) an inhaler.

Try an instant inhaler substitute. Stuck without your bronchodilator and feel an attack coming on? Grab a cup of coffee or caffeinated cola, says Dr. White. Caffeine is very similar chemically to one of the rescue medications.

Tap liquid relief. If you're minus both your inhaler and a caffeinated beverage, drink hot water. Dr. White says that it can soothe the chest.

Work the phone. If an attack hits while you're away from home and you can get to a phone and a drugstore, call your doctor and have her call in your inhaler prescription so you can pick it up at the pharmacy. Depending on the distance, it may be faster and safer than trying to reach your inhaler at home.

Steer clear of car storage. Extreme heat and cold can ruin inhalers, so don't stash yours in your car.

Any way that you can change your environment to minimize exposure to triggers is one more way to keep asthma from controlling your life. Allergy and asthma experts recommend these breath-saving strategies for common home-front triggers.

Freshen that fur. Bathe your pet (or have someone else do it) once a week to minimize dander.

Get into hot water. Wash all bedding (including pillows), clothes, and stuffed toys in hot water at least once a week to control dust mites. Investing in mite covers may help as well.

Clean the carpet weekly. Dust mites love that sheared plush even more than you do.

Cut wet-air woes. Use a dehumidifier to dry out damp basements and bathrooms, favorite haunts of molds and fungi.

Ban the bugs. Get rid of cockroaches with boric acid and traps.

Hang out with the healthy. Avoid contact with people who have colds or the flu to reduce your chances of infection.

Clear the air. Don't smoke, and don't allow it in your home.

Making breathing easier when you're away from home can be a challenge. Try these tips for travel comfort.

In with the good air, out with the bad. Before starting a long car trip, turn on the air conditioner or heater and open the windows for 10 minutes before climbing in. This helps remove dust mites and molds that lurk in the ventilating system, carpets, and upholstery.

Time your travel. Steer clear of car travel when pollution is heaviest in the daytime. Air quality is better in the early morning and late evening.

Get "flight insurance." On international flights that allow smoking, request a seat as far as possible from the puffers. If your asthma is sometimes severe enough to require additional oxygen, you may feel the need at 35,000 feet. Make arrangements with the airline well in advance for supplemental oxygen.

Pack it in. When you travel, keep your inhaler in your purse or carry-on—not in checked baggage that is out of your reach and can go astray.

Be a picky eater. If you have an asthma reaction to certain foods, be wary of in-flight meals. No one on board will know what's in those premade dishes, so if you can, eat at home and take some snacks with you on the plane.

Signs and Symptoms

The warning signs of asthma can vary from person to person, and from attack to attack. If you've already been diagnosed with asthma, a

smoking rate of registered nurses. And L.P.N.'s have less formal education and tend to make less money.

This smoking "gap" mirrors the overall relationship between income, power, and smoking, regardless of gender. The lower someone's socioeconomic status, the higher their smoking risk.

Many women also use smoking as a reward. They work at a paying job all day, sometimes two jobs, then go home and work all evening. Smoking presents a time-out or respite from those demands. The cigarette industry capitalizes on this with ads that show a powerful image: a woman in a garden . . . alone . . . being still . . . smoking.

Overall, the incidence of women smokers 18 and older is declining. But for females under 18, the numbers are going up. So what we're seeing is a transient dip in smoking among grown-up women, which will be more than made up for by the next generation.

Expert consulted
Barbara A. Phillips, M.D.
Professor of pulmonary and critical-care
medicine
University of Kentucky Medical Center
Lexington

Indigestion. It can bring on the tight-chest feeling that marks asthma.

Sinus infections. You can't breathe freely, so these painful pretenders can be misinterpreted.

Nasal congestion. Trying to breathe through a blocked-up, stuffy nose is like trying to suck a milkshake through a wet paper straw, notes Dr. White. Open your mouth to make breathing easier.

Bronchitis. Its coughing, wheezing, and chest tightness can closely mimic asthma.

"The bottom line is, if you're having chest discomfort and trouble breathing, have it checked out," advises Dr. White.

Who Do I See?

A primary-care physician is often the first and only professional consulted. If a specialist is needed, it's usually an allergist/immunologist or a pulmonologist (lung doctor). If you think you have the symptoms of asthma, you should seek treatment, says Dr. Frieri. Postponing care is dangerous; permanent harm may be done to your lungs.

Unlike time-pressed general practitioners, a specialist can take 40 minutes or more to obtain a detailed personal history, says Dr. Frieri. "When giving your personal history, you need to focus on all the factors that may be contributing to asthma: the environment at work and home, the presence of cats or dogs, what a woman uses for cleaning, whether or not she has kids, and so on. Then there are conditions like hay fever, ear infections, and sinusitis. Does she sneeze, wheeze, or cough? And what's the family history of respiratory problems with parents and grandparents?"

drop in the peak flow reading is a sure sign of an attack. Here are some of the other most common symptoms: labored breathing or wheezing; chronic cough, especially at night; fast breathing; shortness of breath; and chest tightness or discomfort. Symptoms of allergic rhinitis, such as fatigue, a scratchy throat, headache, head congestion, or itchy, watery eyes, often occur along with asthma flare-ups.

Don't Panic!

Some fairly minor conditions can make you wrongly suspect that asthma is filching your air. Dr. White mentions these.

What Can I Expect?

During a physical exam, the doctor will concentrate on the upper and lower airways, looking into your ears, nose, and throat and listening to your chest for any signs of wheezing. This may be followed by a pulmonary function test called spirometry: You breathe into a calibrated instrument that measures things like your lung capacity and how much air you exhale in 1 second. This detects any obstruction or restriction in your breathing.

You may also get a chest x-ray to pinpoint an abnormality in your lungs or take an allergy test to find out what substances are triggering allergic reactions.

Emotional as well as physical reactions can be a real issue for women with asthma. "When you have asthma, it feels like you're suffocating," notes Dorothea Lack, Ph.D., clinical assistant professor in the psychiatry department at the University of California, San Francisco. "The memory of a past attack sets up an anticipatory anxiety that can snowball into a new attack," she observes. And in the midst of that attack, the fear of imminent death is overwhelming.

Those anxious feelings can be among a woman's biggest challenges with asthma because of their circular link with the disease, according to Dr. Lack. An attack can trigger panic, panic can make the attack worse, and round and round it goes.

Adding to the tension, asthma medicines can cause anxiety-like side effects. Dr. White's own study of more

AN OLD ENEMY RETURNS: TUBERCULOSIS

We don't think about tuberculosis much anymore. It's a disease we'd thought we'd conquered—until recently.

After 1953, when national surveillance of tuberculosis (TB) began, the number of reported cases steadily decreased. Yet, starting in 1985, the incidence of the disease began to increase and peaked in 1992. Experts think that this may have happened as a result of the AIDS epidemic, which has left so many people with suppressed immune systems. Fortunately, improved TB-control programs have again put the disease on the decline. There were only 18,361 cases in 1998—the lowest rate since 1953.

Tuberculosis is an airborne infection, which means it can be spread through coughing, sneezing, laughing, or even singing. But you would need prolonged exposure to an infected person before you came down with the disease. It usually attacks the lungs, but it can also affect other organs and tissues.

The symptoms of TB range from prolonged coughing, including coughing up blood; fever; chills or night sweats; lethargy; weakness; unexplained weight loss; to loss of appetite. People at higher risk for contracting the disease are those who, like teachers, health-care workers, and prison guards, interact with infected persons or high-risk populations; the poor and medically underserved; people with suppressed immune systems; and the elderly. If you have reason to think that you may have been exposed to TB or are experiencing TB symptoms, see your doctor immediately because, untreated, it can spread to others.

To detect tuberculosis, doctors use either a Mantoux skin test, in which a small amount of tuberculin is injected into the top layers of skin on the forearm, or a tuberculin tine test, a skin test using multiple punctures that contain the testing material. The results are obvious 2 to 3 days after the test, with definite raised bumps on the skin an indication of positive results. Your doctor may also order chest x-rays and sputum tests.

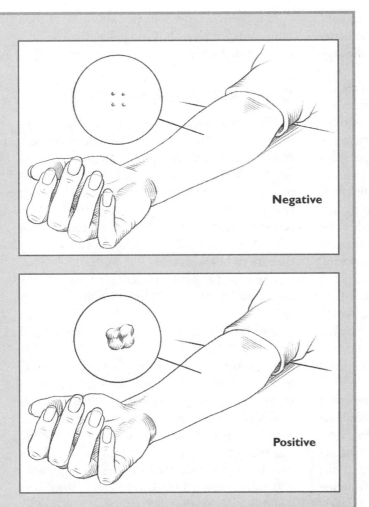

If your test comes back positive, it doesn't mean an end to daily life as you know it. Most TB, more than 90 percent, can be cured with medications, but they have to be taken regularly for 6 months and often longer. Newly approved drugs combine the three main medications into one pill or require less frequent doses.

Incorrectly or incompletely treated, however, TB could progress into multidrug resistant tuberculosis (MDR TB), which does not respond to two or more of the primary treatment drugs, and this resistance spreads with the disease. Response rates of MDR TB plummet to less than 50 percent.

than 1,800 people with asthma showed that roughly 60 percent experienced various side effects from their medication, including shakiness and jitteriness. As a result, up to one-third of adults skipped or reduced doses.

"Often, a patient will come in appearing to have an anxiety disorder, and then you find out that they're taking a bronchodilator for their asthma," reports Dr. Lack. "That's when you see if their medication can be adjusted, and you start them on relaxation training."

Since you can't be deeply relaxed and anxious at the same time, she recommends these keys for calming down during an asthma attack.

Listen and learn. With commercially available relaxation tapes, you can learn to use imagery to quiet the panicky feelings that contribute to an asthma episode.

Practice, practice. Listen to relaxation tapes once a day for 30 days to practice techniques like visualizing, tensing and relaxing your muscles, and deep breathing.

Maintain for a month. Practice relaxation techniques daily for a month, advises Dr. Lack, and you'll be able to practice less often and still call up the relaxation response when needed. "You won't get instant results, so stick with it," she urges.

Conventional Wisdom

While there is no cure for asthma, the closest thing is good old allergy shots, says Dr. White—assuming the asthma is mostly related to an allergy.

The goal is to lower your number of triggers. "The more triggers you can eliminate, the better you can tolerate the ones you still have," she says.

Allergy shots work like vaccinations: You're injected with the substance that provokes the problem, in small, increasing doses over several months. Maintenance doses can then continue for several years. As you build immunity to the trigger allergen, you substantially reduce your misery.

While controller and rescue drugs are effective at quieting inflammation and opening airways after the fact, they may be replaced in the future by medicines that prevent the problem in the first place. Today, inhaled steroids of several types (though steroids can also be taken in pill or liquid form) are the main defense in controlling inflammation. And for acute attacks, bronchodilators in several different classes all ease the muscles around airways so that normal breathing can resume. Among the newer entries are leukotriene inhibitors.

What's coming up? A nonspecific allergy shot called anti-IgE could conceivably control all allergies and asthma by suppressing the allergic reaction. It's been "far more effective in asthma control than I ever imagined," in clinical trials, reports Dr. White. It's a few years away from introduction, though. Also exciting and in development are two drugs that would interrupt the inflammation process even earlier than anti-IgE.

In the meantime, however, experts advise that you follow your doctor's instructions closely and work with your physician to stay on top of your needs. "Asthma therapy is a very fluid thing. You don't just go on medication and stay there for a year," explains Dr. White. If you can anticipate flare-ups, such as just before a menstrual period or when you know you'll be outside during a high-pollen time, talk with your doctor about temporarily boosting your controller medication, she suggests.

"The people who don't pay attention to their symptoms," warns Dr. Gruchalla, "are the ones who can end up in the emergency room."

Great Alternatives

"You can chase asthma symptoms forever, but the key is to treat the causes," says Beverly Yates, N.D., a naturopathic physician practicing in Seattle. While supporting the benefits of steroid medications to handle severe attacks, she reports that reliance on natural medicine can lessen—sometimes even erase—the need for inhalers and pills. Work with your doctor to find alternatives that are right for you.

These supplement and herb strategies get the nod from Dr. Yates to help lessen the impact of asthma.

Get fat(ty). Expand your intake of omega-3 fatty acids by eating cold-water fish like salmon and mackerel, extra virgin olive oil, sunflower seeds, and pumpkin seeds. Dr. Yates recommends a five-to-one balance of omega-6 fatty acids (as found in red meat) to omega-3's. She suggests eating these foods at least once a week, and preferably three to five times a week. But if you decide to stick with supplements, aim for 200 milligrams of omega-3, she advises, and maintain your regular diet. (If you eat an average Western diet, you're probably getting enough omega-6's.)

Keep going with ginkgo. This Asian leaf helps block constriction in the bronchial tubes. About 200 milligrams per day is recommended. As with any herb, don't expect immediate improvement. "Herbs, as medicinal foods, take time," says Dr. Yates. "I usually say to patients, 'Give me a month for every year you've had the problem to see results.'" She recommends, however, taking a holiday from supplements—a week off for every week on. Do not use with antidepressant MAO-inhibitor drugs, aspirin or other nonsteroidal anti-inflammatory medications, or blood-thinning medications.

Breathe easier with evening primrose. Especially for women whose symptoms flare up just before their periods, Dr. Yates recommends taking 1 teaspoon of evening primrose oil twice daily during the premenstrual week to reduce airway inflammation. As an alternative, Dr. Yates suggests taking 1,500 to 3,000 milligrams of evening primrose oil capsules, divided up throughout the day, with food.

Magnify magnesium. Calcium can be aggravating for some people with asthma, reports Dr. Yates, and these same people are often low in magnesium, which may help relax the smooth muscle of airways. Up to 400 milligrams a day can be helpful, she says, but if you have heart or kidney problems, check with your doctor before taking magnesium doses of more than 350 milligrams. Also, magnesium may cause diarrhea in some people.

Calm with coleus forskohlii. There's some evidence that this herb may be as effective at quieting inflammation as some prescription asthma drugs, without jittery side effects. The usual dose is 50 milligrams two or three times a day. Because it may enhance the effects of medications for asthma or high blood pressure, with negative results, do *not* use coleus forskohlii without medical supervision, and always talk with your doctor before adjusting your asthma prescriptions.

Dr. Yates also advocates two other measures to keep air flowing freely: massage and yoga.

Massage. The chest and upper respiratory cavity can benefit from massage because it helps the body clear out waste products that asthma helps build.

Power breathing. Yoga's breathing exercises are a terrific tool, avows Dr. Yates. "If an attack is stress-related, you could use your breath to calm things down before trouble starts."

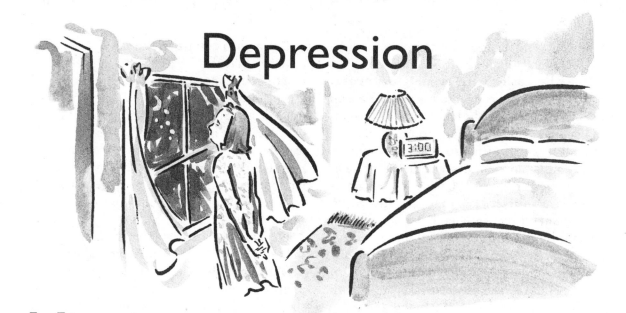

Depression

Marilyn Monroe struggled with it. So did Tammy Wynette. Natalie Wood and Princess Diana both fought to resist it. Even Carmen Miranda, singing Brazilian sambas with a smile on her face and a basket of fruit on her head, had to fight against its smothering pall.

Depression. It's so widespread that it's sometimes called the common cold of mental illness. One out of every four women will have a bout of major depression during her lifetime. That means she'll have feelings of sadness and despair, inconsolable misery, and guilt that last for more than 2 weeks and interfere with her work, her relationships, and even her eating and sleeping.

Some women will face a different challenge: a milder but longer-lasting form of depression called dysthymia (a Greek word meaning "ill humor"), which can make life seem dull, gray, and continually sad. It generally goes on for more than 2 years and may end up developing into full-blown depression.

Unlike the common cold, however, depression can't have its way with you if you don't want it to. You have an effective storehouse of weapons that you can use to fight back.

Risk Factors

A woman whose mother or father suffered from depression is two to three times more likely than normal to become depressed herself, so a family history of depression is obviously a strong risk factor. But women accumulate even stronger risk factors during their lives that have nothing to do with genetics.

For example, three out of four people who develop depression can trace it to some major stress point in their lives—the death of a spouse, the loss of a job, a divorce, or an illness. "It's not uncommon for people who are seriously ill to be depressed, and sometimes their depression goes undiagnosed," says Carol Landau, Ph.D., professor of psychiatry and behavior at Brown University School of Medicine in Providence, Rhode Island. "And although they have good reasons to feel sad and depressed, clinical depression is a serious illness." They need treatment. "Treatment improves your quality of life, no matter what. It can help you see that, even when things are rough, you do have some choices in your life," she adds.

Another high-risk group comprises women who say that they are in unhappy, unsupportive marriages. They are 25 times more likely to be depressed than women who say that they are happily married, suggesting that a stressful relationship may be a much stronger risk factor than family history. But that doesn't mean bad relationships necessarily cause depression, says Bonnie Strickland, Ph.D., professor of psychology at the University of Massachusetts at Amherst. "Women who are already depressed may be more likely to perceive the negative side of their relationships. Or they may be choosing inappropriate partners. Or depression may exacerbate the stress of marriage. It's certainly a question that needs to be addressed."

Finally, having had one episode of depression greatly increases your risk of having another. "Without appropriate treatment, about half of the women who are clinically depressed will experience another episode or more," says Dr. Strickland.

Prevention

As with any illness, avoiding depression altogether is far preferable to having to fight your way from its dark night of the soul. While there is no way to guarantee that you'll never become severely depressed, you may be able to lower your risk.

First of all, look after your general health. That means get enough sleep, eat nutritious meals, and exercise regularly. "Your brain is part of your body, so keeping your body healthy is keeping your brain healthy," says Peg

BIPOLAR DISORDER

All of us have our ups and downs, but people with bipolar disorder have higher ups and lower downs. They have periods of depression, with its typical symptoms, and periods of mania. Mania often appears as an expansive or irritable mood, inflated self-esteem, little need for sleep, talkativeness, distractibility, or a tendency to do pleasurable things that can have painful consequences, such as going on expensive shopping sprees or having an extramarital affair. Some forms of bipolar disorder also cause agitation, paranoia, hallucinations, or rage. Most people with bipolar disorder have plenty of "normal" time in between periods of depression or mania.

Like depression, bipolar disorder is caused by an imbalance of brain chemistry, and it can run in families. It's usually treated with drugs. Lithium remains a popular "antimanic" drug, but other, newer drugs also can help; so may some antidepressants and antipsychotics. Keeping a regular schedule that includes regular times for sleep and exercise and avoiding caffeine, alcohol, marijuana, or other mood-altering drugs can also help.

Nopoulos, M.D., assistant professor in the department of psychiatry at the University of Iowa in Iowa City.

Medical illnesses often run hand in hand with depression, says Michelle Nostheide, a social worker at the National Mental Health Association in Alexandria, Virginia. So living a healthy lifestyle should be your number one priority.

Your number two priority should be to live an active lifestyle. Do you like riding roller coasters? Is spending hours at museums your idea of a good time? Doing the things you like to do and surrounding yourself with people who enjoy doing them with you will help you feel good about yourself, Nostheide says. So be active in the world. Be curious, get involved, read. The more productive you are, the better chance you'll have of preventing depression.

Once you start feeling symptoms of depression, however, such as changes in sleep patterns, changes in your appetite, difficulty concentrating, fatigue or loss of energy, or feelings of worthlessness and helplessness, see a professional, recommends Dr. Nopoulos. Don't expect to be able to cure yourself, she says, just as you wouldn't expect to treat yourself for bronchitis.

Signs and Symptoms

There are many levels to depression, from mild, which allows you to function in more or less normal fashion, to severe, which causes deep and persistent feelings of sadness or despair that interfere with your work, friendships, family life, and physical health.

Not only do severely depressed people tend to feel helpless and hopeless but they also tend to blame themselves for having these feelings. They may sleep fitfully, or they may sleep too much. They may lose their appetites, or they may overeat. But no matter how the symptoms manifest themselves, depressed women tend to feel overwhelmed and exhausted, and they may stop participating in certain everyday activities altogether, says Ellen Leibenluft, M.D., chairperson of the unit for affective disorders in the pediatrics and developmental neuropsychiatry branch at the National Institute of Mental Health in Bethesda, Maryland. Some may also have thoughts of death or suicide. (For more information, see "Suicide: An Epidemic among Women?")

SUICIDE: AN EPIDEMIC AMONG WOMEN?

As with many things, women who attempt suicide do it differently from their male counterparts. Men are more likely to choose violent, irreversible means—using a gun or jumping from a high window—while women prefer drug-and-alcohol combinations, drug overdoses, or carbon monoxide poisoning. Women are about twice as likely as men to attempt suicide but are less likely to complete the deed. They may stop or be discovered before they are dead.

Women with untreated severe depression are at high risk. And among those being treated for severe depression, the time of highest risk is during the first 3 weeks after hospitalization, says Rhoda Olkin, Ph.D., professor of clinical psychology at the California School of Professional Psychology in Alameda.

"People who are severely depressed often don't have the wherewithal to kill themselves," she explains. "It's when the depression starts to be slightly alleviated that people have the energy to try to make the attempt."

Most people are suicidal for no longer than 48 hours at a time, although several such periods may pass before a person pulls out of the mood altogether.

Signs that someone is contemplating suicide may include the following:

Tuning out or turning off. She becomes withdrawn and uncommunicative.

Don't Panic!

Keep in mind that everyone feels sad on occasion. It's natural and emotionally healthy to grieve over upsetting events. These feelings of grief can be extreme, but they tend to become less intense on their own as time goes on. "Allowing yourself to recognize and express all your emotions, whether it's sadness, anger, hope, or happiness, lets you be authentic," Dr. Strickland says. "It can enhance your connection with others and increase self-esteem." Sadness is not self-absorbing or isolating in the way depression is.

Making final arrangements. She begins putting her affairs in order, giving things away, changing her will, or talking about going away.

Risk taking or self-destructive behavior. She may start doing things that could easily end in injury. Reckless driving is a good example.

Sudden elevated mood. A sudden change in mood from gloomy to sunny can precede a suicide attempt.

Direct or indirect statements about suicide. It's not true that people who talk about suicide never do it. They do. Even jokes about suicide should be taken seriously.

Ask her, "Are you thinking of suicide?" Contrary to popular belief, you aren't putting ideas into a person's head. You may have opened the door to honest communication and voiced your concerns.

Then ask, "Do you have a plan? A method? A means? When were you planning to do it?" Concrete plans indicate an immediate crisis.

If it seems to you that someone you know is contemplating suicide, do not leave the person alone, says Dr. Olkin. Take charge, offer support, make sure that she has no means available to hurt herself. If it appears to be an emergency, take her to a crisis center, a hospital emergency room, a mental health center, her psychiatrist, or her family doctor.

Also, keep in mind that even if you are depressed, most depression can be successfully treated. "With the recent advances in both psychotherapy and antidepressant medication, there is always hope, no matter how hopeless it feels," Dr. Landau says.

Who Do I See?

If you have a family doctor, you can certainly see or call her to tell her your concerns. Some family doctors have experience treating depression, and those who don't will most likely refer you to a psychiatrist. Psychiatrists are able to prescribe medications for depression, and many also provide psychotherapy, or talk therapy.

You can also talk about your problems and learn new ways to approach them with a psychologist or a licensed clinical social worker. Many women with depression who need medication will go to see both a psychiatrist and a psychologist, who work closely together on her case.

What Can I Expect?

Everyone's experience of depression is different. You may not realize that you're depressed but may go to your regular family doctor because of bothersome symptoms such as general fatigue or vague aches and pains. Getting an accurate diagnosis may very well be the first step to feeling better. "For most people, it's a relief to get a name and label on what they are experiencing," Dr. Strickland says.

Your doctor may prescribe antidepressants, but don't expect immediate results. They take time to work, and sometimes you'll have to try several medications before you find the one that's right for you. "You can't really know if a drug is going to work for you until you've taken it for 8 or even 12 weeks," Dr. Leibenluft says. Women who are so depressed that they're suicidal may be hospitalized for part of this time. And those who are anxious as well as depressed might be given a faster-acting tranquilizer, such as alprazolam (Xanax).

How long you'll need to take these drugs depends in part on your medical history, Dr. Leibenluft says. "Usually, if you've had two or more previous episodes of depression, especially if they were severe, your doctor may recommend that you take antidepressants for a longer time." So some people go on and off antidepressants, while some stay on them for years. Sometimes, a drug that has worked well for a few years stops working or doesn't work as well as it did previously, and your psychiatrist may try switching drugs or combining them.

Conventional Wisdom

These days, more and more women who are depressed are given antidepressant medications. That's because these drugs have proved helpful for many people. "It may be necessary to correct chemical imbalances in the brain that cause depression," says Dr. Leibenluft.

There are many antidepressant drugs on the market, and your doctor will ask you lots of questions about your symptoms and general health to determine the antidepressant that seems right for you. About 60 to 70 percent of the people who can tolerate the side effects of antidepressants get better with the first drug they take. Some will need to try a second antidepressant and some, rarely, a third.

Psychotherapy has traditionally also been considered a part of treatment for depression. But in these days of managed care, a woman is lucky if her health insurance pays for more than a few sessions of therapy, says Dr. Strickland. So psychologists scramble to find something that can help in a short period of time, such as cognitive-behavioral psychotherapy, interpersonal psychotherapy, or combinations of the two.

"You're not likely to lie around on a couch talking about your childhood," Dr. Strickland says. "You will try to change your behavior and improve your mood in the present rather than dwelling in the past. In cognitive-behavioral therapy, you'll talk about what you want to change now and how you might do that. The

psychologist will want to know what makes you happy and the conditions that lead you to be depressed. You'll examine your behaviors and thought patterns, including automatic negative thoughts that can influence your mood. You'll learn how to change them."

In the course of interpersonal therapy, you'll discuss your personal and social interactions with others and see how they are having an impact on your mood. Basically, you'll work on improving relationships so that you'll feel better about yourself. Research has shown that both cognitive-behavioral and interpersonal psychotherapy are effective treatments for depression.

Great Alternatives

Women who do more than just take drugs to treat their depression often do better in the long run. They learn how to provide balance, perspective, and meaning in their lives. Here are some additional suggestions for keeping depression at bay.

Cultivate a confidante. One classic sociology study, done in the slums of London, found that among women, the outstanding protective factor against depression was having a close confidante, someone to whom they could express any emotion. "It's this freedom to express a full range of emotions—any kind of emotions—that therapists believe sustains mental health," says Rhoda Olkin, Ph.D., professor of clinical psychology at the California School of Professional Psychology in Alameda.

Create a distraction. Men do this more than women do, and it tends to inoculate them against depression, Dr. Olkin says. Of course, a man's way of distracting himself could be hanging out at the corner barroom, which simply substitutes another problem. Women, instead, tend to brood over their problems. "Learning to distract yourself is actually a part of cognitive-behavioral therapy," Dr. Olkin explains.

Exercise is an ideal distraction, but a good book or movie, a favorite hobby, or a pet can work just as well. Do things you like or used to like, and do them even if you don't feel up to it, Dr. Olkin says. "That will start a positive motion that moves into other areas of your life."

Check your medicine chest. Some medications can cause depression. Among the most common are beta-blockers, used to reduce high blood pressure; a class of antibiotics called quinolones (Levaquin is one); steroid drugs, used for autoimmune diseases (these can cause both depression and mania); large doses of any kind of anti-inflammatory, as might be used to treat rheumatoid arthritis; and benzodiazepine tranquilizers, which are often prescribed to women and include alprazolam (Xanax) and diazepam (Valium). Ask your doctor about the chances that a drug you're taking might be causing your depression. He may be able to switch you to a similarly acting drug that does not have a depressing effect.

Ask your doctor about St. John's wort. This depression-relieving herb has become popular in the last few years. Its main active ingredient, hypericin, helps to regulate levels of the mood-lifting brain chemical serotonin, just like some antidepressant drugs, such as fluoxetine (Prozac), paroxetine (Paxil), and sertraline (Zoloft). But there are some things that you need to know to use St. John's wort safely and effectively. It is

MY MAMA TOLD ME

Why are women more likely than men to get depressed?

Women are twice as likely as men to be depressed, but no one knows why.

Some experts say that women's nervous and hormonal systems respond to life's stressors differently from men's. Some say, too, that women are socialized to repress anger, so they learn to get sad, not mad. That's one reason assertiveness training, which helps women deal effectively with anger-provoking situations, is sometimes part of psychotherapy.

In addition, women are socialized to put on happy faces and take responsibility for the emotional well-being of others, including husbands and children. When things don't go well within their families, women may blame themselves and brood about what they believe are their shortcomings.

Finally, men may simply display their dark moods differently. Some researchers believe that men who are having problems with alcoholism, violence, or other self-destructive behaviors are actually depressed and would benefit from treatment.

So if you count all the guys down at the corner bar or driving around in pickup trucks with cases of beer behind the seats, the numbers actually come out about even.

Expert consulted
Bonnie Strickland, Ph.D.
Professor of psychology
University of Massachusetts
Amherst

not recommended for treatment of severe depression, bipolar disorder (manic-depression), or disorders that involve hallucinations and suicidal thoughts.

Don't take it if you are already taking a prescription antidepressant or other psychoactive drugs. Occasional side effects may include agitation, sleep loss, and increased sensitivity to the sun, which can result in sunburn.

Look for a standardized alcohol-derived extract (the alcohol has been removed) containing 0.3 percent hypericin. Experts usually suggest a typical dose of 300 milligrams three times a day. Expect to wait 4 to 6 weeks before noticing an improvement. It's best to take St. John's wort only with knowledgeable medical supervision.

Fill your exercise prescription. Studies show that regular exercise can work as well as psychotherapy at relieving mild to moderate depression, says Kate Hays, Ph.D., author of *Working It Out: Using Exercise in Psychotherapy*. Try walking, running, or weight lifting for a minimum of 20 minutes, three times a week, she says. Exercise may have both an immediate and a long-term biochemical influence on your mood.

If you simply can't motivate yourself to exercise, try doing a physical activity that you enjoy, and approach it slowly but steadily, says Dr. Strickland.

Load up on fatty fish. The omega-3 fatty acids found in fish oils may help ease the symptoms of bipolar disorder, according to a preliminary study from researchers at McLean Hospital in Belmont, Massachusetts. The fatty acids may inhibit transmission of brain signals that trigger dramatic mood swings that characterize the disorder. The participants in the study took about 10 grams a day of fish oil from capsules.

Fish-oil capsules can cause nosebleeds and easy bruising, however. Don't take them if you have a bleeding disorder, uncontrolled high blood pressure, or diabetes; if you take anticoagulants (blood thinners) or use aspirin regularly; or if you are allergic to any kind of fish. Do not substitute with fish-liver oil, because it is high in vitamins A and D, which are toxic in high amounts.

Connect with the larger whole. Depression can be a signal that you have disconnected from the natural world and the soul nourishment that it can provide, says Sarah A. Conn, Ph.D., a lecturer on psychology at Harvard Medical School and founder of the Ecopsychology Institute of the Center for Psychology and Social Change in Cambridge, Massachusetts. To reconnect, she says, start by spending 5 to 10 minutes a day with "a natural being." This can be a tree, a plant, a grassy corner in a park, even clouds or a view out a window. "Simply observe; pay attention to changes," she says. "Then, start to address your deeper questions: 'What does my heart desire? How can I honor that desire? How does it connect me with the world? How does it invite me into the world?'" The natural world becomes an object of meditation that allows your inner world to emerge, she says.

Tune in to natural rhythms. Depression can also be a symptom of being so caught up in the speed of today's consumer-oriented society that you forget how to slow down, Dr. Conn says. "If we develop an ongoing relationship with the natural world, we can learn a lot about natural rhythms and the way we fit into nature." This might include adjusting your sleep patterns to follow the setting and rising of the sun, walking short distances rather than driving, caring for a garden, or just sitting and being still.

Shed some light on the problem. People who get sluggish and irritable during the winter months may actually have seasonal affective disorder (SAD), a form of depression or bipolar disorder that can be relieved with medications and exposure to real or simulated sunlight, says Dr. Leibenluft. People with SAD usually feel their worst in January and February, when days are already lengthening again, and perk up by March or April. To counteract the effects, take a 45-minute stroll in the morning or at lunchtime. Sunlightsimulating light boxes are also available, but it's best to use these under medical supervision. You may also require more sleep during winter months, as there is some evidence that people who sleep longer have fewer SAD-related symptoms.

Schedule your sleep. Irregular sleep/wake cycles can contribute to the symptoms of depression, Dr. Leibenluft says. So keep yours regular by going to bed at the same time every night and getting up at the same time every morning. The more regular your sleep pattern, the more solid your sleep will be. You especially don't want to go to bed so late at night that you sleep through the bright light of morning. Another reason exercise may be very helpful for depression is that it promotes sound sleep.

Get hubby to help with the housework. Sociologist Chloe Bird, Ph.D., of Brown University has found that the larger a woman's share of household chores is, the more likely she is to feel psychologically depressed, especially if she's employed outside the home.

"Housework is less likely to feel like drudgery and is more highly valued by both partners when it's shared," Dr. Bird says. She suggests that couples divide domestic chores evenly. Ideally, each partner should do slightly less than half. Those women who felt least gloomy handled no more than 46 percent. So give yourself a gift by having a third household member or a maid service do the remaining chores.

CAN SAM-E SUPPLEMENTS MAKE YOU SMILE?

It almost sounds too good to be true. A hot, new nutritional supplement being used for depression, S-adenosylmethionine—or SAM-e (Sammy), for short—promises to work faster than antidepressants, have minimal side effects, and provide other health benefits as well. SAM-e has been used for years in Europe to treat depression, and it definitely shows promise. Still, no large U.S.-based studies have been done to confirm its effectiveness and safety.

SAM-e occurs naturally in your body. It helps spur production of the substances in your brain that regulate mood: dopamine and serotonin. Usually, your body can make all the SAM-e it needs, but depression reduces its levels—hence, the idea to take the compound as a supplement and raise levels back to normal.

You can use SAM-e under medical supervision along with antidepressant drugs or alone for mild-to-moderate depression. For minor depression, the usual dosage is 400 milligrams a day, but you can safely use up to 1,600 milligrams a day, advises Richard Brown, M.D., associate professor of clinical psychiatry at Columbia University in New York City and author of *Stop Depression Now*. The supplement should be taken first thing in the morning, on an empty stomach.

People who have bipolar disorder should not use SAM-e without medical supervision, since any kind of antidepressant can tip them over into a state of mania, cautions Dr. Brown.

You'll want the pills to be enteric-coated to protect your stomach from irritation by preventing them from dissolving until they reach your small intestine. A few good brands suggested by Dr. Brown are Nature Made (by Pharmavite), Puritan Pride, and General Nutrition Center products.

SAM-e has a better chance of working well if you're getting adequate amounts of folate and vitamins B_{12} and B_6 to help it along. Aim for 800 micrograms of folic acid (the synthetic form of folate), 1,000 micrograms of vitamin B_{12}, and 100 milligrams of vitamin B_6, recommends Dr. Brown.

Arthritis

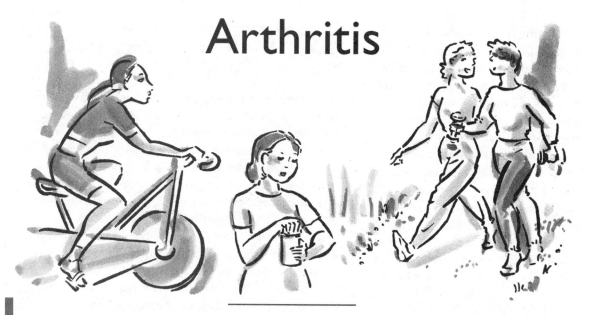

It's not a new problem. Even the dinosaurs had it. But despite its reputation as an affliction of the elderly, arthritis—the catchall term for almost 100 diseases—plays no favorites when it comes to age. Kids, teenagers, and young adults are fair game, too.

The word itself means inflammation or damage to joints, but some varieties of the disease can extend to muscles, skin, and organs. And since women are the favored targets for many forms of this sometimes debilitating condition, new treatment and prevention tools are especially good news for us. "I've worked in arthritis research for more than 16 years, and things are changing," says Leigh F. Callahan, Ph.D., associate director of the Thurston Arthritis Research Center at the University of North Carolina at Chapel Hill. "There's a good feeling about where we are now in treating arthritis."

"We don't see as many wheelchairs in our clinics as in the past," confirms Melanie J. Harrison, M.D., attending rheumatologist at the Hospital for Special Surgery in New York City. "Fewer people are coming in with contracted hands and destroyed fingers."

The reason is that potent new drugs with fewer side effects exist these days. And there is mounting evidence that moderate exercise helps people with arthritis, who currently number some one in six Americans. In addition, acupuncture is gaining ground in pain relief, while naturopathic doctors are using supplements like glucosamine sulfate with good results. More than ever before, when a woman is told that she has arthritis, it isn't the end of active living, but the start of an action plan.

Risk Factors

Despite its variety of forms and names (osteoarthritis, rheumatoid arthritis, gout, and many others), the one thing we don't know about arthritis is what causes it. And that makes pinpointing risk factors iffy.

"We know that some forms are related to genetics. Osteoarthritis is linked to overuse and abuse. And bacteria may be triggers for some forms in some people," explains Teresa J. Brady, Ph.D., medical advisor to the Arthritis Foundation in Atlanta. "We are certain, though, that it's definitely not an inevitable part of aging."

Most common is osteoarthritis, the wear-and-tear form. Cushioning joint cartilage breaks down, causing bone to bump against bone in specific places like your hands, knees, hips, feet, and back. Rheumatoid arthritis, a whole-body autoimmune disease, takes a different toll. Your body's natural immune system attacks its own healthy joint tissue, causing swelling and damage. Following are the factors that can increase risk.

Gender. Some 74 percent of all osteoarthritis, or 15.3 million cases, occurs in women. Rheumatoid arthritis prefers women, too—we're about 1.5 million, or 71 percent, of U.S. cases.

Family ties. Genetics plays a role, especially in rheumatoid arthritis, where a primary risk is having a parent or sibling with the disease, relates Dr. Harrison.

Age. While arthritis strikes all ages, osteoarthritis predominantly targets those over 45.

History of joint damage. Whether it's a tear in a knee ligament that happened while you were skiing, an inflammation, or a repetitive hand motion, injury or chronic strain on a joint can increase your risk of osteoarthritis.

Overweight. Are you overweight, 45 or older, and of average height? Research shows that if you lost 11 pounds or more over 10 years, you would cut your risk for developing osteoarthritis of the knee in half.

Inactivity. There's evidence that exercise not only helps reduce pain but also lessens wear and

WOMEN ASK WHY

Why do joints crack and creak more as people get older?

Inside your joints, wear and tear of cartilage, ligaments, and bones occur as they rub against each other over the years. If your neck cracks when you move it a certain way or your knees crack when you go up or down stairs, it may not be any cause for concern. When a patient says to me, "My knees crack. Do I have to worry about it?" I say, "If it doesn't bother you, no. Don't worry."

If cracking noises are accompanied by other symptoms, such as painful movement, however, it could be a sign of osteoarthritis. Let's say that a doctor examines those cracking knees. When she moves the knees a certain way, you have pain. When she examines your kneecaps, she can feel crepitans, which are the loose bits of cartilage that can cause creaking. And along with that, you have pain when climbing stairs. All these symptoms together could point to early osteoarthritis. If you complain, "My neck cracks," and it doesn't hurt and you have full range of movement, a doctor might just respond by telling you, "Stop cracking it—don't push it." But general cracking and creaking, especially in a younger person, don't have much significance.

Expert consulted
Sicy H. Lee, M.D.
Assistant clinical professor of medicine
New York University School of Medicine
New York City

tear on joints by keeping surrounding muscles strong.

Prevention

You don't have to sit and wait to become a statistic in America's leading cause of disability. Here's how you can avoid or reduce the impact of arthritis.

Get a head start. Joint damage can be slowed down and even prevented in some cases if you get diagnosed and treated early. "Don't listen to old wives' tales about arthritis," cautions Sicy H. Lee, M.D., assistant clinical professor of medicine at New York University School of Medicine and attending physician at the Hospital for Joint Diseases, both in New York City. "Lots of people think that there's nothing you can do about arthritis, and that isn't so."

Find the facts. Because treatment can vary dramatically for different types of arthritis, it's important to know what kind you may have, advises Dr. Lee.

Maintain a fighting weight. You can fight off osteoarthritis by lightening the load on your weight-bearing knees and hips. Being overweight has a domino effect, Dr. Callahan notes. It promotes inactivity, leading to limited joint movement, which fosters joint stiffening.

Get up, get out, get moving. Daily exercise keeps joints flexible, dampens pain, and tones up joint-supporting muscles. If Dr. Brady had osteoarthritis, she would start an exercise plan that would keep her active without aggravating joint pain—such as a plan that includes swimming, walking, or riding a stationary bicycle. But before starting any kind of exercise regimen, work with your doctor to figure out what is right for you.

Feed your health. Experts counsel that a balanced diet helps maintain weight and nourish joints, muscles, and bones. There's evidence that omega-3 fatty acids, the kind found in salmon,

WOMEN ASK WHY

Why is carpal tunnel syndrome everywhere today though it was unheard of 20 years ago?

Twenty years ago, we didn't have a lot of people typing on computer keyboards.

Carpal tunnel syndrome (CTS) is often associated with chronic, repetitive motion of the hands and wrists combined with excessive force. This combination compresses the nerve that supplies feeling to the palm side of the thumb and first two fingers. This nerve passes from your arm to your hand right beneath the carpal ligament, which is part of the carpal tunnel, or canal. The result of nerve compression can be numbness and shooting pain.

So what does all this have to do with computer keyboards? These days, many workers are practically tethered to their computers, sitting for hours at a time. Rather than distributing physical forces across many muscle groups, they're making the same typing motions and using a mouse over and over again—and with too much force. They also don't keep their wrists straight, and they hold their arms in the "action-ready" position even when not typing—all in all, a recipe for trouble.

But computer use is only part of the answer. The other part is the *appearance* of growth in the number of CTS cases because of advances in diagnosis. Better techniques for detecting nerve problems now help correctly identify cases of CTS that before that time may have been blamed on something like insufficient blood supply.

These steps can help alleviate CTS.

anchovies, mackerel, tuna, and sardines, may lower the risk of rheumatoid arthritis.

"C" the light. Vitamin C may help slow down osteoarthritis of the knee, according to one study. Those who ate the most C had less pain and cartilage loss than those eating the least (120 milligrams, or about two medium-size oranges per day).

Be wristwise. A keyboard wrist support isn't a leaning post. Let your hands float over it, like a pianist's, while you type.

Lead with your left. If you're right-handed, you're better off manipulating a computer mouse with your left hand (and vice versa). It eases strain by resting your dominant hand and, for righties, by eliminating the reach to get around the number keypad on the right side of the keyboard.

Perfect your posture. Keep your upper back in contact with your chair to prevent the rounded, hunched shoulders that can result in tighter pectoral muscles. When these muscles tighten, they may compress vessels and nerves as they enter the arm.

Take timeouts. When you're not working the keys, put your hands in your lap or let them hang at your sides to rest muscles and nerves.

Try a trackball. It requires less clutching action than a mouse and lets your hand stay open and more relaxed.

Go with cruise control. When cruising the Internet, move your mouse pad and mouse to your lap and lean back slightly in your chair. This reduces stress on your back, shoulder, wrist, and fingers.

Expert consulted
Margit L. Bleecker, M.D., Ph.D.
Director
Center for Occupational and Environmental
Neurology
Baltimore

Read for relief. Go to school—"Arthritis School." The Arthritis Foundation has a self-help course available in most states to help you eat right and manage pain, among other things. One study of the 6-week course found that it pared pain by 18 percent and saved hundreds of dollars on doctor visits. For information, call the Foundation's National Information Hotline at (800) 283-7800.

Signs and Symptoms

An errant golf swing or a misstep on the stairs can cause temporary woe to a wrist or knee, but beware the complaint that lingers. See your doctor if any of these symptoms in or around a joint persists for more than 2 weeks: pain, stiffness, swelling, and trouble moving a joint.

One of the biggest differences between the two most common forms of arthritis is the kind of swelling that occurs, says Dr. Harrison. "In rheumatoid arthritis, you get a soft swelling—it squooshes, unlike osteoarthritis, where you get bony swelling," says the rheumatologist. Other rheumatoid arthritis cues are a whole-body morning stiffness, flu-like fatigue, fever, and decreased appetite.

Don't Panic!

Not every achy elbow means arthritis, of course. Because the disease takes so many forms, you could have one of the lesser-known types of arthritis. What else might stiffness or fever mean?

Bursitis or tendinitis, both temporary inflammatory joint conditions, says Dr. Brady, can appear like osteoarthritis. They can surface suddenly and stop within days or weeks.

Arthritis-like symptoms very similar to rheumatoid arthritis can also be caused by viruses, according to Dr. Harrison. Two common suspects are parvovirus B19, with feverish symptoms often passed from school-age children to young mothers, and hepatitis C, which can swell the small joints of the hands. The various aches and pains of common flu viruses can also be mistaken for arthritis.

RHEUMATOID ARTHRITIS

Many patients of Melanie J. Harrison, M.D., are looking and feeling better these days and spending less time in the hospital. The reason is that "new drugs and other therapies have changed the symptoms and course of rheumatoid arthritis we see in our clinics," says the attending rheumatologist at the Hospital for Special Surgery in New York City.

This change for the better is especially welcome because of the seriousness of rheumatoid arthritis (RA). "RA is a rapidly progressive disease that can be very crippling over a short amount of time," says Dr. Harrison. And it strikes women up to three times more often than men. Unlike osteoarthritis, which affects joints only, RA is a systemic disease that invades the entire body.

For reasons yet unknown, the natural immune system of a woman with RA starts attacking her body's own healthy joint tissue. Symptoms include fatigue, stiffness (especially in the morning), joint swelling and redness, and lumps under the skin, called nodules. The resulting inflammation and joint damage can lead to severe deformity. Life expectancy can shrink by 3 years in women with RA, and half of RA sufferers can't work within 10 years after the condition starts.

This gloomy picture is brightening, though. "Don't think for a minute that a diagnosis of RA is a sentence," avows Dr. Harrison, a rheumatologist and medical advisor to the Arthritis Foundation in Atlanta. "We have new drugs that seem to alter the course of the disease and a lot of additional treatments that can help with symptoms." The drugs are DMARDs (disease-modifying antirheumatic drugs) that reduce the inflammation and seem to slow the advance of RA—possibly even stop it in its tracks.

"They address the serious effects of RA, such as muscle wasting and joint contraction from disuse," says Dr. Harrison. Physical and occupational therapy techniques, especially aquatic exercises, are effective in strengthening muscles and promoting mobility, she notes.

What's more, there are now products available to ease everyday tasks made difficult by swollen, painful joints, such as ergonomically designed devices to help people button and unbutton their shirts.

The finger tingling and numbness that come with carpal tunnel syndrome can be associated with rheumatoid arthritis, but they can also be unrelated to any medical condition.

Who Do I See?

Your primary-care physician is the one to start and possibly stay with, advises Dr. Brady, as long as she is current on developments in the disease. While an arthritis specialist like a rheumatologist or an endocrinologist isn't necessarily the next step, she says, "You absolutely need someone who stays up-to-date. If your physician says, 'Oh, it's just arthritis, learn to live with it,' that's your cue to get another opinion."

For exercise to ease or reduce symptoms, you may get a referral to see a physical therapist or an occupational therapist.

Seeking out another opinion from an expert in alternative medicine is an option that even the federal government seems eager to explore these days. Dr. Callahan has been involved with a study for the National Institutes of Health, exploring alternative options in arthritis treatment. "We queried physicians and found that 49 percent would recommend some form of alternative therapies," she reports.

What Can I Expect?

Because there is no arthritis cure, treatment focuses on managing the condition. "An appropriate management plan needs to go beyond medications, which are the first things people think about," observes Dr. Brady. "Just as important are self-management strategies, such as losing weight, taking up appropriate physical activity, and trying to take the strain off affected joints."

In addition to these strategies, more common treatments include taking hot baths, using cold packs, protecting joints with braces and splints, and, when necessary, undergoing surgery to replace worn-out joints.

But women with arthritis suffer more than joint pain. They feel the ache of emotional pain as well. "In a very dramatic way, arthritis interrupts your ability to function," says Susan Brace, R.N., Ph.D., a clinical psychologist practicing in Los Angeles. "Little things like cutting with a fork may become impossible. That makes us scared that we might not always be independent."

Dr. Brace recommends the following tactics for handling the psychological impact of arthritis.

Call on your support team. Loved ones need to know that you may be frustrated at not being able to do some things and that this can lead to anger or despair. "It's important to express those feelings and to be heard by people around you," she says.

Come out swinging. "Say, 'I won't be stopped by this.' Don't give up life," urges Dr. Brace. "Arthritis can damage your joints, it's true; but your spirit is made out of something else."

Conventional Wisdom

Medical professionals have made great strides over the past few years in treating arthritis with

MY MAMA TOLD ME
Does cracking your knuckles really give you arthritis?

The easy answer is, as far as we know, no. There are a couple of explanations for that sound, though. One is that cracking knuckles is actually cracking air bubbles in synovial fluid of the finger joints, like cracking air bubbles in bubble gum. Another explanation is that the sound is actually tendons snapping over a little outpouching of bone, which probably makes more sense.

There is no evidence that this practice leads to arthritis. I used to speak to groups about arthritis, and this was a common question. I'd answer by saying, "It was probably your grandmother who told you not to do it, and it was probably because it annoyed her."

While abuse and overuse of a joint can lead to arthritis, knuckle cracking is a "moment in time" pressure on the joint, not a repetitive, ongoing strain. If someone does it a couple of times a day, every day, I wouldn't be concerned. This habit is probably not going to increase anyone's risk of arthritis, given what we know today. It may just annoy those nearby.

Expert consulted
Teresa J. Brady, Ph.D.
Medical advisor
Arthritis Foundation
Atlanta

both drugs and exercise. Here are some of the most current weapons they're using to battle the disease.

Cox-2 inhibitors. These quiet both pain and inflammation but with a big difference from previous medications: They don't cause the stomach upset of their cousins, the nonsteroidal anti-inflammatory drugs (NSAIDs).

DMARDs. This abbreviation is short for disease-modifying antirheumatic drugs. Two of these medications, leflunomide (Arava) and cyclosporine (Neoral) are now FDA-approved to put the brakes on rheumatoid arthritis. Cyclosporine is a drug originally developed to prevent organ rejection in transplant patients. Both actually slow the disease's damage before it becomes irreversible.

Viscosupplements. These substances are replacements for hyaluronic acid, the slippery substance in joint fluid that arthritis takes away. To ease pain in people with mild to moderate osteoarthritis of the knee, viscosupplements are injected directly into the knee joint.

Exercise. "More and more studies show that walking and other kinds of activity can really help people with arthritis," affirms Dr. Callahan. Bicycling, dancing, yoga, and water exercises can all help reduce stiffness and pain.

Great Alternatives

"Glucosamine sulfate can create new cartilage tissue," declares Lorilee Schoenbeck, N.D., a naturopathic physician in Shelburne, Vermont. Citing colleagues who have found x-ray evidence of this phenomenon, Dr. Schoenbeck says that she uses the supplement especially for her patients with affected knees—commonly, skiers. "I have several patients over 40 who had to stop skiing because of osteoarthritic knees," she relates. "With glucosamine sulfate, they can get back to a normal ski season." Here is her recommended regimen.

Give it time. Glucosamine sulfate may take 3 to 6 months to show results with a dosage of 500 milligrams three times a day, says Dr. Schoenbeck. The supplement is commonly available in drugstores and health food stores.

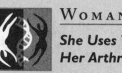

WOMAN TO WOMAN
She Uses Yoga to Control Her Arthritis Pain

Like her mother, Lois S. Hazel has osteoarthritis of the spine. But unlike her mother, this 54-year-old publishing professional in Kintnersville, Pennsylvania, is using yoga as a gentle antidote to her symptoms. Her results include more benefits than she bargained for. Here's her story.

When I was in my late forties, my back pain drove me to an orthopedic surgeon. He advised physical activity to strengthen muscles that support the back and to increase flexibility. I needed an outlet from the stressful marketing job I was doing at the time—something to relax me (I have high blood pressure). Yoga seemed like a good way to achieve all those things.

I tried a beginner's Sivananda yoga class at a nearby fitness center and immediately fell in love with it. Like all yoga disciplines, Sivananda puts the emphasis on breathing, relaxation, and correct posture. The stress relief came almost immediately. After the first class, I could have slept like a baby, yet I felt renewed and calm.

It was the most amazing thing I had ever experienced—like a superdrug with no bad side effects. I went back again and again, and I can still say that after 6 years, I've never been disappointed.

Every once in a while, I have a flare-up, which is common

Try chondroitin. Not all osteoarthritis responds to chondroitin sulfate, another popular remedy. "The only way to know is to try," says Dr. Schoenbeck. About half of her patients with osteoarthritis say that they have less pain when they take between 250 and 500 milligrams of chondroitin sulfate three times a day in addition to their glucosamine sulfate. But, she adds, some of her patients get relief with chondroitin alone, and some report no difference.

Factor in fish. Fish-oil supplements offer the best concentration of anti-inflammatory

with osteoarthritis. It feels like a giant hand reaching in and squeezing around my spine very, very hard. The pain can literally take my breath away. I will gasp, stop what I'm doing, and do some yoga breathing or at least reposition myself to get relief. I'll find a quiet place to do some yoga stretches, and the improvement is always noticeable.

Yoga has also helped lower my blood pressure, and it was a godsend when I had oral surgery recently. I calmed myself before the surgery with yoga breathing, and that helped me get through the procedure with minimum stress.

I like to do things naturally, so I tried glucosamine sulfate and chondroitin sulfate, which I know work well for many people with arthritis. My brother-in-law, a physical therapist, recommended these supplements to me because they worked wonderfully for some of his patients. After 5 months, I saw no change, really, so I just stayed with yoga, plus walking every day and an occasional over-the-counter pain reliever. To keep my back muscles strong, I also do abdominal exercises.

Taking up yoga was one of the best decisions I ever made about my health. When the pain hits, if I just remember to breathe and concentrate the breath into my spine, it absolutely works. I can literally feel that giant hand softening, relaxing its hold.

My mother was severely debilitated by arthritis in her later years, and I don't want to end up the same way. Yoga is helping me take a different path.

bruising as well as upset stomach, so discontinue use if these problems occur.

Reach for relief. A former yoga teacher herself, Dr. Schoenbeck praises the art's gentle stretching as a great way to preserve flexibility and increase blood supply to the joints.

Get needled. Acupuncture, the ancient Chinese practice of inserting fine needles into the body, is winning recognition as an effective pain reliever. Two studies on osteoarthritis of the knee indicated reductions in pain and improvement in walking capabilities.

Chow down on cherries. Just 20 tart cherries a day, according to a Michigan State University study, can ease arthritis pain and inflammation. They contain substances called anthocyanins, which seem to have an antioxidant as well as an anti-inflammatory effect in joints.

Plan on pepper. The red pepper cayenne doesn't just taste hot; it brings warm relief to painful joints. Its chemicals, capsaicin and salicylates, can be rubbed on in the form of capsaicin cream. Always thoroughly wash your hands afterward to avoid getting the cream in your eyes.

Love your joints with ginger. Steep a few slivers of fresh ginger in a tea ball in one cup of freshly boiled water for 10 minutes. Let it cool to sipping temperature and drink up. It may moderate the morning aches of rheumatoid arthritis.

Soothe with green tea. Antioxidant compounds in green tea, according to research funded by the Arthritis Foundation, may ease or even prevent rheumatoid arthritis.

omega-3 fatty acids, according to Dr. Schoenbeck. Her solution to swelling: 1,000 milligrams of fish oil containing EPA (eicosapentaenoic acid, a fatty acid) taken up to three times daily with food. Do not take fish oil if you have diabetes or uncontrolled high blood pressure or if you are allergic to any kind of fish. Since fish oil affects how long your body bleeds when injured, avoid if you have a bleeding disorder, take anticoagulants (blood thinners), or use aspirin regularly. Fish oil may cause nosebleeds and easy

Diabetes

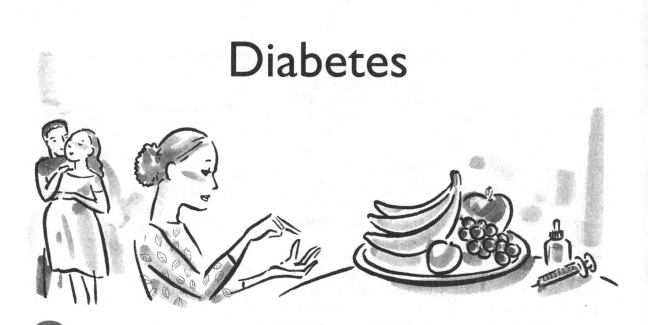

Once upon a time, strict no-sugar diets, rigid weight-loss goals, and demanding medication regimens dominated the lives of those who had diabetes. They were told that they couldn't eat ice cream, they couldn't play sports, and they couldn't have babies. It limited their career options and their freedom. Thank goodness things have changed. Today, it's not only possible but also highly probable that people with diabetes will be able to tame their disease and live full and rewarding lives.

That's not to say that living with diabetes is easy. It complicates almost every aspect of a woman's life—career, marriage, motherhood, menopause. But with today's way of managing this disease, it is possible to achieve and enjoy a balanced, healthy lifestyle.

Unfortunately, of the approximately 8.1 million women in the United States who have some form of diabetes, up to 2.7 million of them don't know they have it and aren't receiving care.

The problem is that if diabetes isn't treated or managed properly, it can damage your vital organs, body tissues, and blood vessels, and can lead to a heart attack, stroke, or kidney, eye, and nerve damage, explains Elizabeth A. Walker, R.N., D.N.Sc. (doctor of nursing science), president of health care and education for the American Diabetes Association.

What goes wrong in your body when you have diabetes? Simply put, you have too much glucose, a type of sugar, in your blood. Your body gets glucose from the foods you eat and uses it as fuel. It is carried in the bloodstream, but it has to get into your cells before it can be expended as energy. Insulin, a hormone made by your pancreas, is the key that opens the door to let glucose into your cells, and it's usually a problem with insulin that leads to diabetes.

This disease comes in three varieties: type 1, type 2, and gestational diabetes. "In people with type 1 diabetes, the problem is decreased insulin in the pancreas, which eventually becomes *no* insulin production," says Melissa D. Katz, M.D., assistant professor of medicine in the department of endocrinology and metabolism at Weill Medical College of Cornell University in New York City. All type 1 patients must take insulin, but only some type 2 patients need to. "Type 2 diabetics produce insulin, but the amount is decreased," she says. "Type 2 patients are insulin-resistant, which means that although insulin is produced, it is not effectively taken up by the body."

Gestational diabetes involves insulin resistance as well, and it usually improves with the delivery of the baby. Diabetes can occur during pregnancy because of the mother's increased weight, which elevates insulin production, explains Dr. Katz.

Risk Factors: Type 1

Type 1, or insulin-dependent diabetes, accounts for 5 to 10 percent of all diabetes. "Both type 1 and type 2 diabetes are multifactorial," says Dr. Katz. The exact cause of type 1 diabetes is not known, but there are some identifiable risk factors.

A parent with diabetes. "The tendency to get type 1 diabetes can be inherited," says Dr. Katz. "Your risk is only slightly increased if you have a diabetic sibling."

A bug. Even if you have inherited the diabetic tendency, other environmental factors, such as illness, must come into play for it to kick in. "Certain viruses or autoimmune responses may be part of the triggering mechanism," says Dr. Katz.

Race. Type 1 diabetes is more common in Whites than in Black or Hispanic people.

Risk Factors: Type 2

If you have type 2, often called adult-onset diabetes, you're not alone. "About 95 percent of people with diabetes in this country are type 2,"

MY MAMA TOLD ME

Can eating too much sugar give me diabetes?

Neither sugar nor carbohydrate, which is broken down into simple sugar, causes diabetes. Diabetes is really an alteration in the way we metabolize sugar—either we don't produce enough insulin, as in type 1 diabetes, or we have a resistance to the effects of insulin, as in type 2 diabetes.

Diabetes is characterized by too much glucose in the blood. Glucose is a sugar that's made by the body when carbohydrates are ingested. Diabetes exists because this metabolic process doesn't work the way it should, not because you have had too much sugar growing up.

Most experts believe that the causes of diabetes are either genetic or environmental. Overweight, physical inactivity, family history, and race/ethnicity are all risk factors for the disease.

Expert consulted
Florence Brown, M.D.
Senior staff physician
Joslin Diabetes Center
Harvard University

says Caroline Richardson, M.D., Robert Wood Johnson Clinical Scholars Fellow and lecturer in the department of family medicine at the University of Michigan Health System in Ann Arbor. You may be at risk if one or more of the following factors apply to you.

Heritage. "There are certain populations where insulin resistance seems to be more prevalent," explains Dr. Katz. Hispanics and Blacks have about two times the rate of type 2 diabetes that Whites have, and Native Americans have a 6.3 percent higher rate than Whites.

Obesity. It seems that the genetic tendency for type 2 must be triggered by an outside force, such as excess weight. "Apple-shaped people with more upper-body fat are predisposed to insulin resistance," says Dr. Katz.

Age. Most cases of type 2 diabetes occur in people over the age of 45, so you should start to pay particularly close attention to any warning signs at midlife.

Previous bouts of gestational diabetes. "A woman who has had gestational diabetes during one or more of her pregnancies is at an increased risk for developing type 2 diabetes later in life," says Dr. Katz. If you've had a baby who weighed 9 pounds or more at birth, your odds are further heightened.

Risk factors for gestational diabetes, which occurs in about 4 percent of all pregnancies, include obesity, a family history of maternal diabetes, and the occurrence of gestational diabetes in a previous pregnancy.

THROMBOSIS

Thrombosis, or blood clotting, is a natural process that happens when you bang your arm or bump your leg, causing a blood clot or bruise to form. If it's normal, the clot will dissolve and your wound will heal. But clot formation inside healthy blood vessels is abnormal and potentially life-threatening.

The threat posed by an abnormal blood clot depends on both its size and its location. An obstructive clot in an artery of your brain, for example, can cause stroke. Blood clots in the coronary arteries to the heart are a major cause of heart attack. Blood clots in the veins to the eye can lead to loss of vision, while a clot that blocks a vein in your lungs can cause shortness of breath and even death.

Some signs of a blood clot include sudden and isolated pain in your arm or leg, followed by skin discoloration, tingling, numbness, or a cold feeling in your extremities; a hard, bluish lump in a vein; sudden or partial blindness in your eye; violent dizziness, or vertigo, that impairs your ability to stand or walk; and shortness of breath and fainting. Other blood clots often produce no obvious symptoms until it is too late.

Research shows that a tendency to have abnormal blood

Prevention

Because the cause of type 1 diabetes is not fully understood and is thought to be both genetic and environmental, prevention may not be possible. There are large studies going on, however, that are designed to discover how to prevent both type 1 and type 2 diabetes. The best way to decrease the risk of type 2 diabetes may be with lifestyle changes, such as maintaining a normal weight, eating a lower fat diet, and getting plenty of exercise, says Dr. Walker.

Get on your feet. "A sedentary lifestyle is thought to contribute to the onset of type 2 diabetes," says Dr. Katz. Regular exercise fights insulin resistance, which makes the onset of type 2 diabetes much less likely. And if you have type 1,

exercise will help keep your blood sugar levels down.

Take off some pounds. "Type 2 diabetes is much more common in obese people," says Dr. Katz. So reducing your body fat is important.

Trim the fat. A diet low in fat may help ward off diabetes. "It is thought that people with a very high fat diet are more predisposed to type 2 diabetes," Dr. Katz says.

Signs and Symptoms

If you're like a lot of women who live very full and busy lives, you're the last person you attend to; your health problems may appear at the end of your to-do list. But there are some signs and

clotting can be genetic, says Alice Ma, M.D., assistant professor of hematology at the University of North Carolina in Chapel Hill.

"There are some clots that also specifically affect women, especially during pregnancy, childbirth, and the month following childbirth," she says. If a woman has a blood clot during pregnancy, she may need to be placed on blood thinners, which are safe for the baby, Dr. Ma adds.

Oral contraceptives may also increase a woman's chance of developing blood clots in her legs and may raise her risk of a pulmonary embolism, which occurs when a clot travels to the lungs. Other risk factors include smoking, a sedentary lifestyle, obesity, and surgery.

The best way to prevent abnormal blood clotting is to eat a balanced diet, get regular exercise, and drink plenty of water, particularly if you are traveling or have been immobile for a long period of time. If you're traveling by car or by plane, for example, make sure that you take time out from your trip to stretch, says Dr. Ma.

People who tend to have problems with clotting may need to be on lifelong anticoagulation that requires them to take blood thinners regularly, either intravenously or orally, Dr. Ma says.

symptoms of diabetes that you should make time to watch out for. Keep in mind that type 1 symptoms usually appear suddenly, while type 2 symptoms may never show up until you develop complications.

You're living in the bathroom. "Polyuria, or frequent or excessive urination, can be a sign of type 1 or 2 diabetes," says Dr. Katz. Polyuria is dangerous because it can worsen the already present dehydration from the disease, she says.

You're chugging water. Polydipsia, or excessive thirst, is another sign of type 1 or 2 diabetes. The thirst is related to the fluid lost because of polyuria.

Your world is fuzzy. Blurry vision can indicate the presence of type 1 or 2 diabetes. "High levels of circulating blood glucose can cause a distortion of the lens," explains Dr. Katz.

You're getting frequent and stubborn infections. Type 2 diabetes can cause repeated or hard-to-cure infections in the body on account of the increased levels of sugar in the blood. Infections typically attack the skin, gums, vagina, or bladder.

You're losing lots of weight. Type 1 diabetes often causes sudden and extreme weight loss.

Don't Panic!

Taken collectively, the symptoms of diabetes are pretty classic, says Florence Brown, M.D., senior staff physician at the Joslin Diabetes Center at Harvard University. "If anything, the problem with diabetes tends to be that the diagnosis is sometimes missed." The symptoms taken separately could point to other ailments, says Dr. Brown. Sudden, unexplained weight loss could point to an overactive thyroid gland. Blurry vision, particularly in those over 40, could be a sign of aging-related changes. And excessive urination could point to a urinary tract infection. If you have only one or two symptoms, you should probably still be checked for diabetes, particularly if you have some of the risk factors.

But even if you discover that you have diabetes, there is no need to panic, says Dr. Brown. It's not that horrible of a diagnosis—after all, there are things that you can do about it.

Who Do I See?

If you've been diagnosed with type 1 or 2 diabetes, there are a number of experts whom you

WOMEN ASK WHY

Why did my mom have to take insulin injections for her diabetes, while the doctor tells me I only need to diet and exercise to control mine?

Today, we know more about the benefits of dietary management and exercise in managing diabetes than we did 20 years ago. We know that people can lose just 10 to 15 pounds and improve their glucose control, whereas years ago, doctors would just automatically use insulin to manage the disease.

The sad thing is that many people think of diabetes as an all-or-nothing proposition. They've been told or they mistakenly believe that they have to lose a great deal of weight and curb their diets to the point of deprivation in order to attain a healthy outcome. Many health professionals talk in terms of 100 percent compliance, meaning that the patient must do everything correctly 100 percent of the time. But that may not be necessary to improve your blood sugar.

According to the American Heart Association and the American Diabetes Association, if people can lose 10 percent of their weight, or an average of 15 pounds, they will improve blood pressure, cholesterol, and blood sugar. The bottom line is, don't be overwhelmed. Focus on small goals. And even if you have to use medication, you may be able to come off it once you lose some weight and begin exercising and eating a healthy diet.

It's important for people to diet and exercise so that they can better utilize the insulin that their bodies make and perhaps put off the need for extra insulin in the future.

Expert consulted
Gail D'Eramo Melkus, Ed.D.
Associate professor and nurse practitioner
Yale School of Nursing

Richardson. Primary-care doctors are usually well-trained at managing type 2 diabetes, and many also treat type 1 patients.

"Some cases of diabetes are more difficult to manage than others," says Dr. Richardson. "If the patient and primary-care doctor both feel that the diabetes management is not working as well as it should, a consultation with an endocrinologist may help."

Nurse educators and nutritionists specializing in diabetes management can address all of the different behaviors involved in managing diabetes, says Dr. Richardson. A nurse educator will help you learn how to check your blood sugar levels, take your medication properly, and monitor your diet.

Whether you have type 1 or type 2 diabetes, you may be prone to secondary symptoms requiring a visit to other specialty physicians. If you have coronary artery disease, you should see a cardiologist, says Dr. Katz. You may also need to see a nephrologist for kidney problems. "I recommend that all diabetes patients see an ophthalmologist twice a year so any possible retinal disease is caught early," she says. Periodic visits to a podiatrist are also helpful because decreased sensation in the feet can lead to unrecognized cuts and infections.

"For patients with type 2 diabetes who do not exercise or walk regularly, the most important consultant might be a personal trainer," says Dr. Richardson. "Personal trainers are experts in helping sedentary patients become

can see for care. You may choose to visit your primary-care physician first. "Most people with diabetes never see a diabetes specialist, who is usually an endocrinologist," says Dr.

physically active." If you cannot afford a personal trainer, you can join an exercise class or exercise with a group of friends for added motivation.

What Can I Expect?

When I first was diagnosed with diabetes, I thought I was dying, recalls former Miss America Nicole Johnson, who has type 1 diabetes. "But once I better educated myself about the disease, I learned that I could control it," she says. Although a diagnosis of type 1 or 2 diabetes will necessitate some lifestyle changes, it is possible to live a happy, healthy life with the disease.

Whether you have type 1 or 2 diabetes, you will need to keep your blood sugar level as close to normal as possible. If you have type 1, and possibly if you have type 2, you will need to take insulin, probably by self-injection. Your physician or nurse will tell you how much insulin you need, when to take it, and what kind you should take. "Instead of injecting insulin, you may also be put on an insulin pump," says Dr. Katz. The size of a beeper, the pump delivers insulin into your abdomen through a small catheter. "The pump gives you a basal level of insulin at all times, but you can program it to give more in preparation for a meal or exercise," she says.

Controlling your blood sugar will require following a meal plan that will tell you when and how much to

IRON-DEFICIENCY ANEMIA

You've probably seen the commercials on television: a young woman or mother complaining that she's fatigued, run-down, or can't get enough sleep—the announcer saying that an iron supplement is the answer to her prayers.

But in reality, iron-deficiency anemia is overdiagnosed, says Suzanne Swietnicki, M.D., of the Mayo Clinic in Jacksonville, Florida. "Iron is overprescribed, in general, in the United States. Largely because of a lot of vitamin ads, people seem to think that when they are tired, they need to take iron. But taking iron can be unhealthy unless you have a reason beyond just feeling tired."

Iron-deficiency anemia, the most common type of anemia, is the lack of iron in the blood. The most common reason for iron deficiency is heavy menstruation, usually lasting longer than 7 days. It can also be caused by blood loss, poor diet, an increased need for iron, or an underlying medical condition. Pregnancy also increases the risk of iron-deficiency anemia. Iron deficiency doesn't always lead to anemia, but it can cause other problems, such as fatigue and weakened immunity.

In most cases, women are not aware that they are anemic. In severe cases, however, you may feel extreme fatigue and weakness, dizziness or fainting, shortness of breath, or heart palpitations. Other symptoms include pale skin, pale nailbeds, and pale lower eyelids.

In addition, several groups of women including those of Mediterranean, Indian, and African-American descent may have a genetic anemia, called thalassemia, which can be misdiagnosed as iron-deficiency anemia.

Health-care professionals don't usually recommend iron supplements unless iron deficiency is confirmed. In fact, excess iron can be harmful because it can lead to liver and heart disease. If you have been diagnosed specifically with iron-deficiency anemia, however, an iron supplement may be prescribed.

The best prevention is to eat a balanced diet containing iron-rich foods, such as meat; fish; poultry; green vegetables, like broccoli and spinach; and legumes, like beans and peas.

eat. "Nutrition is very important in the management of both type 1 and type 2 diabetes," says Dr. Katz. The regimen will likely be somewhat more strict if you have type 1.

A diagnosis of type 1 diabetes will also require you to monitor your blood sugar level. You will do this by pricking your finger and testing your blood with a kit that will indicate your sugar level. You may also need to do home tests if you have a more severe case of type 2 diabetes.

An exercise routine will likely be prescribed for you whether you have type 1 or type 2 diabetes. Exercise helps your body use blood sugar and, therefore, lowers glucose levels in your blood. If you have type 2, exercise will probably be prescribed in conjunction with a weight-loss plan to keep blood sugar levels in check.

On top of everything else, diabetes can worsen changes associated with menopause, such as a lack of sexual desire, vaginal dryness, and pain during intercourse. If you're menstruating or menopausal, you may find that your blood sugar is going haywire.

Coping with diabetes, as with any chronic illness, can be challenging both physically and emotionally. Managing diabetes is a full-time job that calls on your ability to constantly motivate yourself to do the things that will keep you healthy. There are some things that experts suggest you can do to help keep your mind and body in shape.

Don't deny your illness. Most people go through a denial stage when they are first diagnosed, but a long-term state of denial can be dangerous. If you find yourself saying things

WOMAN TO WOMAN

Determination Is Key

Nicole Johnson has lived with diabetes for more than 7 years. As Miss America 1999, Johnson, 26, travels tens of thousands of miles a year, encouraging people to learn more about the disease. Her message to people with diabetes is a simple one: Stay in control and don't give up.

When I first learned that I had diabetes, I was devastated. I thought I was dying.

At the time, I was in college, working a part-time job, juggling extracurricular activities and volunteer work. On weekends, I was starting to compete in the Miss America program, hoping to win scholarships to help pay for school.

When the doctors finally realized that I had type 1 diabetes, I had to drop out of school and stop all my other activities. I learned that to survive, I had to rely on a constant stream of insulin and test my blood glucose regularly.

I was told that I couldn't drink soda and would never be able to eat desserts again. I was afraid I might never be able to marry or have children. I thought a high-pressure career like journalism would be difficult at best. And winning a major beauty pageant? I wasn't the only one who had

like, "One bite won't hurt," or if you stop doing necessary procedures such as testing your blood sugar, you may be in a state of denial. To help yourself get back on track, write down your care plan and goals along with reasons why they are important.

Relieve some stress. The stress of diabetes management can be overwhelming, but there are ways to reduce it. Sharing with members of a support group can help. Sometimes, adding positive things to your life, such as starting an exercise program, taking dance lessons, or volunteering at a charity, can also help.

doubts. Many people told me my goals and dreams were impossible.

For months, I felt fear, self-pity, and anger. Why me? How did I get this? What will happen to me next? There were a million different questions, and as I learned more about diabetes, there seemed to be almost as many answers.

Soon, I made up my mind that even though I might not be able to beat the disease, I wasn't going to let it beat me.

So I read everything I could about diabetes. I found support groups. I learned about the role of diet, nutrition, and exercise in helping to manage my illness. And not only was I able to go back to school, I doubled up on my classes and went on to graduate school.

I worked a part-time job, landed an internship in broadcasting, and returned to pageant competition.

It took me five tries to win the state title that would get me to the Miss America pageant. Some told me that I would never win because of my diabetes. But in 1999, I was crowned Miss America.

I tell people with diabetes that the most important thing that they can do is to be tested and educated. Then, when you have information, you have to take it upon yourself to become an active part of your medical team and to be proactive in your own care.

Don't give up. When you have unexpected highs and lows, keep in mind that your blood sugar level is controlled by outside factors as well as your own efforts. Medications, illnesses, and major life events can all interfere.

Conventional Wisdom

Diabetes is treated with food plans, exercise, oral medications known as insulin sensitizers, or insulin injections. The goal of treatment is to keep blood glucose levels as close to normal as possible.

Besides relying on diet and exercise, people with diabetes have to make time to monitor their blood sugar levels. With diabetes, the doctor and patient set a target blood glucose range, which may be slightly different from the normal range. Performing regular tests helps ensure that you meet your blood glucose goals. "Monitoring your blood sugar and having that information is a powerful tool. It allows you to control your diabetes and not let your diabetes control you," says Dr. Brown.

It is also important for people with diabetes to control the levels of fats in their blood. High cholesterol and triglyceride levels can lead to other serious health problems, such as heart disease and stroke. Blood fats are controlled by some of the same things that control blood glucose levels: healthy eating and exercise.

If following a food-and-exercise plan isn't enough for you to reach and maintain blood glucose goals, the next step in diabetes treatment is to add blood glucose–lowering medications that come in pill form. These oral medications, called insulin sensitizers, are used in conjunction with a healthy diet and exercise to enhance treatment.

Great Alternatives

With the number of people who have diabetes surging, health food stores and experts in holistic medicine are offering a greater variety of supplements to aid glucose management. The following are some of the more common alternative treatments recommended by Jill Stanard, N.D., a naturopathic physician practicing in Providence, Rhode Island.

Gymnema. The leaves of this plant, which grows in tropical forests of central and southern India, seem to help control blood glucose levels. A dose of 400 milligrams a day is recommended.

Bilberry and ginkgo. Both bilberry and ginkgo may improve circulation, lowering the risk of eye damage in patients with diabetes. They are both available freeze-dried or as a tincture. Follow the manufacturer's directions. Do not use ginkgo with antidepressant MAO inhibitor drugs such as phenelzine sulfate (Nardil) or tranylcypromine (Parnate), aspirin or other nonsteroidal anti-inflammatory medications, or blood-thinning medications such as warfarin (Coumadin). Ginkgo can cause dermatitis, diarrhea, and vomiting in doses higher than 240 milligrams of concentrated extract.

Vitamins. "Vitamin C can help prevent the damage to blood vessels that accompanies diabetes," says Dr. Stanard. Take 500 milligrams in the morning and another 500 milligrams later in the day. Take 400 IU of vitamin E daily to help prevent blood vessel damage and help cells use insulin. Niacin contributes to improved insulin activity, and 100 micrograms per day when combined with 200 micrograms of chromium may help normalize glucose levels. Doses above 35 milligrams must be taken under medical supervision.

As with any kind of treatment, you should consult with your doctor or other health professional before using any herbal or alternative treatment.

Heart
Disease

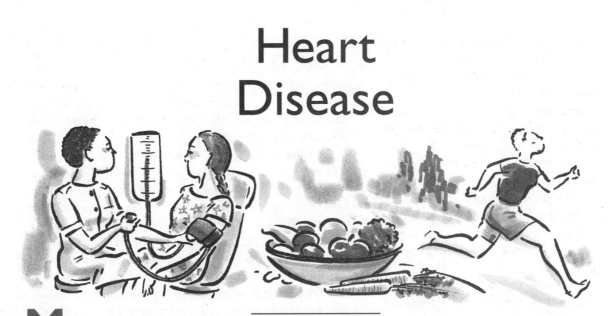

Most women consider breast cancer the greatest threat to their lives and health. But ironically, the greatest danger to our health doesn't lurk in the breast at all—it beats just beneath it.

For every woman killed by breast cancer, cardiovascular disease claims eight.

"Twice the number of women die of cardiac disease—heart attack, heart failure, stroke, all the cardiovascular diseases—as die of all cancers combined," says cardiologist Deborah J. Barbour, M.D., medical director of the coronary-care unit and director of the women's cardiovascular program at Mercy Medical Center in Baltimore. "People just don't know it."

We don't know it because we're used to thinking of heart disease as a male issue. "Our model for heart attacks is not a woman," says clinical psychologist Susan Brace, R.N., Ph.D., who practices in Los Angeles. It's the aggressive businessman keeling over, clutching his heart in the elevator and falling on his briefcase.

The truth is that heart disease is an equal-opportunity illness and has become the number one killer of American women. It appears when consistent exposure to the effects of stress, cou-

pled with high blood pressure, damages the inner lining of the arteries. A sticky blood fat called plaque then begins to accumulate on the damaged areas. Built-up plaque (atherosclerosis, or hardening of the arteries) narrows the arteries and invites blood clots, which reduce or even stop the bloodflow to the heart. The result can be a heart attack or a stroke.

Risk Factors

Heart disease and its awful sibling, stroke, are associated with several risk factors, as identified by the American Heart Association. You're stuck with some, but you can do a lot to change others.

First, here are the ones you can't change.

Age. Around menopause, your risk starts climbing and keeps going up.

Heredity. If a close relative has had heart disease or stroke, your chances of doing the same are increased.

Race. Black women are more likely to get heart disease and stroke than white women.

Health history. If you've had a heart attack or

stroke, you're at higher risk to experience either one at another time.

Here are the factors that you can do something about.

Smoking. Cigarettes skyrocket your risk. Even deadlier is the duo of smoking and birth control pills.

High blood cholesterol. A prime heart disease risk contributor, it is also a co-conspirator for stroke.

High blood pressure. Also known as hypertension, it's the biggest risk factor for stroke, and it's among the top 10 for heart disease.

Inactivity. You may think that a life of leisure is a dream come true, but your heart won't thank you for it.

Overweight. Too much fat, especially around the waist, can weigh you down with cardiovascular problems.

Diabetes. A woman with diabetes has up to seven times the risk of heart disease of one the same age without diabetes. But depending upon the type you have, diabetes can be controlled with insulin or with diet and exercise.

Stress. Though its role in cardiovascular disease isn't clear, unhealthy responses to stress, such as smoking and overeating, are recognized risk factors.

Prevention

Fortunately, if you have some of the changeable risk factors—and it doesn't matter how long you've had them—you can begin modifying and taming them immediately. Here are some places to start.

Snuff cigarettes. "Women smokers come to me asking about herbs and vitamins, and I say, 'Wait a minute,'" reports Sharonne N. Hayes, M.D.,

HIGH BLOOD PRESSURE

You can probably rattle off your height and shoe size, but how about your blood pressure? This measure of how hard blood pushes against blood vessel walls could be a number that saves—or threatens—your life.

For an adult, high blood pressure (HBP), also called hypertension, means that your pressure is 140 over 90 (140/90) or higher. The first number represents systolic pressure, that is, how hard your blood pushes when your heart beats. The second number is your diastolic pressure, which is the measure of the force your blood exerts when your heart is at rest.

Elevated blood pressure, according to the American Heart Association, signals that your heart is working harder than normal to pump blood and oxygen to your organs and tissues. That extra load puts you in extra jeopardy for a host of problems, including hardening of the arteries, heart attacks, and strokes.

Called the silent killer because it has no warning signs, HBP also has no known cause in upward of 95 percent of cases. What we do know, though, is that it more frequently strikes African-Americans, women who take birth control pills, people with diabetes, and those who are obese.

Medications can help control HBP, but there's a better treatment. "Exercise is probably the strongest medicine we have to combat HBP and heart disease," says Janice Christensen, M.D., assistant professor of clinical medicine at the University of Arizona College of Medicine in Tucson. "Most of the drugs available decrease your cardiovascular risk by 20 to 40 percent, but study after study shows that even moderate exercise cuts your risk of heart problems by up to 50 percent." Here are her tips for better blood pressure control.

Move it. Keep weight and blood pressure down by getting up and moving. For women especially, physical inactivity invites higher risk. To keep yourself healthy, get some form of moderate-intensity exercise—such as brisk walking, swimming, or aerobics—for at least 30 minutes most days of the week.

Follow doctor's orders. If you're on a low-salt diet or HBP medication, stick to it; otherwise, pressure can rise.

Do your homework. Because blood pressure rises and falls hour to hour, day to day, home monitors are useful for tracking readings. "Home monitors help you find your average pressure over months and years," says Dr. Christensen. She recommends the commonly available aneroid version, with the familiar stethoscope, arm cuff, and dial gauge, or a digital monitor with an electronic screen display. Ask for a lesson from your doctor or nurse on how to properly use your home monitor. Blood pressure readings will be inaccurate if your cuff is the wrong size, so you should also ask for your doctor's advice on the best size for you. Have your doctor check your machine for initial accuracy, then again annually.

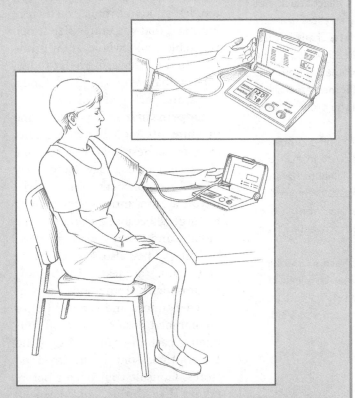

To use a home blood pressure monitor, sit with your back supported and your legs and ankles uncrossed. Place your arm at the level of your heart on a table or desk, and wrap the cuff around the upper part snugly. Some popular digital models will inflate automatically; for others, you will need to squeeze a rubber bulb. Your reading will appear on the display window or dial. Digital home blood pressure machines are portable and easy to use, with the controls and blood pressure readings clearly marked.

director of the Mayo Clinic Women's Heart Clinic. "Your slightly elevated cholesterol's not going to kill you; your 10 pounds overweight won't kill you; but your smoking will." Gender is a minus here, says Dr. Hayes, because the same level of cigarette smoking puts women at greater risk of heart disease than men.

Get off that couch. Movement in the form of exercise tackles almost every preventable facet that underlies heart disease, says Elizabeth Ross, M.D., a cardiologist at Washington Hospital Center in Washington, D.C., and author of *Healing the Female Heart*. "It improves cardiac conditioning and lowers blood pressure, blood sugar, and stress. You couldn't ask for a better prescription."

This menu of heart-healthy benefits is supported by almost 100 studies, which were analyzed recently by two university doctors, one from the University of Toronto and one from Boston University Medical Center. They found that physical activities, such as walking, swimming, and aerobics, help lower blood pressure and prevent the development of high blood pressure, reduce cholesterol levels in the blood, discourage blood clots, and improve blood vessel performance.

Be lighthearted. Exercise also plays a big role in controlling another risk factor: obesity. Maintaining a healthy weight helps avoid the heart-related complications of obesity, according to Dr. Ross. "People who are obese tend to have lower activity levels, elevated cholesterol, diabetes, and higher blood pressure," she says.

WOMEN ASK WHY

Why do you so often hear of men suddenly and without warning dropping dead of heart attacks, but you seldom hear the same about women?

This scenario describes a distinct health problem called sudden cardiac death (SCD). This isn't the "massive heart attack" that we hear about or even a heart attack at all. SCD can be caused by a heart attack, but often it is not. SCD is the result of cardiac arrest: The heart suddenly stops functioning because of a fatal change in the rhythm of its beating, and unexpected death occurs. The reason we don't hear about it striking women as much as men is that it's less common in women. Some researchers speculate that natural estrogen may help protect women against SCD.

In one study at Massachusetts General Hospital in Boston, researchers looked at underlying heart disease in male and female SCD victims. Women seemed less likely to have underlying coronary artery disease: 45 percent, compared to 80 percent for the men. So that suggests that women with coronary artery disease may actually be protected from SCD.

We need to find out how risk factors such as smoking, high blood pressure, and diabetes may differ between men and women. Prevention is key because the survival rate from sudden cardiac arrest is dismal—it ranges from 6 to 25 percent. Anything that can reduce risk is vital.

Expert consulted
Christine Albert, M.D.
Instructor in medicine at Harvard Medical School
Cardiac electrophysiologist at Massachusetts General Hospital

your levels under control. Dr. Barbour's advice is basic and simple: Get your blood pressure and cholesterol checked every year. Your doctor will tell you how low they should be. And if you're on medication, don't stop taking it or make changes without checking with your doctor first.

Favor heart-smart foods. Your mouth helps determine heart health, too. For good nutrition, experts recommend that you emphasize fruits, vegetables, and whole-grain products, and eat fewer high-fat foods, such as baked goods, fried foods, chips, and packaged cookies.

Depressurize. To take some pressure off high blood pressure, experts suggest that you try one clove of garlic a day (stay away from the supplement form of garlic if you are on anticoagulants prior to surgery, because garlic thins the blood and may also increase bleeding). They also suggest trying potassium (at least 3,500 milligrams daily from foods such as baked potatoes and cantaloupe) or a combined dose of 30 to 60 milligrams each of coenzyme Q_{10} and L-carnitine, sold in health food stores. Consult your doctor before taking L-carnitine, and keep in mind that coenzyme Q_{10} can cause a decrease in the effectiveness of the blood thinner warfarin (Coumadin).

Know your numbers. Too much "bad," or low-density lipoprotein (LDL), cholesterol and high blood pressure hurt blood vessels and help heart disease advance, so it's important to keep

Corral cholesterol. Experts offer a wide variety of nutritional options to control cholesterol. One of the newer herbal remedies is guggul, a resin from a tree grown in India. One study there showed a 24 percent drop in cholesterol after a 12-week regimen of 500 milligrams daily. Rarely, guggul may trigger diarrhea, restlessness, or hiccups.

Research also shows benefits from fenugreek, an herb available in seed or capsule form (1 to 2 tablespoons, or two 580-milligram capsules, taken three or four times daily), and a daily teaspoon of ground turmeric, the Indian herb you sprinkle on poultry, fish, and beans (or take a 150-milligram capsule of turmeric three times a day). Watch out for turmeric if you have high stomach acid, ulcers, gallstones, or bile duct obstruction.

Other cholesterol busters include a 3-ounce serving of fish with lots of omega-3 fatty acids, such as mackerel, salmon, and tuna; soy protein (pick your favorite soy product to get 47 grams per day); ground flaxseed (try a tablespoon on cereal, soup, or yogurt); and 500 to 1,000 milligrams daily of vitamin C.

Signs and Symptoms

While both sexes get cardiovascular disease, it's a mistake to assume that it can be diagnosed and treated the same way in each—a mistake that, by postponing care, could end up costing a woman her life.

Heart attack is the most visible sign of heart disease. It means that the vital supply of blood to the heart muscle has been reduced or halted and that immediate medical attention is urgent. "Women really don't

STROKE

"Stroke" sounds ominous but vague. "Brain attack," though, zeroes in on the problem: The brain's supply of blood and oxygen is impaired, and brain cells can die. The symptoms, all sudden, include numbness or weakness of the face, arm, or leg, especially on one side; confusion; trouble speaking or understanding; trouble seeing in one or both eyes; dizziness; loss of balance or coordination; or extreme, unexplained headache.

Stroke is still the third leading cause of death, resulting in many more than 150,000 American deaths annually. It's also a chief culprit in adult disability in the United States. Two million Americans are estimated to struggle with the paralysis, loss of speech, and poor memory that stroke can bequeath, while one million bear little disabling evidence.

Sadly, women are the preferred targets of this cerebrovascular killer, constituting some 62 percent of stroke deaths. Those who smoke and take high-estrogen birth control pills are really in the crosshairs, bearing a stroke risk 22 times higher than average.

"Strokes are very common. People used to tell you that you couldn't do very much: Either you got better or you didn't," says Audrey S. Penn, M.D., deputy director of the National Institute of Neurological Disorders and Stroke in Bethesda, Maryland. "Today, though, prevention and acute treatment are really here."

Here is Dr. Penn's advice to help protect against stroke.

Manage high blood pressure. It's the biggest risk factor for stroke—and a key contributor to heart disease and kidney failure.

Stop smoking, period. Cigarette smoking promotes fatty buildups in your carotid arteries, the main highways for getting blood to your brain.

Get a heart checkup. Undiagnosed heart disease is a big threat since it can produce clots that cut down your brain's bloodflow.

Shake that body. "Exercise is good for everything—your heart, blood pressure, and helping to reduce your stroke risk," says Dr. Penn.

have symptoms as clear-cut as men's," says Dr. Ross. While crushing chest pain is considered the classic red flag of heart attack, the warning signs for women may not wave as vividly.

You need to know when to act. Here's how.

Read the classics. The classic symptoms we most often associate with a heart attack include a feeling of pressure, fullness, squeezing, or pain in the center of the chest that lasts more than a few minutes; pain that spreads to the shoulders, neck, or arms; or chest discomfort accompanied by light-headedness, fainting, sweating, nausea, or shortness of breath.

Beware of *la différence*. Since women are more apt to have symptoms that aren't so classic or typical, according to Dr. Barbour, some other signs you should be aware of include breathlessness; tightness in the chest; sudden, overwhelming fatigue; and nausea.

Tightness or aching in the jaw, teeth, neck, throat, shoulder, or between the shoulder blades is also a warning sign.

Any one of these symptoms doesn't necessarily mean that you're having or about to have a heart attack, but it does mean that you should be checked out by your primary-care physician, advises Dr. Barbour.

Don't Panic!

Any heart attack warning sign may be due to a number of other conditions, some fairly minor. "You don't need to see a cardiologist for every twinge," counsels Dr. Hayes. Sometimes, a feeling of pressure in your chest may be nothing

WOMAN TO WOMAN
Her "Silent Heart Attack" Finally Spoke Up

You can have a heart attack without even knowing it. Just ask Gladys M. Leist, 72, who didn't find out about hers until months afterward. Two more heart attacks later, the retired psychiatric nurse treasures her active, pain-free days. Here's her story.

My children and grandchildren all came to my house in Rochester, Minnesota, for a family dinner about 10 years ago. Right after we ate, I had a little pain in my chest, but I thought it was indigestion. I started feeling really rotten, so one of my daughters, who's a nurse, helped me to the bathroom. I passed out.

When I came to, I remember feeling really, really hot, so I asked my daughter to run some cool bathwater. When I got in the tub, I passed out again, so my daughter called the hospital emergency room. I felt okay after that, so I didn't go to the hospital and didn't really think much about it until I went for my yearly physical at the Mayo Clinic here a few months later. My doctor was looking over all the test results and said, "My gosh, Gladys, you had a heart attack, a silent heart attack. Did you know that?" I didn't.

My mother died of heart trouble when she was 62, so

more than a gassy souvenir of the bean dip you ate before dinner. But if your symptoms concern you at all, see your doctor.

Here are some other examples of conditions that can mimic a heart attack. Heartburn or esophageal reflux-type symptoms, where food and gastric juices flow backward from the stomach, can cause chest pain, says Dr. Hayes. She also notes that many joints, muscles, and their connections within the chest wall can be sources of discomfort.

And according to Dr. Barbour, chest symptoms can also be due to gallbladder disease, ulcers, panic attacks, or a variety of other causes.

partly because of that I've always tried to take care of myself. I never smoked (except when I was 18, for maybe a year) always tried to eat right (lots of low-fat foods, fruits, and vegetables), and I exercise.

That's pretty much what the clinic doctor told me to do, and everything was fine for several years.

Then in 1994, on a visit to my daughter in Iowa, my heart spoke up loudly. On the morning I was planning to drive home to Minnesota, I got up feeling as if something were sitting on my chest. The pain didn't go away, but I still drove the 3½ hours back home. The pain just kept up, and I was sick to my stomach, too. Once I got home, I went to the emergency room at St. Mary's Hospital, where I had surgery called angioplasty to open up a blocked blood vessel.

Then things went pretty well again until last year, when I had another heart attack. I went to the Women's Heart Clinic at Mayo, and they implanted three stents. Those are stainless steel–mesh tubes that keep arteries open. Within a month, I was back to my full activities: I do aerobic exercises, I walk a lot, I use my treadmill at home, I garden, and I play ball with my two grandsons.

I'm not silent about heart disease; I talk to my women friends and family about risk factors, especially smoking, but a lot of them still smoke.

Whether or not we have symptoms, many of us are actually more likely to brush off the threat of heart disease than to overreact, according to research. One study of 200 women ages 41 to 95 done at Stanford University School of Medicine found that only 34 percent knew that heart disease is the leading cause of death in older women.

Who Do I See?

For nonemergencies, the first stop is your family or primary-care physician. "If you have chest pressure, pain, nausea, or shortness of breath when you exercise, you should tell your doctor. These are all concerning symptoms," says Janice Christensen, M.D., assistant professor of clinical medicine at the University of Arizona College of Medicine in Tucson.

If a cardiac problem is suspected, you may be referred to a heart specialist, or cardiologist.

In alternative medicine, options abound—sometimes the same ones offered by conventional medicine. "Heart disease is an area where conventional and alternative medicine are beginning to merge," says Tori Hudson, N.D., a naturopathic physician, professor at the National College of Naturopathic Medicine, and director of A Woman's Time Clinic in Portland, Oregon.

"High-fiber, low-saturated-fat diets with lots of fruits and vegetables, eating soy, the importance of exercise . . . these are all things we naturopathic doctors have been practicing for years," she notes. "Now, clinical research backs us up." Not all heart disease can be treated effectively by a naturopathic physician alone, Dr. Hudson says. "If I have someone with dangerously high blood pressure, I'm calling up my nearest cardiologist and referring her for blood pressure medication before trying herbs and supplements. Then, we'll see if we can gradually reduce her medication while integrating herbal and nutritional therapies."

What Can I Expect?

The physical aspects of cardiovascular disease take many forms, from heart attack to chronic chest pain, and so do the methods to diagnose it. In your doctor's office, a physical exam may start with the familiar cuff and pump to take your blood pressure. From there, depending on your risk factors, health history, and symptoms, you may have an electrocardiogram, a chest x-ray, an exercise stress test, or a nuclear imaging test.

Be wary of the exercise stress test, cautions Dr. Barbour. "Women tend to have false readings from a treadmill workout because women don't have the same response to exercise that men do." Instead, she prefers a stress echocardiogram or a stress test with imaging as a more reliable way to test the heart at rest and under exertion.

Emotionally, heart disease can have a frightful impact. "There's a 'terrified factor' with women who've had heart problems," says Dr. Brace. "They're really scared it might happen again."

A former coronary-care nurse who specializes in treating people with chronic and terminal illnesses, Dr. Brace sees a wide range of women's responses to heart attack. "Some women become more careful in a reasonable way, and some become what we call cardiac cripples: They're afraid to reach for the sugar because they might have another attack and die."

Some level of fear is perfectly normal, Dr. Brace relates, and so is grieving for a healthy heart. Medically, heart attacks are called MIs (myocardial infarctions). "The *infarction* means that part of the heart muscle didn't get blood and died," she says.

The grief response is extremely common in women diagnosed with heart disease, affirms Dorothea Lack, Ph.D., clinical assistant professor in the psychiatry department at the University of California, San Francisco. "There's

WOMEN ASK WHY

Why do they say that flossing my teeth can help my heart?

The connection is the bacteria in plaque, that invisible, sticky film that forms on your teeth. Without daily flossing, brushing, and periodic professional care to remove that plaque, you can develop periodontal (gum) disease, as do three out of four Americans over the age of 35. Gum disease bacteria can gain entry to your bloodstream through injured tissue. Ultimately, these bacteria can contribute to narrowed arteries and blood clots, which can lead to heart attacks.

Our research team at the University at Buffalo School of Dental Medicine was among the first to find a link between plaque bacteria and the risk of heart attack. During one of our studies, we found that people who had one of the more damaging types of oral bacteria had up to a 300 percent greater risk of heart attack than people without the bacteria. Continuing research lets us say with certainty that you cannot be healthy without oral health.

Here are the latest recommendations.

Get a physical for your mouth. At every regular dental checkup, don't just ask if you have cavities. Ask about your

guilt (thinking they caused the disease themselves by not exercising or eating healthfully), denial, shock, rage, depression, and, finally, acceptance."

Of course, different women handle their heart disease differently, reports Dr. Lack, who specializes in the psychology of medicine. Someone who handles life's challenges in a relaxed, accepting way is probably going to do better than someone who is anxious and driven. A litigation lawyer is not going to do as well as a yoga teacher, she observes.

Here's what the two psychologists find most effective in helping women handle heart disease.

plaque accumulation; get a complete probing of your gums once a year.

Ask for flossing feedback. You can be diligent about flossing and not be effective at removing plaque if your technique or flossing material isn't right for you. Show your hygienist your flossing technique and discuss your brushing habits. Ask what you can change to improve your oral health.

Buy right for your mouth. With all the different toothpastes, aids, and flosses on the market, it's easy to be misled. Tartar-control toothpastes benefit some, not all, people; mouthwashes that have an antibacterial effect are available; some floss is coated to resist shredding. Your oral-care program shouldn't be built around advertising. Ask your hygienist and dentist what's best for you.

Like taking a shower and washing your hair, oral health used to be regarded merely as part of your daily routine. Now we know that the prevention of oral disease is far more important than we used to believe.

Expert consulted
Sara Grossi, D.D.S.
Clinical director
Periodontal Disease Research Center
State University of New York at Buffalo

Cry if you want to. Being upset is a normal part of serious illness. Try to accept your feelings.

Be helpless sometimes. "Women caretake other people so much that we think we're not supposed to get sick. There are some things we can't fix or change," says Dr. Brace.

Give yourself positive messages. "The thought process is a key part of rehabilitating a cardiac patient," Dr. Lack avows. People make their own 'audiotapes' that they play over and over in their minds. It's important that they find out what messages they're sending themselves and if they're negative, try to change them, she adds.

Conventional Wisdom

Today, there are reasons to be positive if you're diagnosed with heart disease, affirms Dr. Hayes. Conventional medicine offers several treatment options and procedures, some especially good news for women.

Diagnosis. A noninvasive test known as electron beam computed tomography (EBCT) can detect heart disease in women who have no outward symptoms. The EBCT rapidly scans the beating heart with x-rays in search of problems in the arteries.

Medicines. Taking drugs called statins may reduce a woman's cholesterol and will consequently reduce her chances of having a first heart attack, says Dr. Hayes. An aspirin a day can work as a preventive method for a woman who has already had a heart attack. Long-acting drugs called nitrates and beta-blockers can be taken for chronic chest pain.

Devices and materials. To open the arterial highway for better blood-flow to the heart, doctors can perform a balloon angioplasty, inserting a catheter or tube into a narrowed artery and literally inflating the balloon. To keep widened arteries from reclosing, doctors can implant a stent, a wire-mesh tube. And there have been huge advances in the catheters, metals, and computers used for these and other procedures, says Dr. Hayes. "Arteries that we wouldn't have touched 3 years ago we're doing successfully now. This is a particular advantage for women, because their arteries are smaller than men's."

Surgery. There's a less invasive type of bypass surgery where the incision is made under a breast, reports Dr. Hayes. And for people who are not el-

---

GOING TO EXTREMES

Two diet and exercise plans that mandate extremely low levels of fat intake have documented success in lowering cholesterol and weight levels, but they require big lifestyle changes. Both plans, one created by Dean Ornish, M.D., and the other by Nathan Pritikin, call for limiting fat to as little as 10 percent of daily calories, exercising, and managing stress. Are they the answer for everyone? Probably not.

"For someone with a severe form of heart disease, the Ornish or Pritikin plan is probably okay," observes Beverly Yates, N.D., a naturopathic physician practicing in Seattle, and author of *Heart Health for Black Women*. "But for the average person trying to be preventive, getting that fat intake down to about 10 percent is very tough."

"Ornish and Pritikin have done groundbreaking work," says Elizabeth Ross, M.D., a cardiologist at Washington Hospital Center in Washington, D.C., and author of *Healing the Female Heart*. "But you have to match the intervention with the severity of the disease—and the patient's ability to adapt." While she does recommend the strict low-fat regimens for some patients, Dr. Ross notes that many people are in too much of a hurry to comply with the programs.

Recently, four of the nation's top health organizations, including the American Heart Association, issued "Unified Dietary Guidelines" to help prevent heart disease and other killers. A ceiling of 30 percent of calories from fat is recommended, with the complex carbohydrates of fruits, vegetables, grains, and cereals pegged at a minimum of 55 percent.

---

preventing and treating heart disease: exercise, nutrition, and stress management. "There's a huge variety of things alternative medicine can do here," attests Beverly Yates, N.D., a naturopathic physician practicing in Seattle and author of *Heart Health for Black Women*. Here are some preferred therapies.

Manage your minerals. If a woman is athletic or eats a poor-quality diet high in saturated fats and trans fatty acids, she may need extra magnesium and calcium, says Dr. Yates. Typical dosages are 350 milligrams a day of magnesium oxide and 1,200 to 1,500 milligrams daily of calcium carbonate. People with heart or kidney problems should check with their doctors before taking supplemental magnesium.

Eat your herbs. For women with high blood pressure or high cholesterol levels, Dr. Yates deploys a varying arsenal of herbs: hawthorn, shown to open arteries and improve bloodflow to the heart; ginkgo, for its dual action in strengthening vein tissues and enhancing brain bloodflow; and garlic, which has been shown to help decrease high cholesterol levels and increase "good" high-density lipoprotein (HDL) cholesterol. Dr. Yates also suggests trying citrus fruits and berries for their bioflavonoids, compounds that strengthen blood vessels.

Step up soy. Soy flour, soybeans, tofu, whatever the form, Dr. Hudson says to aim for 47 grams of soy protein a day. That was the average amount, she reports, in a summary of 38 clinical trials showing cholesterol reductions of more than 9 percent through soy protein intake.

---

igible for a bypass because of certain obstacles, such as the locations of their blockages, one investigational technique seems to be promising. The new procedure involves using a laser beam to foster the growth of new blood vessel cells.

Great Alternatives

Alternative and conventional medicine are pretty much in sync on several key aspects of

Go high fiber. Yes, a bowl of oat bran cereal or oatmeal each day can help lower cholesterol levels by 8 to 23 percent in as little as 3 weeks, advises Dr. Hudson. These and other sources of soluble fiber, such as fresh fruits and beans, promote the intestines' ability to excrete cholesterol.

Downplay "bad" fats. Saturated fats, typically animal fats, are associated with higher cholesterol levels. Instead, Dr. Hudson urges, reach for monounsaturated oils, like olive and canola oils, and steer clear of margarine. "Margarine is an unsaturated fat that has been made into a saturated fat," she explains. "Margarine raises the bad LDL cholesterol levels, lowers the good HDL cholesterol, and can therefore increase the incidence of heart disease."

Find "good" fats. For the clot-busting, blood pressure–lowering benefits of omega-3 fatty acids, reach for salmon, tuna, halibut, mackerel, and herring, advises Dr. Hudson.

Osteoporosis

Margaret Atwood, the Canadian novelist, poet, and critic, once said, "The basic Female body comes with the following accessories: garter belt, panti-girdle, crinoline, camisole, bustle, brassiere, stomacher, chemise, virgin zone, spike heels, nose ring, veil, kid gloves, fishnet stockings, fichu, bandeau, Merry Widow, weepers, chokers, barrettes, bangles, beads, lorgnette, feather boa, basic black, compact, Lycra stretch one-piece with modesty panel, designer peignoir, flannel nightie, lace teddy, bed, head."

An exhaustive list, but she may have missed one item: a plaster cast for those with a tendency toward brittle bones.

The disease of "porous bone," osteoporosis, can strike at any age but prefers postmenopausal women. That's because estrogen, which has a starring role in maintaining bone strength, begins to dwindle around menopause, making you more susceptible. Osteoporosis is a stealthy disease and has no symptoms of its own. In fact, the first clue that your bones are fragile may not come until you break one, usually in the wrist, hip, or spine, during a bump or fall. In time, it can make your bones so brittle that you find yourself hunched over with a dowager's hump.

All in all, not a pretty picture, but not an inevitable one either. In fact, the outlook for this disease is improving all the time.

"The media picture of the older woman is of one bent over and disabled," notes Karen A. Roberto, Ph.D., professor and director of the Center for Gerontology at Virginia Polytechnic Institute and State University in Blacksburg, Virginia. While osteoporosis can disfigure and disable, that's absolutely not the picture of everyone with the disease, she says. "We have new treatment options, and there's new hope."

The hope is that osteoporosis, which sneaks around our skeletons like a cat burglar, can be caught before it makes off with the strength and support of our bones.

Risk Factors

Although there's nothing we can do about some of the major risk factors for osteoporosis, others are well within our control. So while it may be impossible to make this disease disappear from the face of the Earth, each of us can make some changes to help keep it from becoming a scourge in her life.

Here are the risk factors we're just plain stuck with, according to the Osteoporosis and Related Bone Diseases unit of the National Institutes of Health.

Gender. Eight out of 10 Americans with low bone density or osteoporosis are women. In their lifetimes, fully half of all women over age 50 will have broken bones as a result of the disease.

Age. It's true that risk increases as the years roll on: Time steals bone strength and density. The lowered estrogen levels of menopause, combined with age, are "the biggest influences on what happens to a woman's bones," according to Ethel S. Siris, M.D., director of the Toni Stabile Center for the Prevention and Treatment of Osteoporosis at Columbia-Presbyterian Medical Center in New York City.

Body size. If you're small-boned and thin (under 127 pounds), you're at greater risk than bigger women.

Race. Caucasian and Asian women have been thought to be at higher risk than African-American and Hispanic women. A study from Columbia University, though, suggests that ethnic background is a less important factor than many believed.

Family and personal history. You're more susceptible to breaking a bone if one of your parents has a

BAD TO THE BONE: STEROIDS

Remember the schoolyard retort "Sticks and stones may break my bones, but names will never hurt me"? There's one name that may: steroid-user.

Corticosteroid drugs like prednisone (Deltasone) or dexamethasone (Decadron) are often prescribed for people with rheumatoid arthritis, asthma, lung disease, and other chronic ailments. But even as they help with the symptoms of those diseases, they can be paving the way for osteoporosis.

"We have to be especially watchful with people who are taking steroids, because we know that the medication can cause bone loss," says Diana L. Anderson, Ph.D., director of the osteoporosis center at St. Paul Medical Center in Dallas. Some 20 percent of the people who come to her center, she reports, are taking some form of steroids, increasing their risk of fractures.

And the risk can be big. According to the National Osteoporosis Foundation, taking corticosteroids is among the top 10 risk factors for developing the bone-sapping disease. The bone loss from steroids can be swift, especially in the first 3 to 6 months of treatment. "If you take steroids, you need to be aware of the effect on your bones," says Dr. Anderson. Most of the men treated at the St. Paul Osteoporosis Center are referred by their rheumatologists because of steroid usage, she reports. Both women and men who have had heart or lung transplants are often referred, according to the director, because some of their medications can also rob bone.

Bones fall prey to steroids for two reasons: First, the drugs chip away at the body's bone-making power, and second, they impede the absorption of calcium, a vital bone-building nutrient.

Here is Dr. Anderson's bone-healthy advice for women who take steroids.

Know your steroid status. Talk with your doctor about your medications and the effect that they may have on your skeleton.

Remember the two Ms. Your higher risk means that you should be managed and monitored carefully.

history of fractures or if you've had a fracture as an adult.

Here are the risk factors that you can do something about.

Sex hormones. Due to low estrogen levels, an abnormal absence of menstrual periods, including a premenopausal halt in menstruation due to anorexia, bulimia, or too much exercise, can boost risk. So can normal or early menopause.

Bone-depleting diet. Have you made a lifelong habit of skimping on calcium and vitamin D? You could be in trouble.

Medications. Drugs used to treat chronic medical conditions such as rheumatoid arthritis and seizures can batter bones. Other risk boosters include thyroid hormones, glucocorticoids, anticonvulsants, and antacids with aluminum.

Smoking. If you still need a reason to quit, think about this: By smoking, you double your risk of an osteoporosis bone break. The habit has been linked to earlier menopause, bone cell damage, and blockage of new bone.

Excessive drinking. Heavy alcohol use is not a healthy habit, especially in the eyes of the National Osteoporosis Foundation (NOF). Drinking too much will increase your risk of developing the disease.

Inertia. "If you're physically active, you avoid the extra bone loss that highly sedentary people get," advises Dr. Siris. So get moving.

High blood pressure. In a study of 3,676 women ages 66 to 91, doctors found that the higher the blood pressure, the greater the amount of bone loss in the hip, which means an increased risk of fracture there.

REAL-LIFE SCENARIO

She Won't Get Her Bone Density Checked Because She's Scared of What She'll Find Out

Jo, 55, knows all about osteoporosis. She's made it her business to know. Both her mother and her grandmother suffered terrible leg and rib fractures from the disease after they went through menopause, and she has no intention of ending up the same way. So she has read every bit of literature she could find on the subject, has been adding extra calcium to her diet for years, and does weight-bearing, bone-building exercise religiously. But now that she's gone through menopause herself, her doctor has recommended that she get her bone density checked, and she has adamantly refused. As far as she's concerned, she has done everything as "natural" as she can to protect herself, and if she's going to end up like her mother and grandmother anyway, she doesn't want to know until it happens. Should her doctor just give up?

In Jo's case, it's what she might *not* find out that's disturbing. Without a bone-density test, Jo and her doctor can't know exactly what her bone mass picture is now, and they'll have nothing to compare it with in the future.

Far from giving up, her doctor should tell Jo why this test is so important: It gives a baseline reading. It gives knowledge. And the doctor can use that knowledge to Jo's advantage in future tests to detect bone loss, can prescribe medications, and can recommend changes in exercise or diet—all to help slow down or even halt osteoporosis.

Prevention

You *can* beat the odds of getting osteoporosis, say experts. These are the leading strategies, according to Felicia Cosman, M.D., clinical director of the NOF.

Reduce your risk. If you have one or more of the risk factors that can be changed, change it. If you smoke, stop. Cut down on heavy

So while Jo is smart to take extra calcium and do weight-bearing exercise, she's hurting herself by avoiding the test. Her doctor may be able to win her over by explaining how simple, fast, and noninvasive a bone-density test is.

The preferred bone-density test, and the one that's most precise, is a DEXA (dual-energy x-ray absorptiometry). There's nothing scary, no enclosure, no pain; the test is totally nonthreatening, and you often can keep all your clothes on.

Here's what happens: You lie on a regular doctor's exam table in your street clothes (as long as you're wearing no metal, like a buckle or bra fastener). An arm called a scanner is positioned above you, and it moves back and forth over you, from your neck to your lower abdomen. While this happens, a technician is usually in the room with you, watching the images that the scanner feeds to a computer screen. This equipment is very sensitive and high-tech.

After 15 minutes on the table, you're done. A DEXA test is quite safe: The scanner emits less radiation than one chest x-ray. There's no lead-lined room or special radiation requirement because the DEXA test is so low-dose.

To a great degree, osteoporosis is preventable. What Jo doesn't know can hurt her, and her doctor should try even harder to convince her to get a DEXA test.

Expert consulted
Diane L. Anderson, Ph.D.
Director of the osteoporosis center
St. Paul Medical Center
Dallas

Concentrate on calcium. Bone-building calcium comes from an array of dairy foods (nonfat or low-fat), calcium-fortified soy milk and juices, and supplements. Don't rely on pills alone, though, to get your 1,200 to 1,500 milligrams daily. "It's important that your diet plus any supplement provide at least 1,200 milligrams of calcium every day," advises Dr. Cosman.

But not just any calcium supplement will do. Read the label to find the elemental calcium content, says Dr. Cosman. That's the important number to know if you want to meet your daily need. A 1,000-milligram calcium carbonate pill, for example, may have just 400 milligrams of elemental calcium content. For best absorption, look for calcium citrate.

Dig into "D." Because vitamin D helps the body absorb calcium, it's a grade-A part of avoiding osteoporosis. Get 400 IU per day in a multivitamin, a vitamin D supplement, or a calcium supplement. Dr. Cosman suggests taking even more vitamin D if you're over 65 (but keep it below 2,000 IU). Vitamin D and calcium are a powerful pair: They've been shown to significantly reduce the risk of hip and other fractures in women over age 65.

drinking. If you're taking any medications that may damage bone, talk to your doctor about possibly reducing dosage or changing medications (but don't make any changes without consulting your doctor first). If you have low estrogen, think about hormone-replacement therapy (HRT). Get your blood pressure under control. And of course, if you don't exercise, get moving.

Stand up for your bones. Aerobic exercise done while standing appears to yield the most bone benefits, according to Dr. Cosman. Tennis, a treadmill workout, walking, stair-climbing, and low-impact aerobic dance are all recommended. Add in a muscle-strengthening routine with free weights or an exercise video and repeat three to five times per week. You'll help keep bones and muscles strong, boost co-

daily had higher bone densities than those who abstained. Exactly how alcohol helps is still a question mark; it may increase estrogen or stimulate the body's production of calcitonin, a bone-friendly hormone.

Get tested. For women at or beyond menopause who have one or more risk factors or who have had a fracture, the cornerstone of prevention is three letters: BMD. They stand for bone mineral density, also called bone mass, and having it measured is a must, especially if you have a family history of osteoporosis. Dr. Siris recommends that you have your BMD tested when you turn 65 or if you're postmenopausal, whichever comes first.

"Just as a mammogram gives you a baseline for detecting breast cancer, a BMD test is your foundation for detecting and preventing osteoporosis," says Diane L. Anderson, Ph.D., director of the osteoporosis center at St. Paul Medical Center in Dallas. The object is to detect the disease before a fracture occurs, predict your chances of a future break, and monitor rates of bone loss. Several types of machines are used to measure bone density, but the undisputed leader is DEXA (dual-energy x-ray absorptiometry).

"DEXA is the gold standard of bone-density testing," says Dr. Anderson, who describes the process as painless, noninvasive, and brief: 15 minutes. With very low-dose radiation, it scans your spine and hip to take "pictures" of these areas where osteoporosis can have the gravest consequences.

Other devices take bone-mass measurements

ordination, and probably reduce your risk of falling, she says.

Drink to your health? Moderate amounts of alcohol—say, one glass of wine a day—may actually be good for your bones (except for women at high risk of breast cancer), reports Dr. Cosman. In a study of 188 postmenopausal women, researchers found that those who drank at least the equivalent of about one glass of wine

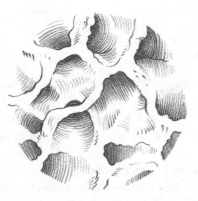

In healthy bone, the network of numerous bone fragments is large and connected, giving strength and stability.

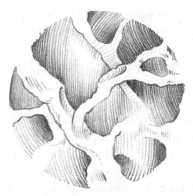

This bone, riddled with osteoporosis, shows bone fragments that are sparse and not well-connected.

in your wrist, heel, or finger, and an ultrasound version takes readings at your heel, shinbone, and kneecap.

A handful of medications are available for preventing osteoporosis, some fairly new, but they are for postmenopausal women only, according to Dr. Siris.

Signs and Symptoms

Are you peering a little higher over the steering wheel lately? Do you have a backache that doesn't go away? Or have you had a broken bone after age 40? These are all warning signs that osteoporosis could be doing its bone-zapping work.

Shrinking stature. Up to an inch of height loss is common among those ages 60 to 80, but if you are younger or have shrunk more than that, it could be due to a spinal fracture caused by osteoporosis. Such fractures can be gradual or can strike suddenly. "You may have sudden, severe pain with a vertebral fracture that gets better over several weeks," observes Dr. Siris. More common is a gradual break in a vertebra— "It kind of squishes down on itself," she says— and either one can make you shorter.

An aching back. Chronic, nagging back pain can be a warning sign of a fractured vertebra. "The break changes the contour of the back, and you're not aligned properly," notes Dr. Siris.

A fracture from a fall. If you slip on the stairs and break your wrist, the fracture might not be due to osteoporosis, but it could be. The NOF estimates that osteoporosis causes more than 1.5 million fractures every year. Weakened bones are simply more susceptible to breaking than strong ones. And if you've had an osteoporotic fracture after age 40, you're twice as likely to have another as someone who hasn't had one at all.

"Many middle-aged and older people think, 'Well, I get older and I fall,'" says Dr. Anderson. "But it isn't the falling down that really causes the fractures. It's the osteoporosis."

Naturally, preventing falls is a prime objective if you have osteoporosis. Here are some everyday tips that can help.

Slip into shoe safety. Stick with supportive, low-heeled shoes, indoors and out; rubber soles increase traction. Avoid walking in socks, stockings, or slippers.

Walk wisely. When sidewalks are slippery, keep on the grass. Step carefully on highly polished floors, especially when they're wet.

Clean up your rooms. Clear the clutter, especially on floors, that invites bumps and stumbles.

Keep floor fashions secure. Use area rugs and carpets with nonskid backs.

Head off bathroom hazards. Put safety first with a rubber bath mat in the tub or shower, and install grab bars nearby.

Cut the cord. Let a cordless phone cut out those headlong rushes to answer calls.

Don't Panic!

These pains and problems may trigger false fears of osteoporosis, according to Dr. Siris.

Intermittent back pain. The most likely cause is a muscle sprain or possibly arthritis. Osteoporosis itself doesn't hurt, so there's no painful alarm to warn of thinning bones. "If a bone breaks suddenly because of osteoporosis, then of course there's pain," observes Dr. Siris. But the disease doesn't declare itself until that break.

Curving upper back. "Some women come to me because they think they're starting to get a curved back, the dreaded dowager's hump, and they're terrified," Dr. Siris says. What many actually have is a slight bend to the upper back from poor posture or a muscle condition unrelated to osteoporosis.

Who Do I See?

Since osteoporosis is a "woman's disease," the first health professional to bring up the topic may be a gynecologist. "Gynecologists are becoming more responsible and responsive about

PAGET'S DISEASE: LEGACY OF THE *MAYFLOWER*

Along with its cargo of Pilgrims and dreams, the Mayflower may also have brought to America a genetic legacy that deforms bones. It's called Paget's disease, named after the English physician who first studied it, Sir James Paget.

Like osteoporosis, Paget's disease involves bone cells called osteoclasts that remove old bone so that other cells can build new bone. Unlike osteoporosis, which can affect the entire skeleton, Paget's osteoclasts zero in on the skull, spine, pelvis, or legs, creating enlarged bones that are weaker than normal. Pain, deformities, fractures, and arthritis can follow.

"In Paget's, the osteoclasts at affected sites aggressively remove bone," relates Ethel S. Siris, M.D., director of the Toni Stabile Center for the Prevention and Treatment of Osteoporosis at Columbia-Presbyterian Medical Center in New York City. "That requires the bone-building cells to come marching in in great numbers and quickly, haphazardly, lay down new bone." The resulting new bone is bigger but flimsier than usual. And the outcome in more severe cases can be an enlarged skull, sometimes with hearing loss from affected nerves; a bowed leg; or a curved spine. What's the

educating their patients, as are some internists," says Dr. Cosman.

As the NOF works to spread awareness, women themselves are taking the lead. "We're telling women that if you're menopausal—and especially if you have any of the risk factors—you should talk to your primary-care physician about getting a bone-density test," says Dr. Cosman. Often, it's this patient-to-doctor inquiry, and not vice versa, that leads to testing.

Osteoporosis doesn't "belong" to any one medical specialty, so if an expert is needed, there are three main types who may be called on. One, like Dr. Cosman, is an endocrinologist, who

Mayflower connection? Paget's is very common in England, present in other parts of Europe, and rare in Asia and Africa.

Affecting about 2 percent of Americans over the age of 50, Paget's can run in families, says Dr. Siris, and research is pinpointing genes that may be responsible. Viruses are also suspected in the ailment. Women and men are equally affected by the disease, which can be very mild. Many people with the disorder don't know they have it.

Osteoclasts aren't the only thing that Paget's disease and osteoporosis have in common. "A lot of the drugs that some people think are new for osteoporosis were actually being used years ago for Paget's," says Dr. Siris. Calcitonin and bisphosphonates such as alendronate (Fosamax) or risedronate (Actonel), which work on shutting down overzealous bone removal, were the drugs of choice as long as 25 years ago.

Today, blood tests, x-rays, and bone scans tell physicians whether Paget's is at work and where. "This disease doesn't strike an array of places in the skeleton like osteoporosis," says Dr. Siris. "Where it's detected is where it is." While research moves forward to identify just what causes Paget's, drugs and exercise therapies can help allay pain and the progress of the disease. "A lot of primary-care physicians still say, 'Forget it, there's no treatment,'" she says. "That's just not true."

deals with hormone-related conditions. Another is a rheumatologist, who concentrates on diseases of joints and connective tissue. Finally, orthopedists are doctors who correct skeletal problems surgically.

What Can I Expect?

If you can avoid fractures, you'll evade the pain potential of osteoporosis. "If you've never broken a bone," says Dr. Siris, "you can expect that with proper evaluation and intervention you'll be able to maintain good bone health as you grow older."

But if you're in that half of women over age 50 who have an osteoporotic break in their lifetimes, the picture changes. You may recover to as good as new from a first spinal fracture, according to Dr. Siris, but your risk of future fractures zooms. A hip break requires surgery, whereas a broken arm or wrist can be put in a cast.

Emotional fractures can't be detected by a machine, but they can be as shattering as a broken bone, says Dr. Roberto. "Osteoporosis affects every aspect of a woman's life, from physical pain and disability rolling right into self-esteem and self-perception."

After 15 years researching the psychological and social aspects of the disease, Dr. Roberto finds that women's feelings about osteoporosis move through three stages: denial, information-seeking, and coping.

Denial, or a dismissive attitude, often comes with the second fracture: "The first fracture, most women manage; the second fracture can begin a spiral into fear, depression, and stress," she says.

In the information-seeking stage, the woman herself gathers all the material she can about osteoporosis. Dr. Roberto says that family and friends need to be included in this information loop, too. "We've found that when a woman has a visible fracture, like a broken hip, the family is usually helpful and understanding. But when it's a vertebral fracture, which you can't see," she relates, "the attitude can be 'Mom looks the same; what's the problem?'"

Finally, coping comes as a woman readapts to the reality that there are things she can do and things she can't, says Dr. Roberto. One woman who loved marathon shopping days parcelled her outings to one store per day, with rest days in between. Others, who had been skiers or golfers, took up less vigorous activities. "Our runners became our walkers," she says.

Based on interviews with hundreds of women with osteoporosis, Dr. Roberto offers these coping strategies.

Find strength in numbers. Support groups can be a great source of comfort and assurance. If your doctor can't help you locate one nearby, write to the National Osteoporosis Foundation, Attn.: Support Groups, 1232 22nd Street NW, Washington, DC 20037-1292 or visit the foundation's Web site at www.nof.org.

Cultivate calm and quiet. Relaxation techniques like meditation and visualization can help ease fear and stress.

Opt for options. When pain alters your plans, find a distraction: Read, talk to a friend on the phone, work on a craft project.

Be frank with family. Some older women with osteoporosis have a particular emotional stab: They can't pick up their grandchildren for fear of breaking a bone. Letting children and adults in the family know what you're experiencing helps them understand.

Conventional Wisdom

Advances in detecting and treating the disease help make it far from inevitable. Here are some of those strategies.

Determining density. In the last few years, techniques to measure bone density have multiplied, says Dr. Cosman. While the DEXA test of the hip and spine is considered the best, other

WOMEN ASK WHY

Why is a fractured hip so serious for an older woman?

A fractured or broken hip means surgery, and to some extent, that's why it's so serious: the complications of surgery and of being immobilized.

At the National Osteoporosis Foundation, we have a single statistic that points out just how grave this can be: An average of 24 percent of hip fracture patients age 50 and over die in the year following their fractures. Just as alarming, about 25 percent of older women with hip fractures require placement in a nursing home because they never regain the independence that they had prior to the fractures. When you consider that women have a hip fracture rate two to three times higher than men and that 80 percent of Americans with osteoporosis are women, it's clear that this poses a considerable threat to our gender.

Older people should stay active to maintain health, but a hip fracture can keep them bedridden for a week or two. Subject them to surgery, and there's a great toll from that: They can get pneumonia, heart disease, or infections, and all of this contributes to the death rate in the year after the fracture. The majority survive, but quality of life can be severely af-

tests can still be useful in predicting the risk of fracture.

Some "peripheral" tests, like those found at health fairs, can be helpful screening tools, notes Dr. Anderson. "They may tell you if you have osteoporosis or a bone density that should be looked at with a DEXA, but not all of these tests are equal in their ability to predict the risk of fractures."

Hormone power. For postmenopausal women, hormone-replacement therapy with estrogen or other hormones is still a standby in reducing the risk of osteoporotic fractures. But questions about side effects and links with cancer remain unresolved.

fected. Hip fracture is a leading cause of admission to nursing homes.

Actually, when we say "hip fracture," we're really talking about a break in the thighbone, or femur. The top of the femur, called the proximal femur, is where "hip fracture" occurs—it's all the same bone. That bone is what fits into the socket of the hip, like an upside-down L—the short piece is actually in the hip and the long piece is the thighbone. So what most people call a broken hip, doctors call a proximal femur fracture. And a fracture along any part of the femur is a major problem; it always requires surgery.

From my clinical experience, I can report a common scenario: Women in their seventies and eighties who are fully functional and having a good quality of life fall and fracture their hips. Many of them just never get back to life as before because the older you get, the harder it is to recover from a trauma. Put a 20-year-old down for 2 weeks, and she pops back up, but this is less and less likely as people get older.

Sadly, statistically, a hip fracture is what's going to take many older women down.

Expert consulted
Felicia Cosman, M.D.
Clinical director
National Osteoporosis Foundation

Pharmacy factor. New drugs with fewer side effects are now available to prevent and treat osteoporosis. They include raloxifene (Evista), a selective estrogen receptor modulator (SERM) shown to increase bone mass in the spine and hips and reduce the risk of vertebral fracture by up to 50 percent. A 3-year study of 7,705 post-menopausal women that produced those results also suggested a stunning effect on breast cancer: Raloxifene reduced the risk of invasive breast cancer by 75 percent.

Also making a difference are alendronate (Fosamax), which is especially effective for reducing spine and hip fractures, and a companion drug called risedronate (Actonel). Calcitonin, a hormone that slows bone loss and modestly builds spinal bone density, is a common treatment for women at least 5 years beyond menopause.

Great Alternatives

Calcium and vitamin D: There's no contest and no controversy here between conventional and alternative medicine. These are the big guns in the battle to keep bones strong, agrees Lorilee Schoenbeck, N.D., a naturopathic physician in Shelburne, Vermont.

Once a patient's bone-density test indicates osteopenia (reduced bone mass that isn't yet osteoporosis), Dr. Schoenbeck tailors these options to her individual needs.

Boost calcium benefits. To ensure that the calcium you take is readily absorbed into your system, Dr. Schoenbeck suggests that you look for calcium citrate supplements. Shoot for 1,000 milligrams as your total daily intake of calcium if you're premenopausal and 1,500 milligrams a day if you're postmenopausal. These amounts include any calcium that you get from your diet.

Be diligent about D. If you diligently slather on the sunscreen in summer or stay indoors all winter, you could be shielding yourself from the sun's vitamin D. If you fall into either of these categories, Dr. Schoenbeck insists that vitamin D supplementation is essential. Women who already have reduced bone density should get up to 800 IU of vitamin D daily.

Crank up the K. Keep eating dark leafy greens such as lettuce, broccoli, and spinach. Their high vitamin K content helps your body produce osteocalcin, a protein building block for bone.

Remember magnesium. Help your bones absorb calcium by getting this important mineral in foods like bananas and baked potatoes with skins. If eating a dozen potatoes is enough to drive you bananas, Dr. Schoenbeck recommends supplements of 500 milligrams a day. (Many calcium supplements include magnesium, but if you take a combination supplement, be sure you are not exceeding 2,500 milligrams of calcium.) Because this is a high amount of magnesium, you should check with your doctor before taking supplements if you have heart or kidney problems; also, supplemental magnesium may cause diarrhea in some people.

Hip, hip, ipriflavone! Derived from the isoflavone daidzein, found in soy, this supplement has been studied extensively in Japan, Italy, and Hungary, where it's used to prevent and treat osteoporosis. "Because it's synthesized, you really can't get it by eating soy," advises Dr. Schoenbeck, so ask your practitioner if it's an appropriate option for you.

Ipriflavone is really exciting, says Dr. Schoen-beck, because research indicates that it slows bone loss without the potential problems of estrogen. A dosage of 200 milligrams three times a day is her recommendation for women who shouldn't use hormone-replacement therapy or for those who do use it but want additional bone help. (If you can't find an ipriflavone product, look in the bone-health-supplement section of a health food store and read the labels to see if it's an ingredient.)

It's probably not a good idea to take isoflavone supplements instead of ipriflavone products, even if you're just taking a small amount of isoflavones. It looks like you get the most health benefits from eating whole soy foods, which have many other components in addition to isoflavones. The isoflavones seem to be very important but not the whole story, and if you take them in isolation from the other components in soy, they may even be harmful under some circumstances.

Extend your exercise. Take weight-bearing workouts a step further, advises Dr. Schoenbeck, with extension exercises like yoga and stretching to help maintain good posture.

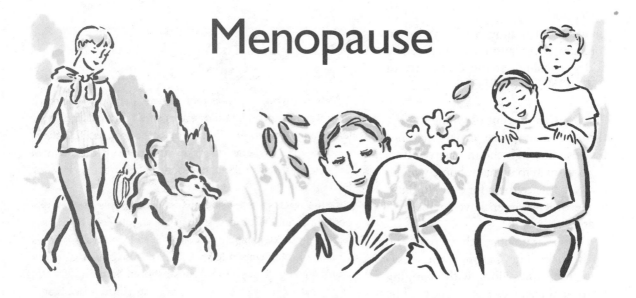

Menopause

No more birth control! No more tampons or pads! No more premenstrual syndrome!

Once upon a time, we called it the change. It was a landmark that signaled the end of the best and most productive years of our lives. We avoided talking about it and tried not to think about it. But not anymore.

Most of the millions of women who will reach menopause over the next decade will still have a third of their lives ahead of them. As far as they're concerned, "the change" no longer means an end to anything. Instead, it heralds a new beginning.

Consider that in a recent Gallup poll of 750 women between the ages of 45 and 60, more than half viewed menopause as a fulfilling stage of life; 60 percent did not associate menopause with feeling less attractive; and a whopping 80 percent expressed relief over the end of menstruation.

"Culturally, we're beginning to look upon menopause as the start of a new life. You're free from your children and many other obligations. You can start a new career, go back to school, travel, open up a business. You are not going to be a hunched-over little old lady pushing a vol-

unteer cart," says Mary Leong, M.D., director of gynecology at the Nassau County Medical Center in East Meadow, New York.

No one is pretending that *everything* about menopause is pleasant. All of the well-known side effects still happen to women, including hot flashes, mood swings, and vaginal dryness. But these days we can openly discuss these side effects and get far more information about how to deal with them.

Turning Down the Heat

It starts with a flush of warmth in your chest, then intensifies and quickly moves into your neck, face, and head. Your heart starts to beat faster and faster, and sweat forms on your skin as your body tries to cool off. As quickly as it comes, it can go, but it can last up to several minutes. It's a hot flash, and for many women, these sporadic moments of burning within are what menopause is all about.

"When you talk about symptoms, what actually causes women to come in to see a doctor are the hot flashes. It's the number one complaint about menopause," says Susan Johnson, M.D., professor of obstetrics and gynecology at the University of Iowa College of Medicine in Iowa City.

About 75 percent of women going through menopause experience hot flashes, although the intensity differs from woman to woman. Some women may experience them for only a month, while other women have them for 5 years.

While annoying, they pose no health risks. They're simply the sensation that comes along with changing hormonal balances in the body. "The only reason to treat hot flashes is if they bother you and you have trouble sleeping," Dr. Johnson says.

If you find the flashes unendurable, you can talk to your doctor about hormone-replacement therapy. But Dr. Johnson suggests that there's lots you can do to control your body's thermostat yourself.

Add soy to your diet. Soy contains phytoestrogens, natural substances that act very much like the estrogen your body makes. Some women find relief from hot flashes by eating soy-based foods such as soy milk or tofu. "There is pretty good evidence that soy provides relief, but it won't work for everybody," she says. Start with two 8-ounce glasses of soy milk a day. Once you get used to that, add tofu or other soy products to your diet. Don't expect immediate results. It can take from 6 to 8 weeks for you to feel its effects.

Take a deep breath. According to the North American Menopause Society, deep

HRT: SHOULD YOU OR SHOULDN'T YOU?

When a woman enters menopause, her body begins to slow down its production of estrogen. That can cause problems ranging from hot flashes to osteoporosis. To relieve those symptoms, she can take hormones in the form of drugs, a treatment called hormone-replacement therapy, or HRT.

Some doctors prescribe HRT as commonly as they dispense aspirin. Yet others, such as Susan Johnson, M.D., professor of obstetrics and gynecology at the University of Iowa College of Medicine in Iowa City, aren't so sure that every woman going through menopause should be on it. "By and large, estrogen is safe, and it's a good solution for some women. But that doesn't mean everyone should be taking it," she says.

Before you decide whether hormone-replacement therapy is right for you, you'll need to know some facts. Here is what experts have learned from their research.

- Short-term HRT helps alleviate menopausal symptoms such as hot flashes and vaginal dryness.

- Long-term use of HRT may not reduce the risk of heart disease, as once thought. A major study found that HRT did not reduce the risk of heart attacks in women who already had heart disease before taking HRT. Another showed an increased risk of heart attack within the first year of starting HRT. Given that HRT no longer seems to prevent heart disease and may cause harm short term, HRT should not be prescribed for the express purpose of preventing heart disease and heart attacks in healthy women. It may be appropriate for women at increased risk of heart disease if other benefits outweigh the

breathing can reduce hot flashes by 50 percent. Take six to eight slow, deep abdominal breaths per minute. Practice for 15 minutes each morning and night, and breathe deeply when you feel a hot flash coming on.

risks. Moreover, women who already have heart disease and have been on HRT for a year or two don't necessarily need to discontinue its use if they're doing well.

▶ Long-term use of HRT is the standard care for the prevention and treatment of osteoporosis.

▶ Long-term use is associated with increased risk of breast cancer. However, more women die every year of heart disease and osteoporosis-related conditions than breast cancer.

Unfortunately, all the data doesn't point to an easy answer. Assuming that HRT will prevent osteoporosis ignores other factors, such as diet, physical activity, obesity, and smoking, all of which contribute to the development of disease.

Each woman, in conjunction with her doctor, must make up her own mind about hormone-replacement therapy. Consider these questions when deciding.

Long term or short term? There are two reasons to take HRT: for short-term relief of menopausal symptoms and for long-term prevention of heart disease and osteoporosis. Studies haven't shown any health risks associated with short-term (5 to 10 years) HRT, Dr. Johnson says. If you take it for disease prevention, however, you'll have to take it for the rest of your life.

What are your risks? Depending on a woman's individual health risks, HRT may or may not be a good choice. People at a higher-than-normal risk for heart disease and osteoporosis should consider HRT, while those at higher risk of breast cancer probably should not. Dr. Johnson recommends that you weigh your risk of each disease before making a decision.

Stay cool. Do your best to stay in cool areas during the day since heat or a dramatic temperature change can trigger a hot flash. During the summer, remain in air-conditioned rooms or use fans to keep your internal temperature from rising. During the winter, be careful not to turn the heater up too high.

Steer clear of triggers. For some women, certain foods or even situations can bring on a hot flash. Take note of what you ate or did right before a hot flash came on, so you can avoid it in the future. Caffeine, alcohol, and spicy foods are all common hot flash triggers.

Slumber in coolness. If you experience night sweats, turn the thermostat down or open a window when you go to bed. Make sure that the room is cool, yet comfortable. Wear light, comfortable night clothes and place a fan by your bed.

Go natural. Wear clothing made of natural fibers, such as cotton. Natural fibers allow heat and moisture to escape instead of trapping them against your skin.

Layer it on. Dress in layers, such as T-shirts under sweaters or long-sleeve shirts. Or wear vests and cardigans so that when a hot flash occurs, you can peel your clothes back off in layers to cool yourself down.

No one is quite sure how deep breathing works to help you. It may slow your metabolism, regulate your body temperature, or even control the brain chemicals associated with hot flashes.

In the Mood

Your body temperature isn't the only thing that can suddenly switch from one extreme to the other during menopause. You may also notice sudden mood changes. Some women report being very short-tempered and even somewhat depressed.

Even women who have experienced mood swings from premenstrual syndrome all their lives note that these are a bit more intense. "They find it is much more noticeable than it used to be," says Lisa Domagalski, M.D., a gynecologist and assistant clinical professor at Brown University School of Medicine in Providence, Rhode Island.

Experts aren't sure what links mood changes to menopause. It could be an estrogen connection, or it may have something to do with mood-altering brain chemicals, such as serotonin. Part of the difficulty may lie in sleep deprivation due to hot flashes and night sweats.

If your mood changes last a long time or impair your ability to work or function, or if you feel that you are slipping into a deep depression, see a doctor immediately. She will help you explore options such as medication and therapy. If your mood changes are causing you (and those around you) only minor grief, try the following strategies to get your emotions back on an even keel.

Walk or exercise often. In a study at Texas A&M University College of Medicine in College Station, women who walked 20 minutes reported significant improvements in mood. "Walking and exercise naturally increase the body's endorphins, chemicals in the body that make you feel good. That's where the 'high' that people get from running comes from," Dr. Domagalski says. People who exercise regularly have a much easier transition during menopause in general, she adds.

REAL-LIFE SCENARIO

What She's Not Doing to Protect Her Bones

At age 67, Anne's grandmother broke her hip. Afterward, tests showed she had osteoporosis. That fracture was only the first of many. At almost exactly the same age, Anne's mother fell and broke her shoulder. Same diagnosis. Now 49 and approaching menopause, Anne is determined to avoid the same fate by getting plenty of calcium and exercise. Each day she takes 600 milligrams of calcium carbonate first thing in the morning and last thing before bed. Since she skips breakfast, she makes sure to eat *real* (she hates the low-fat stuff) yogurt along with her salad at lunch. She loves cheese and eats it freely—heck, she has a great excuse! Though petite and only 110 pounds, she never gains weight, which she credits to her addiction to running and her abstinence from alcohol. Diet soda is her drink of choice, at least a six-pack a day. Naturally, she was surprised to find out at her annual checkup last week that she's now 5 feet 3½ inches tall—½ inch shorter than she was a year ago. Should she be concerned?

Anne should be concerned. Her loss of height may be a symptom of bone loss. But she's already on the right track with her focus on weight-bearing exercise, calcium intake, and awareness of her risk. Some small mistakes in her daily routine, however, are subtracting the benefits of her bone-protecting strategies. With only a few changes, Anne should be able to preserve her bones, which would make her less likely to share her mother's and grandmother's fate.

First off, Anne should switch to calcium citrate. The calcium she takes, calcium carbonate, is the least absorbable type.

When buying her calcium citrate or any calcium product, Anne must check the back label for the number of mil-

Practice relaxing. In the early 1970s, Herbert Benson, M.D., at the Harvard Medical School devised the "relaxation response." This tension-releasing technique can help you

ligrams of elemental calcium—the amount of pure calcium in each pill. For instance, there is only 20 percent of elemental calcium in each milligram of calcium carbonate. If the amount of elemental calcium or calcium is not given on the back label, when she takes 600 milligrams of calcium carbonate, she's really only getting 120 milligrams of calcium.

It's also important to take calcium supplements with meals. Calcium needs stomach acid to dissolve and be absorbed by your body. The only time you have stomach acid is when you eat. By taking calcium supplements without food, Anne is not absorbing any of it.

Anne should also space out her calcium intake better. You can't absorb more than 500 milligrams at a time. Anne should evenly divide her needed 1,200 to 1,500 milligrams over three meals, in either food or supplements. The best way to do so is to make sure that she eats calcium foods with every meal or at least takes supplements. And by not eating breakfast, Anne is missing a great opportunity to get calcium at the start of her day.

Finally, Anne must cut back on her diet soda fixation. Soda contains caffeine and phosphoric acid, both of which cause the body to excrete calcium. At the least, Anne should cut back to only two cans of soda a day, perhaps substituting fat-free milk or calcium-fortified orange juice the rest of the time.

Expert consulted
Michael T. DiMuzio, Ph.D.
Assistant professor at Northwestern University
Evanston, Illinois
Director of the Osteoporosis Prevention
*   and Research Centers at Highland Park*
*   Hospital*
Highland Park, Illinois

ings of relaxation for you, perhaps a word like *calm* or *serene*. Repeat the word in your mind every time you exhale. Practice this for 20 minutes once a day or 10 minutes twice a day as well as anytime you feel your mood begin to change.

Reward yourself. If you're feeling down and blue, don't sit there and brood about it. Do something that makes you happy. Take a bubble bath, treat yourself to a massage, buy yourself a treat. With all that's going on in your life and your body, you deserve to nurture yourself, Dr. Johnson says.

Solving a Sexual Problem

Thanks to Mother Nature's birth control, your sex life can flourish after menopause. But there is one physical change that you'll have to overcome. The drop in estrogen that occurs during menopause may cause the lining of your vagina to thin. During this thinning process, the vagina can become shorter, narrower, and drier. For some women, these changes make sex unpleasant and even painful.

Vaginal dryness isn't a barrier to sex, but simply a physical change that you'll have to adapt to, says Beverly Whipple, R.N., Ph.D., professor of nursing at Rutgers College of Nursing in Newark, New Jersey, and president of the American Association of Sex Educators, Counselors, and Therapists. You may want to discuss hormone-replacement therapy with your doctor, but you have many avenues to keep your sex life sizzling during menopause and for years after.

through mood swings or periods of anxiety, Dr. Johnson says. Sit or lie down in a comfortable position and breathe deeply. Relax all your muscles. Think of a phrase or word that evokes feel-

Peri Who? The New Kid on the Block

We either have the cramps and mood swings of menstruation or the hot flashes and sleepless nights of menopause. Not much of a choice, is it? But guess what? There's actually a time when we can have all the symptoms at once!

It's called perimenopause.

The name itself means "near the end of menstruation." It's the time when your estrogen levels begin to decline, which triggers the symptoms of hot flashes, mood swings, and irregular periods, says Dori Becker, M.D., a physician at Highland Park Hospital in Highland Park, Illinois. While your body isn't producing as much estrogen as it did, it still produces some, so you still have all the symptoms associated with menstruation to deal with, too. Perimenopause lasts until you reach menopause, which happens when you have gone a full year without a period.

Perimenopause can start in your forties and can last up to 5 years, possibly even longer, Dr. Becker says. Because they're still getting periods, many women don't think of their symptoms as part of the process of menopause. Or they think they've reached early menopause. Both are misconceptions.

Women have always gone through perimenopause, of course. But giving it a name validates what a lot of women experience at this time of their lives. "I am really pleased that there is more press about this. My friends and patients are at this age and are noticing that things are beginning to change," says Wendy Fader, Ph.D., a licensed psychologist and certified sex therapist in Boca Raton, Florida.

Love to love. According to Dr. Whipple, having sex generates estrogen, even during menopause. Studies have shown that women who have sex two or more times a week maintain twice as much estrogen in their bodies as women who don't. As a "natural" estrogen-replacement therapy to help keep the vagina lubricated, continue to have sex regularly, either with a partner or by yourself, advises Dr. Whipple.

Use water-based lubricants. Over-the-counter lubricants make sex comfortable for both partners. When buying a lubricant, make sure that it is water-based like K-Y jelly, not oil-based, Dr. Whipple says. Oil-based lubricants take longer to dissolve and can make a comfortable breeding ground for germs. They can also cause latex-based products, such as condoms, to develop small holes and deteriorate.

Shake up your routine. You and your partner might have to get a bit more creative in the bedroom. You may need more foreplay before sex, or you might want to try other sexually pleasing acts that don't always include intercourse. Just like everything else in life, your sexual practices may need to change, and the people who do best are the ones who roll with the changes instead of fear them, says Karen Donahey, Ph.D., director of the sex and marital therapy program at Northwestern University Medical Center in Chicago.

Sexually Transmitted Disease

If you've made it past the age of 26 without contracting a sexually transmitted disease (STD), you've been either very lucky or very prudent. Nearly two-thirds of all cases in the United States occur in people who are younger than that. But no matter what your age, if you're still chasing after those wild oats and having unprotected sex—even with seemingly "nice" guys—your risk for getting an STD is as high as any 18-year-old's.

STDs are transmitted by close intimate contact—through sexual intercourse or oral sex. The organisms causing them are found in semen, vaginal secretions, saliva, or the skin around the genitals or mouth. These organisms can be of all sorts—bacteria, viruses, even protozoans, which are somewhat similar to the microscopic critters that live in pond water. All of them can invade your sexual organs, and most of them can also invade your mouth, throat, and anus. Some of these organisms, such as the corkscrew-shaped bacteria of syphilis or the tiny virus that causes AIDS, can spread throughout your entire body. And many can be transmitted to your baby if you have the infections while you're pregnant.

Risk Factors

The more sex partners you have, the more likely you are to pick up any kind of STD. But even if you have only one sex partner, if that partner has unprotected sex with others, you're still at increased risk. "I've seen women who didn't realize that their husbands were having affairs until they came down with STDs," says Shirley Glass, Ph.D., a psychologist practicing in Baltimore. In fact, there's evidence that men may be less safety-conscious about sexually transmitted diseases than women may like to believe. One study found that men who'd had a previous STD were almost three times more likely to engage in unprotected sex than men who had never had one. Women, on the other hand, were more likely to use protection if they'd had a previous infection.

Common vaginal infections such as trichomoniasis (which is itself an STD), bacterial vaginosis, and yeast vaginitis make you more likely to develop an STD if you're exposed to it. That's because these infections, minor as they may seem, disturb the natural defense mechanisms of

SYPHILIS

The English and Italians called it the French disease, the French called it the Italian disease, the Russians called it the Polish disease, and in Spain, where it was first recognized, it was called the disease of Haiti. We call it syphilis.

Syphilis starts with the appearance of a small, painless ulcer, called a chancre, on the spot where the bacteria entered your body. The chancre lasts for 1 to 5 weeks and then heals on its own. In the meantime, however, the bacteria spread throughout your body. Some time later, you may have a secondary outbreak in the form of lesions, swollen glands, hair and weight loss, slimy white patches in the mouth, muscle aches, and fever. It's possible to get syphilis just by touching someone who has these lesions. Eventually, the lesions go away, and about one-quarter of people appear to be healed. Another one-quarter have antibodies to syphilis but show no symptoms.

In the remaining half of the people with syphilis, the infection appears a third time, as long as 5 to 40 years after the initial infection, and can cause extensive brain damage, mental illness, and death. Good reason to get your penicillin within a year of your first exposure.

your vagina and cervix, so these infections should be treated promptly.

And if you have one STD, chances are higher that you also have a different one along with it.

Prevention

Despite impressive advances in treatment, prevention is still your best bet. And prevention can be summed up with one of two words: *abstinence* or *condoms*. Short of not having sex at all, condoms are the most effective method for preventing transmission of STDs, says Mary Lake Polan, M.D., Ph.D., professor and chairperson of the department of gynecology and obstetrics at Stanford University School of Medicine.

"The spermicide nonoxynol-9 has been said to be somewhat effective in the prevention of STDs, but it's not as good as condoms." Using a spermicide in combination with a latex condom may be more effective than condoms alone.

Remember, however, that although using a condom reduces your risk for STDs, it does not eliminate the risk entirely. You can still pick up infections orally or from areas of skin that are not covered. Male and female condoms work equally well at preventing most diseases, but the female condom has a slight advantage when it comes to preventing genital herpes and warts, since it keeps a bit of skin around the outside of the vagina from coming in contact with the penis.

As for other birth control devices, don't put your faith in them when it comes to preventing disease. "Diaphragms and cervical caps provide little or no protection and should not be used to prevent an STD," Dr. Polan says.

Some STDs can be knocked out with drugs, but others simply cannot. These include those caused by viruses: human papillomavirus, which causes genital warts; human immunodeficiency virus (HIV), which causes AIDS; herpes; and sexually transmitted forms of hepatitis (types B and C). Most of these viral infections persist in your body for the rest of your life, but that does not necessarily mean that you will be ill for life, says Anne Rachel Davis, M.D., assistant professor of obstetrics and gynecology at New York Presbyterian Hospital in New York City.

Health problems caused by STDs tend to be more severe and more frequent for women than for men because women often don't develop symptoms that cause them to seek treatment until the disease has gained a stronghold, Dr. Davis says. By that time, infection may have spread to the uterus and fallopian tubes and developed into pelvic inflammatory disease, a major cause of infertility and ectopic pregnancy (pregnancy in the fallopian tubes, which can be fatal if not diagnosed and treated promptly). And sometimes the symptoms of an STD are mistaken for a disease not transmitted through sexual contact. For instance, pelvic inflammatory disease, caused by chlamydia or gonorrhea, can be confused with endometriosis.

Some women mistakenly believe that if they simply get a Pap test each year, it will reveal if they have an STD, but that's a potentially harmful misunderstanding, says Amy Hughes, M.D., professor of obstetrics and gynecology at Medical College of Georgia in Augusta. It simply isn't true.

What's more, many women—and their gynecologists—follow a don't-ask, don't-tell policy. During an office visit, neither patient nor doctor brings up the subject of possible exposure to an STD. That, too, can cause serious problems down the road.

Signs and Symptoms

Symptoms vary according to which STD you have, but they often include vaginal discharge, odor, or itching, and may include pain or pressure. If you have herpes, you may develop blisters in and around your vagina and feel as if you have the flu. If you have genital warts, you'll develop painless, small, fleshy growths. If your infection develops into pelvic inflammatory disease, you'll have pain in your pelvic area and possibly a fever.

Don't Panic!

If you're experiencing symptoms, there's no need to immediately point a finger at a sexual partner. There are other possible explanations

GONORRHEA

An estimated 800,000 new cases of gonorrhea occur in the United States each year. The early symptoms are often mild, and many women who are infected have no symptoms at all. If symptoms do develop, they usually appear within 2 to 10 days after sexual contact with an infected partner, although some people may be infected for several months without showing any signs of the illness. Initial symptoms in women include a painful or burning sensation when urinating and a yellow or bloody vaginal discharge. More advanced symptoms indicate that the disease has progressed to pelvic inflammatory disease and include abdominal pain, bleeding between menstrual periods, vomiting, and fever. Men usually have more symptoms than women, with discharge from the penis and a burning sensation during urination that may be severe.

Gonorrhea can be diagnosed with several different tests. Doctors often choose to use more than one because results can be inaccurate. Because penicillin-resistant cases of gonorrhea are common, other antibiotics are sometimes used to treat the disease, most often ceftriaxone (Rocephin), which a doctor can inject in a single dose. Since gonorrhea can occur together with chlamydia, doctors usually prescribe a combination of antibiotics, such as ceftriaxone and doxycycline (Doxycin).

If you have gonorrhea, your sex partner should be treated as well, even if he has no other symptoms.

GENITAL HERPES

If you have genital herpes, join the crowd. About one in four U.S. adults have herpes, and as many as 500,000 new cases are thought to occur each year. Once you get herpes, it's forever. There's no cure for this viral infection.

Most people who are infected with herpes never develop symptoms. When symptoms do appear, they vary widely from case to case. The first symptoms usually appear within 2 to 10 days of exposure to the virus and last an average of 2 to 3 weeks. Early symptoms may include itching or burning; pain in the legs, buttocks, or genital area; vaginal discharge; or a feeling of pressure in the belly. Within a few days, small red bumps appear at the site of infection that may later develop into blisters or painful open sores. Over a period of days, the sores crust over, then heal without scarring. Some people also develop fever, headache, muscle aches, and swollen glands in the groin area.

There are two types of herpes viruses, genital and oral, but the oral type can also cause genital herpes, and genital herpes can infect the mouth.

Recurrences are more likely to happen if you're under stress, ill, or menstruating.

Herpes can be accurately diagnosed only by viral culture, which means that your doctor must take scrapings from your sores when they first appear. If you get tested after your sores are no longer active, the results may be negative even though you have the virus.

It's possible to infect someone with the virus even when you have no sores. That's because the virus can reactivate without causing sores. It's important to avoid direct contact with skin that contains the virus. Since recurrent outbreaks are not always apparent, you should always wear a condom if you or your partner is infected with the herpes virus.

Antiviral drugs such as acyclovir (Zovirax) can help people with a first or a recurrent outbreak of herpes. The medicine interferes with the virus's ability to reproduce.

for your discomfort. "Both urinary tract infections and yeast infections can mimic the symptoms of an STD," says Dr. Polan. These symptoms include painful urination, increased frequency of urination, and vaginal itching.

"Dermatological reactions to clothing or certain chemicals or perfumes can also cause problems similar to those of an STD, especially itching," adds Suzanne Trupin, M.D., clinical professor in the department of obstetrics and gynecology at the University of Illinois College of Medicine in Urbana-Champaign and coauthor of *Sexually Transmitted Diseases: Problems in Primary Care*.

But if you think that you may have contracted one of these infections, it's best to see your doctor to confirm the medical reason for your discomfort, especially if you have pelvic pain or a fever. "Many STDs have no symptoms, and that's really the biggest problem," says Dr. Polan. "With no symptoms, there's no way to know if you have an STD except for a culture, and cultures are often inaccurate. That's why prevention is so important. Although some STDs are difficult to diagnose, if they are caught early, many can be cured with today's modern antibiotics."

Who Do I See?

Gynecologists traditionally treat female STDs, but don't presume that if you have something, your doctor will find it on her own, Dr. Hughes says. Tell her about your symptoms or concerns so she can do the proper tests and examination.

What Can I Expect?

If you suspect that you have an STD, you may undergo a microscopic examination of your vaginal secretions, or you may have a culture to see what organisms are causing the problem. Some of these diseases require careful examination of the cervix with a lighted magnifying tube, a procedure called colposcopy. If you have reason to suspect that you've been exposed to HIV, you will need to have a blood test to look for antibodies to that disease.

If your tests confirm the presence of one of these illnesses, you will most likely feel a range of emotions in addition to the possible physical discomfort. If an STD takes you by surprise, you may feel enraged, violated, and betrayed—and perhaps angry with yourself for allowing yourself to be exposed to the illness. But no matter how angry you feel, take time to stop and think calmly about what has happened. "One important aspect of the emotional response is trying to determine how the STD was acquired in order to prevent a future occurrence," says Dr. Trupin.

If you're diagnosed with AIDS, you'll probably have much stronger feelings. "Most women feel the same sort of emotions as others with potentially terminal illnesses—hopelessness, grief, anger, and denial—but with the added social stigma that HIV carries," says Dr. Trupin. "The most common emotions that women with HIV/AIDS face are depression and anxiety."

GENITAL WARTS

Genital warts are flat lesions or small, fleshy, cauliflower-like bumps that can grow in and around your cervix, vagina, and anus, or, in men, on the penis and scrotum and in the urethra. The warts are usually painless, but they may itch. They are caused by the human papillomavirus (HPV). Several strains of the virus have been linked to cervical cancer, but these strains do not always produce visible warts. It's possible to have your warts analyzed to see which strains of virus you have.

You can get these growths through direct contact with someone else's warts, but the virus can also be spread through bodily fluids such as semen or vaginal secretions.

The warts are diagnosed by a doctor's visual examination and are removed by the use of chemicals, freezing, burning, or a laser. The warts return at least 30 percent of the time, however, so you may need more than one treatment.

Getting regular Pap tests can reveal the presence of pre-cancerous or cancerous cells caused by HPV. A biopsy is warranted if the warts are brown or black, if they look unusual in some way, if they are larger than a thumbnail, if they are red and scaly, and—regardless of the nature of the warts—if a woman has an abnormal Pap test.

Some women even contemplate suicide, she adds. But an AIDS diagnosis is no longer a death sentence. In many cases, new medicines have helped slow HIV's progression to AIDS. "It may be very helpful to talk to women who have gone through the same problems," advises Dr. Trupin. "There are a number of national and local support groups that can be very useful in coping with different aspects of the disease."

Conventional Wisdom

Doctors use a whole arsenal of drugs and treatments to try to knock out STDs. The

HIV/AIDS

While just 7 percent of AIDS cases in 1985 were attributed to heterosexual sex, that number rose to 23 percent in 1998.

Of the infections among women, 75 percent are due to heterosexual sex and 25 percent to injection-drug use. Still, women account for only 30 percent of new infections. And of that percentage, Black women account for 64 percent, while Hispanic and White women account for 18 percent each.

A woman can contract HIV if her HIV-infected partner is an IV-drug user or bisexual or has been in the past. Two new studies suggest that bisexual risk behaviors among Black men may be fueling the spread of HIV infection to Black women in some parts of the country. One study, done in New York City, found 20 percent of Black men reporting bisexuality, compared to 4 percent of White men.

Women are also more vulnerable to getting HIV if they have some other sexually transmitted disease or if they have anal sex. It is also possible to contract HIV from oral sex.

Male-to-female transmission of the virus is eight times more efficient than female-to-male transmission, so men are much more likely to spread the virus to women than women are to men.

The average time between the initial infection and the appearance of symptoms that could lead to a diagnosis of AIDS is 8 to 11 years. This time varies greatly from person to person and depends on health status and behavior. Many people don't have any symptoms for many years or have mild symptoms of swollen lymph nodes and fever. Then, as AIDS develops, they experience weight loss, fatigue, diarrhea, and development of opportunistic infections that take advantage of their bodies' ravaged immune systems.

If you think that you're at risk for having HIV, get tested. Current tests for HIV are among the most accurate medical tests available.

If you test positive, you can take drugs that may downgrade HIV from a death sentence to a chronic disease, including AZT (Retrovir), also known as zidovudine or azidothymidine, and protease inhibitors like ritonavir (Norvir) and saquinavir mesylate (Invirase).

choice depends entirely on which STD you have and, sometimes, how long you've had it. For instance, if you've had syphilis for less than a year, it can be cured with one dose of penicillin. Those who have had it longer will need additional doses.

Women with genital herpes may take an antiviral drug, such as acyclovir (Zovirax), to lessen the severity of an initial outbreak or to reduce the number of recurrent outbreaks. Women with genital warts can have them removed with chemical-peel creams, laser surgery, freezing, or cauterization. Women with HIV infection can take a combination of antiviral drugs, usually zidovudine (AZT) and protease inhibitors. In some people, these help to stop the virus from multiplying.

In most cases, if you have an STD, so does your sexual partner. He needs to be treated for the same problem.

Great Alternatives

Once your infection has been brought under control, you can use alternative medicine to help maintain vaginal health and to rebuild your immune system, says Jody Noe, N.D., a naturopathic physician in Brattleboro, Vermont. Here's what she suggests.

Adopt a healthy diet to strengthen immunity. Our bodies' response to any infection depends on the ability of our immune systems to gear up to fight it, and that requires good nutrition. It's important to get adequate amounts of all the vitamins and minerals, especially vitamins A, C, E, and B complex, and the minerals zinc and selenium. It is also crucial to stay away from too much sugar and to balance adequate amounts of high-quality protein with carbohydrates. Whole grains, fish, beans, lots of vegetables, and fruit all fit this bill.

If you have a viral infection, consider trying N-acetylcysteine (NAC). This nutritional supplement, available in health food stores, may act as "a general antiviral," Dr. Noe says. She recommends that people who have AIDS or hepatitis B or C take 1,000 to 2,000 milligrams a day of NAC. People with recurrent herpes infections may also benefit from taking this amount. Check with your M.D. before taking cysteine. In high doses, cysteine can cause kidney stones in people who have cystinuria. Since it may inactivate insulin, use with caution if you have diabetes. Cysteine may also deplete zinc and copper, so if you're supplementing cysteine or N-acetylcysteine for more than a few weeks, take it with a multivitamin/mineral supplement that supplies the Daily Value of these minerals.

Don't douche unless your doctor recommends it. Studies show that women who

CHLAMYDIA

This sexually transmitted disease gets its name from the Greek word for "cloaked." And chlamydia, caused by the *Chlamydia trachomatis* organism, lives up to its name. Often, it initially has such mild symptoms that a woman does not know she is infected. If left untreated, the chlamydial infection may lead to pelvic inflammatory disease (PID). PID can result in scarring of the fallopian tubes, which can then block the tubes and make conception difficult or impossible. Often, men also have no apparent symptoms and can unknowingly pass the infection along to their partners.

Chlamydia can set up shop not only in your reproductive organs but also in your mouth, throat, eyes, anus, and lymph nodes.

The best way to diagnose chlamydia is for your doctor to get a sample of secretions from your genital area for laboratory analysis.

Chlamydia can be knocked out with antibiotics, often azithromycin (Zithromax) or doxycycline (Doxycin). Your sex partners must be treated, too. Penicillin (Robicillin VK), which is often used for treating some other sexually transmitted diseases, is not effective against this one.

douche are actually more likely to develop pelvic inflammatory disease than those who don't, perhaps because the process disrupts the balance of protective organisms in the vagina, allowing faster growth of unfriendly organisms. Instead of douching, see a doctor if you develop an unusual discharge or smell.

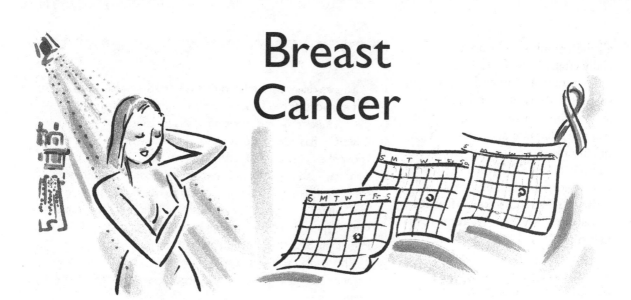

Breast Cancer

Our breasts are not getting the attention they deserve.

Hard to imagine, isn't it? Female breasts seem so important in our culture. They're ogled, glorified, and vilified. They're displayed in the movies, accentuated in clothing design, and used to sell products. When Brandi Chastain, a defender for the U.S. women's national soccer team, hammered the game-winning shot past the Chinese goalie in the finals of the 1999 Women's World Cup, then joyously ripped off her jersey, they even made the news. Sometimes, it's easy to wish they weren't the focus of so much attention.

But there remains one kind of attention that they absolutely need and don't always get. Incredibly, even in this age of tremendous public awareness of breast cancer, some women still shrug off self-exams, mammograms, and other important screening tests.

"There is this unfortunate idea that if my breasts aren't causing me problems in my day-to-day life, if they're not causing me pain, then I don't need to get them examined regularly. Unfortunately, breast cancer doesn't bother most women until it's at a fairly advanced stage," says A. Marilyn Leitch, M.D., a surgical oncologist and professor of surgery at the University of Texas Southwestern Medical Center at Dallas.

That's why vigilance and early detection play such important roles in the battle against breast cancer.

Risk Factors

Few other places in the world have rates of breast cancer higher than those in the United States. Other than skin cancer, it is the most common form of malignancy diagnosed among women in this country, affecting 175,000 of us and claiming 43,000 lives each year. Only lung cancer is more lethal. Since 1973, the number of breast cancers diagnosed has increased about 2 percent annually, although much of that increase is the result of better methods of detection.

Doctors aren't certain what makes the breast so susceptible to cancer, but a number of factors are known to increase a woman's risk of developing the disease, including the following.

Age. The risk of breast cancer increases gradually as a woman gets older. It is rarely diagnosed in women under age 35, but all women age 40 and over are at increased risk. Most cases occur in women over age 50, and the risk is particularly high among women over age 60.

Family history. If your mother, sister, daughter, or at least two other close relatives, such as cousins, have a history of breast cancer, especially at an early age, you may be at high risk yourself, says Dr. Leitch. When checking your history, don't neglect your father's family. Even if he hasn't had the disease himself, if his mother or sister had it, he may carry a breast cancer gene. Risk assessment and genetic testing may be appropriate if you have a significant history of breast cancer on either side of your family.

Certain breast changes. A previous diagnosis of benign conditions or more than two breast biopsies are associated with a higher risk of cancer.

Late childbearing. Women who had their first children after the age of 30 have a greater chance of developing breast cancer than women who had children at a younger age.

Estrogen exposure. Women who began menstruating before age 12, experienced menopause after age 55, never had children, or took birth control pills or hormone-replacement therapy for a number of years may also be at higher risk. That's because these factors increase the amount of time that a woman's body is exposed to estrogen. And the longer you are exposed to estrogen, the more likely you are to develop breast cancer.

REAL-LIFE SCENARIO

She Doesn't Trust Her Doctor's Diagnosis

One week after Renee's 45th birthday, she had a mammogram done. She expected nothing but good news, of course, so it was like a splash of cold water when she got word over the phone that something slightly unusual had turned up in her x-ray. Within a week, she had a needle biopsy done. Fortunately, she ended up with a clean bill of health. The diagnosis relieved Renee's apprehensions for a while, although she had a moment of panic when a little blood leaked from her nipple after the biopsy. The doctor told her it was a normal side effect of the procedure. But now, a month later, a little more blood has leaked out, and she's getting panicked again. Does she have reason to be?

Bloody discharge is common after you've had a breast procedure done. But it should go away. So if it is still occurring a month later, I would certainly want to investigate that. It's not something that Renee or her doctor should ignore. She should make a follow-up appointment with her physician. If she doesn't feel satisfied with the answers she receives during that visit, she should definitely seek out a second opinion. And for that opinion, I would highly recommend that she go to a physician who has a lot of experience with the biopsy procedure that caused the discharge in the first place.

Expert consulted
Deborah Capko, M.D.
Breast surgeon and associate medical director
Institute for Breast Care at Hackensack
   University Medical Center
New Jersey

Risk factors are important, but paying too much attention to them may be misleading, as the odds that any one of them will trigger breast cancer is less than 1 percent, says Deborah Capko, M.D., breast surgeon and associate medical director of the Institute for Breast Care at Hackensack University Medical Center in

New Jersey. In fact, many women with known risk factors do not get breast cancer. And many women who have none of these factors develop the disease. Doctors are hard-pressed to explain this paradox. That is why diligence is so critical.

"Most women who don't have a family history of breast cancer feel that they can let self-exams and mammograms slide a bit because they're not at risk," Dr. Capko says. "The truth is that most women who get breast cancer do not have a family history or any of the other risk factors."

Prevention

There are no known surefire ways to prevent breast cancer, Dr. Capko says. But the following steps may help slash your risk.

Slim down. Weight control is one of the few modifiable lifestyle factors that may reduce a woman's risk of breast cancer, Dr. Capko says. Researchers suspect that excessive weight—more than 20 percent above your ideal range—sparks increased production of sex hormones that are thought to promote breast tumors. So if you're overweight, try shedding a few pounds. In fact, just trimming 150 calories per meal—the equivalent of a slice of cheese pizza, five gingersnaps, or a 1/2-cup serving of vanilla ice cream—and eating one fewer snack per day can help you begin losing up to a pound a week. That may not sound like much, but in 6 months, you'll be nearly 24 pounds lighter, says Maria Simonson, Sc.D., Ph.D., director of the Health, Weight, and Stress Clinic at the Johns Hopkins Medical Institutions in Baltimore. Trimming

> ### STOPPING THE TIME BOMB: PREVENTIVE MASTECTOMY
>
> Tricia Marrapodi knew it was only a matter of time. Her mother had died of breast cancer at the age of 44. Although Tricia was just 17 when it happened, she decided what she wanted. She would have a preventive mastectomy—her breast tissue would be surgically removed and replaced with saline implants, significantly reducing her chances of developing breast cancer. But a doctor persuaded her to wait until she was 30. By then, he told her, she would be better prepared both physically and emotionally for the ordeal.
>
> So Tricia waited. Then, at age 27, her twin sister, Kelly Munsell, told Tricia that she had found a lump in her breast. A month later, Kelly underwent a mastectomy and began chemotherapy treatments for her cancer. Because she and Kelly are identical twins, Tricia's doctor estimated that her chances of developing breast cancer were more than 90 percent. Tricia knew the time had come. She had a double mastectomy at age 28.
>
> "I feel I made the best decision, because of the peace of mind it has given me," Tricia says. "I still have a 2 percent chance of getting breast cancer because I still have some residual breast tissue. But my high risk before surgery had been a terrifying prospect. I feel as if a heavy burden has been lifted from my shoulders."

visible fat off meats can save you about 60 calories per meal. Over a year, that can add up to 22,000 calories—and about 6 1/2 pounds that you don't have to worry about gaining.

Run for your life. Regular exercise, such as walking, swimming, gardening, or vigorously doing housework several times a week, can dramatically slash your risk of breast cancer even if you start late in life.

When researchers at the Mayo Clinic followed 1,806 postmenopausal women (whose average age was 75) for 11 years, they found that those who were moderately active had a 50 per-

Even though researchers have found that prophylactic mastectomies can reduce a woman's chance of getting breast cancer by up to 90 percent, most doctors consider this kind of surgery a radical option—even for women who have a long family history of the disease or who carry one of the two genes known to promote breast cancer.

"If we're going to do such drastic surgery, we want to be sure that the risk of developing breast cancer is very significant and high," says A. Marilyn Leitch, M.D., a surgical oncologist and professor of surgery at the University of Texas Southwestern Medical Center in Dallas. "So for somebody who is going to have a bilateral preventive mastectomy, my preference is for them to go through genetic testing and counseling."

But preemptive mastectomies aren't just for healthy women at risk. Some who have had cancer in one breast opt to have the other one removed as well.

"Once a woman has experienced breast cancer, she knows what is involved with the surgery and its effects. If she makes the decision, after careful thought, that she wants to have a preventive surgery on the other breast, then we will do that," Dr. Leitch says. "But we don't do that surgery very cavalierly. We do it only after a lot of thought and counseling."

cent lower risk of breast cancer compared to sedentary women. Previous studies among those 40 or younger found similar effects among premenopausal women.

Exercise probably diminishes your breasts' exposure to cancer-promoting hormones, especially estrogen, says Leslie Bernstein, Ph.D., professor of preventive medicine at the University of Southern California School of Medicine in Los Angeles. Based on these studies, she suggests that women of all ages include a regular exercise program of 30 to 40 minutes a day as part of a healthy lifestyle.

Milk it for all it's worth. Sip on a warm mug of 1% milk with ¼ teaspoon almond extract at bedtime, suggests Holly McCord, R.D., nutrition editor for *Prevention* magazine. Milk fat contains an intriguing substance known as conjugated linoleic acid that fights breast cancer cells in test tubes and animals.

Defy it with D. Women whose diets contain higher amounts of vitamin D appear to have less risk of breast cancer. To ensure that you get the recommended level, make a multivitamin a part of your daily routine, McCord suggests.

Tea up. Green tea brims with antioxidants that block cancer by preventing damage to DNA, a cell's blueprint for reproducing itself properly, says McCord. Tests suggest that one of these compounds, EGCG, is 100 times stronger than vitamin C and 25 times stronger than vitamin E at protecting DNA. Although tests are ongoing, green tea inhibits the formation of cancer cells in animals. And in Japan, where people routinely drink two to three cups a day, cancer is less common and generally occurs at a much older age than in the United States. Green tea and its extracts (sold in capsule form) are available at most health food stores.

Go fishing. Order salmon whenever you find it on a restaurant's menu, McCord suggests. Salmon is rich in omega-3 fats, and research suggests that women with higher tissue levels of omega-3's have lower rates of breast cancer.

Flip a veggie patty. Flavorful vegetable burgers and sausages are better main-course choices than meat because they don't form compounds called heterocyclic amines when cooked.

WOMEN ASK WHY

Why do mammograms have to hurt so darned much?

During a mammogram, the breast is compressed between an x-ray plate below and a plastic cover above. This flattens out the breast so that as much tissue as possible can be imaged. It may seem painful, but in the big scheme of things, relative to other procedures, I really don't think it's that uncomfortable. I think the discomfort has more to do with anxiety and with fear of the results.

I highly recommend that women go to a center where the technicians do nothing but mammograms. They tend to have a bit more expertise and compassion than people who do a variety of x-ray studies and only occasionally do mammograms. The technician is more likely to talk you through the procedure, answering your questions and addressing your concerns. That gives you more sense of control and involvement, and it personalizes your care.

If you are uncomfortable during the procedure, let the technician know, and she should try her best to work with you. If she doesn't, then I would ask for another technician or find somewhere else to have your mammograms done.

Another thing women can do to lessen their discomfort is to schedule their mammograms so that they occur sometime during the 10 days after their periods normally begin. The breasts seem to be less tender during that time, and there's no chance of pregnancy.

Expert consulted
Emily Conant, M.D.
Associate professor and chief of breast
*   imaging*
The Hospital of the University of Pennsylvania
Philadelphia

Booze, you lose. Consuming more than two alcoholic drinks a day may elevate estrogen levels, promote cell division, and increase your risk of breast cancer, Dr. Capko says. So if you imbibe, don't overdo it. Drink no more than one 12-ounce bottle of beer, 4-ounce glass of wine, or 1-ounce shot of hard liquor daily.

Stay in touch. If you know the shape and texture of your breasts by sight and touch, you're more likely to detect changes. In fact, 90 percent of the time, breast masses are found through self-exams. That's why it's so important to *really* do a monthly self-exam and not just think about it, Dr. Capko says. Do it at the same time each month. If you are premenopausal, do it 5 to 7 days after your period ends. By that time, your hormones will have stabilized and you'll get a better sense of your breasts' natural size and shape.

Begin with a visual inspection, says Dr. Capko. Stand before a mirror with your hands at your sides. Raise your hands and clasp them behind your head. Look for any changes in the size or shape of your breasts as well as for nipple discharge, redness, puckering, or dimpling. Then, press your hands firmly on your hips with your shoulders and elbows pulled forward; again, look for any changes.

Following this visual exam, check your breasts by touch. It's important to follow a definite pattern to ensure that you examine yourself thoroughly for any lumps. You may want to do it in the shower with soapy water so

These compounds may be a major reason why women who eat lots of red meat and well-done meat seem to get more breast cancer, McCord says.

that your hands slide smoothly, suggests Dr. Capko.

Squeeze it in. Even though you're not fond of the process, an annual mammogram after age 40 is one of the best ways to detect and get breast cancer treated in its earliest stages, Dr. Capko says.

Ask about tamoxifen. Ask your doctor to help you calculate your risk of developing breast cancer in the next 5 years (the National Cancer Institute offers computer programs that simplify this process). If your risk is at least 1.7 percent, which is considered a moderately high risk, ask your doctor about taking tamoxifen (Nolvadex), a drug that can cut your risk by 50 percent, Dr. Leitch suggests.

"For tamoxifen to be appropriate, the woman has to have a certain level of risk," Dr. Leitch says. "It's not something that a doctor would just give to any woman."

That's because there are some rare but significant risks associated with tamoxifen use, including potentially fatal side effects such as pulmonary embolism and uterine cancer. So be certain that you fully understand the pros and cons of this medication, given your level of risk for breast cancer, before taking it, recommends Dr. Leitch.

Signs and Symptoms

It can't be stated often enough: In its earliest and most treatable stages, breast cancer usually doesn't cause pain, and there may be no symptoms at all, so annual mammograms are ex-

PERFORMING A BREAST SELF-EXAM

Follow a definite pattern during breast self-exams, and do them the same way every time so that you become familiar with the way your breasts feel. One of the basic examination patterns is a circular shape, in which you move your fingers from the outer portions of your breast toward the nipple using small circles. But there are other patterns to use. To examine your breasts with the vertical pattern, slide your hand up and down in vertical lines from one side of your breast to the other. To try the wedge pattern, start from the nipple and work your fingers out to the edge of your breast and then back toward the nipple again. Continue until you have gone around your entire breast.

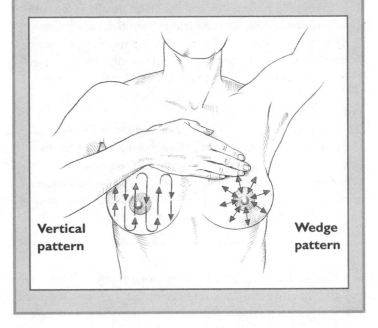

Vertical pattern

Wedge pattern

tremely important. But sometimes, early symptoms do occur. The National Cancer Institute advises that you see your doctor if you notice any of the following:

- A lump or thickening in or near the breast or in the underarm area
- A change in the size or shape of the breast

BREAST PAIN: WHAT DOES IT MEAN?

"Probably 70 to 75 percent of women experience breast pain at some point in their lives. Often, it's associated with hormonal changes that occur in the breast during the menstrual cycle. Many women also get breast pain in their forties as they approach menopause. Again, it's all due to hormones—they're completely out of control. You may have constant pain in the breast in the form of a feeling of fullness, burning, or throbbing. Hormonal influences on the breast are truly incredible," says Deborah Capko, M.D., breast surgeon and associate medical director of the Institute for Breast Care at Hackensack University Medical Center in New Jersey.

Cysts and mastitis, a painful condition usually associated with breastfeeding, also can trigger sensitivity and tenderness. Arthritic conditions in the ribs and sternum are other possible sources of breast pain. And medications such as birth control pills can cause pain. But breast pain, particularly if it correlates with your menstrual cycle, is rarely a symptom of breast cancer.

Certainly, keep track of your pain, record its comings and goings in a notebook, if you like, and mention it to your doctor, Dr. Capko says. But in most cases, warm compresses and over-the-counter pain relievers or anti-inflammatory medications such as acetaminophen or ibuprofen, used as directed on the label, will alleviate the problem.

- Nipple discharge or tenderness, or a nipple that has inverted back into the breast
- Ridges or pitting of the breast (the skin looks like the peel of an orange)
- A change in the way the skin of the breast, areola, or nipple looks or feels (for instance, warm, swollen, red, or scaly)

Don't Panic!

The vast majority of breast lumps are not cancerous, says Emily Conant, M.D., associate professor and chief of breast imaging at the Hospital of the University of Pennsylvania in Philadelphia. "More often than not, what you're feeling is an area of normal breast tissue or a benign lump," she says. Common benign causes of breast lumps include cysts, fibroadenomas, or areas of fibrosis. But don't let the medical names frighten you. These lumps are all harmless. Your doctor will probably conduct imaging tests, such as mammography or ultrasound. In some cases, a biopsy or a needle aspiration, which draws fluid out of the area of concern with a syringe, is necessary to confirm these benign diagnoses.

Even if the growth is cancerous, often the diagnosis is still hopeful, Dr. Leitch says. In fact, women now have more treatment options and hope for survival than ever before. Ninety-nine percent of women whose breast cancer is detected early are still alive 5 years after diagnosis, and 98 percent survive 10 years or more.

In addition, the death rate from breast cancer has tumbled in recent years. A woman's estimated lifetime risk for dying of breast cancer is less than 4 percent. In comparison, a woman's lifetime risk of dying of heart disease, stroke, diabetes, or complications of osteoporosis hovers near 40 percent, Dr. Capko says.

If you're concerned about disfigurement, you should know that breast-conservation surgery has become an option in all but the most advanced cancers, Dr. Capko says. Even those women who have total mastectomies, or complete removals of the breasts, lymph nodes, and surrounding tissue, are often able to get immediate reconstructive surgery, helping to blunt the psychological blow of losing a natural breast.

Finally, rather than panicking, try as best as you can to maintain a positive attitude, suggests Patricia Gordon, M.D., director of radiation oncology at the Century City Hospital in Los Angeles.

"Attitude plays an enormous role in one's ability to recover from breast cancer," Dr. Gordon says. "Mind over matter is extraordinarily important. Having a positive attitude, having a loving family, having a significant other all contribute to an enhancement of well-being. And a sense of well-being will help you through the process of treatment."

Who Do I See?

If you develop any suspicious signs or symptoms, start with your gynecologist, suggests Barbara Fowble, M.D., a radiation oncologist at Fox Chase Cancer Center in Philadelphia.

Keep in mind that benign lumps often feel different from cancerous ones. Some doctors examine the breast in only one position, which makes it more difficult for them to get a complete sense of size, shape, and texture of a suspicious lump. So when you go in for the breast exam, make sure that your doctor checks your breasts in at least two positions, such as lying down with your arms raised up over your head and then standing or sitting upright, Dr. Capko suggests.

WHEN A LUMP ISN'T BREAST CANCER

Notify your doctor about any new lumps that you notice or feel in your breasts. Although cancer is always a possibility, in most cases, these lumps will be harmless. Here's a closer look at a couple of common noncancerous conditions that you may develop.

Benign fibroadenomas are firm, movable, fibrous breast lumps, of any size. These painless growths, which may feel like small, rubbery marbles and are firm to the touch, usually form from the fibrous supportive tissue of the breast. But they can also arise from the tissues in the mammary glands, the 15 to 20 milk reservoirs that radiate outward from the nipple. They most commonly occur in women before age 30 and may enlarge at certain times during the menstrual cycle. Although these lumps are harmless, most physicians will urge you to have them surgically removed—at least the first time they occur—to rule out cancer.

Fibrocystic breast disease is a condition in which numerous cysts form in both breasts, accompanied by lumpiness and breast pain. It usually affects women over 30 and dissipates after menopause. If you develop severe discomfort, your doctor may prescribe drugs such as tamoxifen (Nolvadex) to curb cyst formation. In addition, you may be able to ease the symptoms if you avoid consuming caffeine, alcohol, and saturated fats.

What Can I Expect?

If, after a careful physical exam, your doctor suspects that there is something abnormal in your breast, she may order further tests such as a mammogram or an ultrasonogram, a test that uses high-frequency sound waves to help determine if a lump is solid or fluid.

If those tests raise further suspicions, then your doctor may recommend that you have a biopsy. This can be done with a special needle, or the surgeon may opt to cut out all or part of the lump. A pathologist will examine the tissue under a microscope to check for cancer cells.

If it turns out to be cancer, there's a good chance that you'll be deluged by fear, anxiety, anger, and resentment. "Women's breasts are very important emotionally. After all, our society puts a lot of emphasis on a woman's breasts. So when you tell a woman that she has this cancer, she's thinking about all of the losses she faces: her breasts, her womanhood, her life," Dr. Capko says. "A lot of people might say, 'Oh look at the big picture. Your breast isn't that important; it's your life that matters.' It all goes together. I don't think it's fair to flippantly suggest, 'Oh, you need a mastectomy,' because the fear of losing a breast is overwhelming."

When a woman learns that she has breast cancer, her first response may be a desire for treatment, any treatment, immediately. Resist that impulse, Dr. Capko urges. Keep in mind that breast cancer is seldom a medical emergency. Your treatment options or odds of survival probably won't change if you take a few days to let the news sink in.

"What I tell a patient is, 'You're going to have questions. You're probably not going to understand fully what I've just told you. And there are a couple of things that you're going to start doing,'" Dr. Capko says. "'First, you're going to read everything you can about breast cancer. Second, you'll probably mention your diagnosis to a few close friends and family members. As soon as you do that, anybody you've ever known is going to call you with advice. They're going to tell you about the best doctor. They're going to call you with suggestions of all the things you need to do.

"'So you really need to filter that information,

MY MAMA TOLD ME

Will standing too close to a microwave give me cancer?

Microwaves have really helped some people eat better on the run. From heating up last night's hearty leftovers to zapping a side of veggies to go along with that bagel, they've given women an extra minute to eat their more nutritious, quickly cooked meals.

And the meals *are* more nutritious. In addition to reheating a healthy food item, microwaving can retain the vitamins and minerals in vegetables.

Yet, for all its advantages, microwaving still makes us a little nervous. Notice how we talk about "nuking" our food when we put it in that oven. So what's the story? Are those invisible rays harmful? And do the ovens leak?

Microwave ovens are designed to keep their energy waves enclosed. Although some people may be concerned that leaking microwaves could injure a person standing in front of an oven, that's highly unlikely. To be certain that your microwave oven is safe, check the seals around the door to be sure that they're intact and in good condition. If you can slide a piece of paper between the door and the oven, the seal has deteriorated, and you should have it re-

---

educate yourself about the disease, and work with your doctor to determine the best course of action for you. And that's going to take some time.'"

Conventional Wisdom

Treatment will depend on the size of your tumor and whether it has spread to the lymph nodes or other parts of your body. But in general, your treatment will likely include surgery, radiation, chemotherapy, or various combinations of these cancer fighters, Dr. Capko says.

Breast cancer surgery dates back to medical antiquity and remains a fundamental treatment

placed. If you're still concerned, have a repairman check it for you.

When using microwave ovens in your office or elsewhere, stand away from them while they're operating.

And, if you're concerned about microwaves' effect on foods—just what *is* going on with all those excited molecules?—minimize your concern by microwaving only in glass, ceramic, or microwaveable-plastic containers. Those old margarine tubs and plastic wrap may melt and possibly leach chemicals and other foreign molecules into your food. (Plastic wrap covering a dish or bowl but not touching the food is all right for trapping steam.)

There's also no evidence that food chemistry can be altered by microwaving. The truth is that a microwave oven is a useful appliance for reheating leftovers in appropriate microwaveable containers, heating microwaveable dinners in their specially designed packages, cooking some foods from scratch (oatmeal, vegetables, potatoes, or poached fish or chicken), or even making yourself a quick cup of herbal tea or hot cocoa.

Expert consulted
Barbara P. Klein, Ph.D.
Professor of food science and human nutrition
University of Illinois
Urbana-Champaign

for the disease. But the days of automatically doing a total mastectomy are long past. A lumpectomy—removal of the tumor only, followed by radiation—is far more likely now.

Radiation therapy, also called radiotherapy, uses high-energy rays to kill cancer cells and stop them from growing. Your doctors may also suggest placing radioactive implants into your breast. In some cases, you may receive both types of treatment. Radiation therapy, alone or in conjunction with chemotherapy or hormonal therapy, may also be used before surgery to destroy cancer cells and shrink the tumor. Despite the effectiveness of radiation, some women are apprehensive about undergoing it, Dr. Capko says.

"They just have visions of what it can do to you," Dr. Capko says. "They don't understand that it is limited to the breast itself. They don't understand that the equipment that is used is very sophisticated and ensures that the radiation gets directly centered on the breast. They fear that receiving radiation will cause cancer somewhere else in the body. That's just not true."

In fact, the typical side effects of a 5-day-a-week, 6-week course of radiation may be limited to a sunburnlike burn on the treated breast, fatigue, and the loss of underarm hair near the treated breast, Dr. Fowble says.

Chemotherapy, which involves a combination of anti-cancer drugs, is a standard treatment for premenopausal women whose breast tumors are greater than 1 centimeter in diameter. Because these drugs travel throughout the bloodstream, they are often able to destroy cancerous tissue that other forms of treatment can't completely wipe out. It is also a treatment that scares many women because of its reputation for having nasty side effects, including hair loss, nausea, vomiting, and loss of appetite. But in many cases, these side effects can be controlled or even eliminated.

"Without question, we are making giant advances in the management of the side effects of cancer treatments. There are medications that counteract chemotherapy's side effects to the point that most women experience little or no nausea or vomiting," Dr. Gordon says.

In the future, there may be no need for surgery, radiation, or chemotherapy. In fact, researchers are working on a number of vaccines

Breast cancer is a disease most of us associate only with women. In fact, we are 100 times more likely than men to develop this disease. Our breasts are constantly being bombarded with estrogen and other hormones that can trigger tumor growth.

But it's important to remember that men have some breast tissue as well and occasionally can develop cancer there. In fact, about 1,300 men each year develop the disease. When men do get breast cancer, it often isn't detected until a later stage than it would be in women, simply because men aren't screened for it as vigilantly as we are.

It wouldn't be a bad idea for men to examine their breasts on a regular basis, just as they should be examining their testicles. Like women, men should also be aware of the warning signs of breast cancers, including a lump on or near the breast, bleeding from the nipple, and swollen lymph nodes under the arm. If they develop these symptoms, they should see a doctor as soon as possible.

Expert consulted
Emily Conant, M.D.
Associate professor and chief of breast
*   imaging*
The Hospital of the University of Pennsylvania
Philadelphia

that may eradicate breast cancer and other forms of cancer.

Among the most promising is a vaccine developed by James McCoy, Ph.D., a former staff immunologist at the National Cancer Institute. Dr. McCoy's vaccine is autologous, meaning that it is made from a person's own cancer cells.

"It's not a preventive vaccine. It is a treatment," Dr. McCoy says.

The process begins when a surgeon removes a sample of the person's tumor, freezes it, and ships it to Dr. McCoy's laboratory in Atlanta. There, the specimen is used to create the vaccine. The initial treatment is given to individuals during a 2-week visit to the lab.

So far, the best results have occurred among people who have breast cancer. All of those women in Dr. McCoy's studies who have Stage I and Stage II breast cancer—two of the earliest stages of the disease—have been in remission for 5 years. In other words, they have no detectable signs of cancer and will likely stay that way.

"It looks as if when there isn't a large tumor present, the vaccine activates the immune system and keeps the cancer from recurring," Dr. McCoy says.

Although the vaccine is less effective against more advanced tumors, it also appears to help one in five of those women.

"I suspect that vaccines and genetic engineering are the ways that breast cancer is eventually going to be cured," Dr. Capko says.

Great Alternatives

Traditional Chinese medicine is a good complementary treatment for breast cancer and may help prevent the disease altogether, says Nan Lu, O.M.D., doctor of traditional Chinese medicine and founder of the Breast Cancer Prevention Project at the Traditional Chinese Medicine World Foundation in New York City.

According to traditional Chinese medicine, the root cause of breast cancer is the stagnation of vital energy, or *chi*, in the meridians (energy pathways) that run through the breast area, and the malfunction of one or more of three major organs—the kidney, stomach, and liver. This stagnation and dysfunction, explains Dr. Lu, are caused primarily by chronic negative emotional energy that has built up over time. In the view of ancient Chinese medical tradition, when energy stagnates over time, a small seed can progress to a cancerous mass.

"Chinese medicine has at least a 500-year history of dealing with breast cancer," says Dr. Lu, author of *Traditional Chinese Medicine: A Woman's Guide to Healing from Breast Cancer*. "As long as energy can flow freely through the meridians, and the five major organs—liver, heart, spleen, lung, and kidney—function in harmony, then a tumor can't form."

Practitioners of traditional Chinese medicine look for warning signs, such as the sudden appearance of red veins in the heels of the feet, that suggest energy flow in the body is blocked. If it is, you could be at risk for breast cancer until you get your *chi* back into balance.

Dr. Lu and other traditional Chinese healers use a variety of methods to balance *chi*, including acupuncture, acupressure, massage, herbs such as angelica root or Chinese ginseng, and *qigong*, a self-healing system that uses movements and postures to stimulate energy flow in the body.

"It can make your whole life change," Dr. Lu says. "It is not uncommon in China for women to recover from breast cancer by practicing *qigong*."

Foods such as broccoli, cauliflower, garlic, eggplant, mushrooms, pineapple, and watermelon can help improve the energy function of the liver—the major organ that controls women's health—and can help prevent breast cancer, Dr. Lu says.

For more information about traditional Chinese medicine and its role in preventing breast cancer or its recurrence, write to the Traditional Chinese Medicine World Foundation, 396 Broadway, #502, New York, NY 10013.

Reproductive Cancer

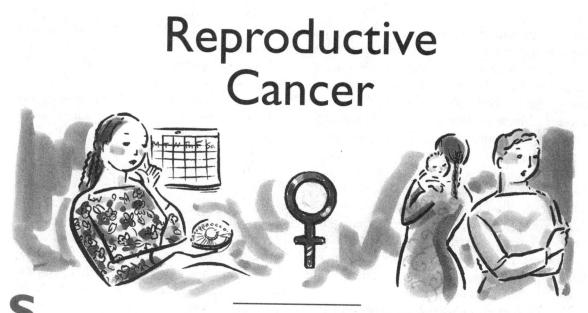

Serious illness is always worrisome, but it's especially so when it involves a woman's reproductive system. "Many women see their wombs as being tied up in who they are as females," says Yvonne Thornton, M.D., clinical professor of obstetrics and gynecology at the University of Medicine and Dentistry of New Jersey in Morristown and author of *Woman to Woman*. And since an estimated 37,400 cases of endometrial cancer and 25,200 cases of ovarian cancer are expected to be diagnosed this year, the worry is warranted.

Risk Factors

Simply being a woman puts you at risk for cancers of the reproductive organs. But there are other factors that can up the ante.

Age. Most ovarian cancers occur in postmenopausal women, half of them appearing after age 65. So your risk increases with each year, says Dr. Thornton.

Fertility drugs. "There may be a link between superovulation—the acceleration of ovulation that is usually the result of fertility drugs—and ovarian cancer," says Dr. Thornton.

A small family tree. If you had one or no children or you started your family later in life, you may be more likely to get ovarian cancer, says Joanna Cain, M.D., professor and chairperson of the department of obstetrics and gynecology at Hershey Medical Center of Pennsylvania State University in Hershey.

Family history. Has your mother, sister, or daughter been diagnosed with ovarian cancer? If so, you have an increased risk. Dr. Cain says that 5 to 10 percent of women whose close female relatives had ovarian cancer will also get the disease.

Obesity. A woman who is 30 pounds overweight has a tripled risk for endometrial cancer, and 50 extra pounds increases her risk tenfold.

Estrogen sans progesterone. When it's not coupled with progesterone, estrogen-replacement therapy increases your chances of developing endometrial cancer, says Dr. Cain. Taking the two together, however, actually decreases your risk. If you are taking estrogen and you experience bleeding or an abnormal discharge, see your doctor right away.

Talcum powder. If you've been exposed to talc—which was sometimes contaminated with asbestos until that was banned 20 years ago—either from direct application or from sanitary pads, your chances of developing ovarian cancer may be higher because talc may have a carcinogenic effect on the ovaries.

Prevention

Although oral contraceptives have long been maligned for *causing* cancer, they have actually proved to have a protective effect against hormone-related cancers that affect the uterus or ovaries, says Dr. Thornton. Birth control pills keep you from ovulating, so you're less likely to experience a cancer-causing malfunction, explains Lisa Domagalski, M.D., a gynecologist and assistant clinical professor at Brown University School of Medicine in Providence, Rhode Island. The Pill also ensures that you'll have a regular period each month, and the action of shedding the endometrium every 4 weeks makes conditions in your uterus less cancer-friendly.

"You don't have to take the Pill for long to enjoy its effects," adds Dr. Thornton. "If you take the pill from ages 20 to 21, you will still be reaping the protective benefits when you are 50."

If for some reason you can't take birth control pills—say you're a smoker or you have a history of migraine headaches—there are other ways to reduce your risk of ovarian cancer, says Beth Karlan, M.D., director of the Gilda Radner

OVARIAN CYSTS

The first thing to know about ovarian cysts is that they are actually part of what an ovary does normally. "Forming a cyst is often one of the normal consequences of ovulation," says Laurie Swaim, M.D., an obstetrician/gynecologist at Houston Women's Care Associates in Texas.

Cysts are just fluid-filled structures. They generally form and fade away during the menstrual cycle as a matter of course. Problems arise only when a cyst ruptures or grows too fast. And even when a cyst ruptures, the fluid is usually reabsorbed by the body with no further complications. "As a precaution, we might decide to observe the woman in the hospital for 24 hours," Dr. Swaim says, "but that's often the extent of it."

Of course, sometimes a cyst is more than just a cyst. While the presence of an ovarian cyst in a young woman is rarely cause for concern, the older a woman gets, the more worrisome any cyst becomes. That's because the risk for ovarian cancer rises with age. "You don't play around with a cyst in a woman over 35 or so. That's when an ultrasound is in order," says Dr. Swaim.

Ovarian Cancer Detection Program at the Cedars-Sinai Medical Center in Los Angeles. If you don't want to have any more children, you may have a procedure called tubal ligation, in which your tubes are tied, resulting in sterility. "Research shows that it can reduce your risk of ovarian cancer by up to two-thirds. The mechanism is unclear. One possible reason is that tubal ligation may inhibit the upflow of carcinogens into the abdomen," she explains.

Here are some other tips for prevention.

Get to the gynecologist. "Cancer can strike at any time, like lightning," says Dr. Thornton, "so it's important to screen for it with an annual pelvic exam." Even if you've had your children and gone through menopause, you need to get an annual gynecologic checkup.

Ask for a CA-125 test. If you have other signs of ovarian cancer, blood tests can be done to screen for CA-125, a tumor marker that may indicate the presence of ovarian cancer in the beginning stages. "If I'd had this test as part of my annual exam, my cancer would have been caught before it spread throughout my entire pelvis," says Charlene Lynn, 58, a nurse in Houston, who was diagnosed in April 1998. Researchers at the Massachusetts General Hospital in Boston have concluded that regular CA-125 testing could save up to 5,000 lives each year. "I will yell from the top of the roof, 'Get a CA-125!'" says Lynn.

Watch your weight. Methods of preventing endometrial cancer are a bit more difficult to pinpoint. "Since we don't know what causes it, keeping in the best health you can is the best advice I can give," says Dr. Thornton. For one thing, that means staying slim—because a large number of women with endometrial cancer are overweight. Excess fat equals excess estrogen, and high estrogen levels put you at risk for both endometrial and ovarian cancer, she explains.

Eat whole foods. Another way to fend off endometrial cancer is to eat unprocessed fruits and vegetables, whole grains, and foods containing omega-3 fatty acids, recommends Katrina Claghorn, R.D., an oncology dietitian for the University of Pennsylvania Medical Center in Philadelphia. These whole foods may help boost your immune system and fight off reproductive cancers. "There seems to be a correlation between a high-fat diet and ovarian and endometrial cancers," she adds. So try to keep

---

ENDOMETRIOSIS

Endometriosis could be called the case of the wandering womb. For 10 percent of women between ages 25 and 50, endometriosis causes patches of uterine (or *endometrial*) tissue to migrate to locations outside the uterus. Strange as it sounds, these misplaced bits of womb, called endometrial implants, respond normally to female hormones, regardless of their location. When it's time for menstrual bleeding to occur, the implanted tissues begin to bleed as well.

Blood seeping from implants gets absorbed by other organs in the area—the ovaries, rectum, bladder, appendix, or even the lungs. This leads to irritation and the development of adhesions, dense internal scar tissue that can eventually build up to connect one organ with another. Severe menstrual cramps are the most common symptom, but pelvic pain, painful intercourse, and infertility—alone or in combination with each other—can also signal endometriosis.

Unfortunately, since the troublemaking bits of endometrial tissue are scattered within the abdominal cavity—and because symptoms associated with endometriosis could actually be signs of other problems—a surgical procedure called a laparoscopy is what's necessary to make an accurate diagnosis.

But before they do diagnostic surgery, most gynecologists would recommend that you try medications for 3 to 4 months, says Laurie Swaim, M.D., an obstetrician/gynecologist at Houston Women's Care Associates in Texas. "Since

---

your binges on ice cream and french fries to a minimum.

Signs and Symptoms

The number one symptom of endometrial cancer is abnormal—meaning, unscheduled—bleeding. That makes this type of cancer blessedly easy to detect, says Laurie Swaim, M.D., an obstetrician and gynecologist at Houston

any surgery carries risks, we would rule out other possible causes, like infection or sexually transmitted diseases, then assume it's endometriosis and treat it medically."

As treatment for endometriosis, doctors often recommend contraceptive pills taken either continuously, to stop menstruation altogether, or as they would be for birth control, to help lighten menstrual flow and lessen the chance of backup. Synthetic hormones such as danazol (Danocrine) or leuprolide (Lupron) have also been used to treat severe endometriosis. While they can help relieve pain, both of these drugs have potentially problematic side effects, ranging from weight gain and deepening of the voice to hot flashes, depression, and osteoporosis.

Surgery can also constitute treatment for endometriosis. Adhesions or implants can be removed, cauterized (burned), or vaporized with a laser during laparoscopy, a procedure sometimes called belly button surgery because the small primary incision is made near the navel. In some cases, though, implants are too large or the organs involved are too delicate for laparoscopy, so *laparotomy*, or abdominal surgery, is the procedure of choice.

When endometriosis doesn't respond to medication or conservative surgery or when implants or adhesions recur, hysterectomy (removal of the uterus and ovaries) is an option. Women who have experienced crippling pelvic pain for years may find that this drastic-sounding measure brings the best and most reliable relief.

Women's Care Associates in Texas. Bleeding between periods isn't normal and should be checked out. "And postmenopausal bleeding of any kind needs to be investigated right away," she says. Even seemingly simple spotting should be brought to the attention of your gynecologist.

"Endometrial cancer can occur before menopause as well," says Dr. Cain. If you're bleeding heavily between periods, have continued heavy periods, or experience a very foul-smelling discharge, see your doctor, she adds.

Ovarian cancer, on the other hand, is quite a bit more difficult to discover. "Women aren't usually diagnosed until their cases are very advanced," says Dr. Swaim.

The problem is that there is no specific list of symptoms associated exclusively with ovarian cancer. Symptoms mimic everyday womanly complaints—cramping, bloating, abdominal swelling. "We cope and continue," says Dr. Karlan.

"I experienced some early morning nausea and a slight change in my bowel habits, but I was going through a divorce, so I blamed it on my emotions," recalls Lynn.

"We need to begin finding ovarian cancer when it's in Stage 1—where cures can be effected most successfully," says Dr. Karlan.

There are ways to distinguish normal discomfort from the kind that should take you to your gynecologist. Troubling symptoms are constant, daily, and progressive, says Dr. Karlan. Pelvic pressure, bloating, urinary frequency, and constipation or any other change in bowel habits that lingers for a month should get your attention. "You know your own body," she says. "If you notice that suddenly your clothes fit tightly around your middle, have someone examine you."

Don't Panic!

The unexpected bleeding that can be a sign of endometrial cancer can also be a symptom of many other female complaints, ranging from the mild to the more serious. If you are premenopausal, you could have a polyp, a cervical infection, or fibroids, says Dr. Swaim. Don't let fear stop you from seeing your doctor.

Postmenopausal women do have more reason to worry about unscheduled bleeding. But even so, something harmless and correctable, like skipped or changed hormone-replacement medication, can often be to blame for spotting. "It's easy to test for endometrial cancer," Dr. Swaim assures. So get it checked out.

Symptoms that could mean ovarian cancer could also mean a host of other, non-life-threatening problems. Abdominal swelling could indicate fibroids, pregnancy, or a benign pelvic mass. Cramping or one-sided abdominal pain could be caused by a cyst or irritable bowel disease. Urinary frequency could be due to a bladder or urinary tract infection. Before you panic, see your doctor, then get treatment for whatever it is that ails you.

Who Do I See?

Any unusual bleeding should be evaluated first by your regular gynecologist. "As general gynecologists, we can treat most endometrial cancers," says Dr. Domagalski. If your case is more severe, you will most likely be referred to a gynecologic oncologist, a gynecologist specially trained in surgery and cancers of the female reproductive tract.

And be sure to ask if the doctor is board-certified, recommends Dr. Thornton. Certification

FIBROIDS

The slow-growing tumors commonly known as fibroids get called by the wrong name more often than not. The correct term for these common growths is *myomas*—the root of that word relating to muscle, specifically the uterine muscle where these tumors appear.

Fibroids seem to develop without any particular inspiration: Their cause, other than the simple presence of the female hormone estrogen, is somewhat of a mystery. A study conducted at the Mario Negri Institute of Pharmacological Research in Milan showed that women who frequently consume beef have 1.7 times the risk of fibroids. Eating a lot of fish, on the other hand, *lowers* a woman's risk by 30 percent.

The incidence is overwhelmingly common: One-fourth of all women have fibroids, with that rate rising to one-half in black women. While that sounds like a lot of women with "female problems," the fact is that the vast majority of fibroids keep to themselves, never causing the slightest complaint.

"So many women have them and don't even know it, because in so many women fibroids just aren't an issue," says Karen Meyer, N.P., L.M.W., a nurse practitioner and licensed midwife at the Pacific Fertility Center in San Francisco. Most

means your doctor has chosen to take national standardized oral and written tests in her field and can use the initials F.A.C. (for Fellow of the American College of the particular specialty). For example, F.A.C.O.G. stands for Fellow of the American College of Obstetricians and Gynecologists.

If your gynecologist decides that your symptoms suggest ovarian cancer, it's important that you choose a specialized doctor even *before* diagnostic surgery, says Dr. Karlan. "You want to have a gynecologic oncologist present at the initial surgery. It is very impor-

fibroids exist quietly during a woman's later reproductive life (they are most common around age 40) and then shrink away as estrogen levels drop at the time of menopause. Mild cases of fibroids may require no treatment other than close monitoring (of size and discomfort levels, for example) by you and your gynecologist.

Unfortunately, not all fibroids are silent. When fibroids grow large or multiply, they cause symptoms that are hard to miss and usually require medical treatment. Pressure on internal organs can lead to chronic pelvic pain. Fibroids can change the shape of your endometrium (uterine lining), often causing menstrual irregularities and frequent or extremely heavy periods, says Meyer. Other obvious indications that you may have fibroids are abdominal swelling, pain during intercourse, and urinary frequency or constipation.

Surgery is the most reliable way to end the heavy bleeding and possible anemia that come with large or multiple fibroids. For younger women who want to bear children, a procedure called myomectomy can remove the fibroids without removing the entire uterus. This type of abdominal surgery is complicated, however, and the growths do have a chance of recurring. If a woman with fibroids is already finished building her family, hysterectomy can be a sensible option that brings welcome relief.

What Can I Expect?

If you see your gynecologist because of unusual bleeding, she will most likely order an endometrial biopsy, which sounds worse than it is. She'll perform the procedure in her office. She'll use a thin catheter to retrieve a sample of endometrial tissue from the inside of your uterus. "You'll feel one giant menstrual-type cramp, and then it will all be over," says Dr. Swaim. No local anesthesia is used because there is no way that a doctor can numb your uterus, she says, and the procedure is so quick that general anesthesia is unnecessary.

If the test results reveal endometrial cancer, you will need surgery to "stage" the disease—that is, to discover how involved the cancer is and to determine the best course of treatment. Along with abdominal surgery to examine your uterus, your surgeon will probably want to biopsy some nearby lymph nodes as well. Further surgery, perhaps to remove your uterus, and chemotherapy may also play a part in your treatment.

tant that all visible tumor be removed the first time."

In addition to an M.D., you may choose to see a psychologist or a social worker to deal with the stresses you are facing pending or after a diagnosis of reproductive cancer, says Dr. Cain. "Because your entire family will be affected, I also suggest that you all attend counseling or group therapy together," she says. And an R.D. can help you with nutritional support. To promote general wellness, you may want to consult a naturopathic physician.

A suspicion of ovarian cancer will most likely lead directly to a trip to the operating room. There, a gynecologic oncologist will remove the mass and send it to a pathologist. If they think it is an early cancer, the surgeon will also remove one ovary, nearby lymph nodes, and tissue from neighboring organs to screen for cancer cells that may have spread.

A diagnosis of cancer of the reproductive organs presents emotional on top of physical challenges. "Women often think, 'I won't have a life without my uterus,'" says Dr. Thornton.

"Because of what women have learned about Gilda Radner's death, a suspicion of ovarian cancer will elicit a greater emotional response than endometrial cancer," says Dr. Domagalski. Radner, a comedienne of *Saturday Night Live* fame, died of ovarian cancer in 1989 at the age of 42.

"But when a woman is diagnosed with endometrial cancer, she may still assume the worst," says Dr. Domagalski. "Once she discovers how curable it is, she feels a sense of relief. With both endometrial and ovarian cancer, women just want it over with as soon as possible."

Conventional Wisdom

Most endometrial cancer is caught fairly early and surgically treated with hysterectomy, explains Dr. Domagalski. If the cancer is more advanced, the doctor may also decide to remove the ovaries, the fallopian tubes, the upper part of the vagina, or nearby lymph nodes. Sometimes, a period of radiation treatments, hormone therapy, or chemotherapy will follow.

The primary treatment for ovarian cancer is the surgical removal of the tumor, says Dr. Cain. If the case is more severe, one or both ovaries, nearby organs, and lymph nodes will be removed as well. Unfortunately, many cases of ovarian cancer are not cured by surgery alone, so chemotherapy is usually prescribed.

Great Alternatives

If you've been diagnosed with a cancer of the reproductive system or you want to reduce your

REAL-LIFE SCENARIO

Her Unusual Bleeding May Be More Than a "Heavy" Month

Four months ago, Rose, 39, started having unusually heavy menstrual periods. She thought nothing of it at the time, but the same thing has happened every month since then. She has also been bruising more easily, and her gums have started to bleed. When she mentioned her symptoms to a friend who is a nurse, her friend suggested she see a doctor right away. In the same breath, the friend rattled off the names of several life-threatening diseases, such as leukemia and aplastic anemia. Rose wasted no time. She went straight to her family doctor, who passed her directly to a hematologist. But after blood work had been done, the doctor tried to calm her. She had something called von Willebrand's disease—nothing to worry about. Well, she can't help herself. She's worried. Should she be?

The scenario above is a very common presentation for von Willebrand's disease. Although not everyone with this genetic abnormality has symptoms, often women with this problem experience nosebleeds, easy bruising, heavy menstrual flow, excessive or unusual bleeding from the mouth or gums, and occasionally, gastrointestinal or urinary tract bleeding.

chances of a future diagnosis, these alternative or complementary therapies may help boost your immune system.

Gulp some green tea. A number of studies performed in China and Japan indicate that people who regularly drink green tea have a lower incidence of cancer. The protective effects are thought to come from the antioxidants in the tea, says Helen Healy, N.D., a naturopathic physician and director of Wellspring Naturopathic Clinic in St. Paul, Minnesota.

Pop some selenium. The mineral selenium, which is found naturally in meat, dairy foods,

Von Willebrand's disease is the most common inherited bleeding disorder. It occurs when von Willebrand factor, a substance needed for clotting that's normally present in the blood, is lacking or abnormal.

Although it is a lifelong condition, von Willebrand's disease is easily manageable. Depending on the form of the disease (there are three types), treatment may consist of nasally administered desmopressin acetate (DDAVP) or a blood product called cryoprecipitate.

Any woman with symptoms that suggest von Willebrand's disease should be sure to get an accurate diagnosis—even if she has learned to live with the problem. That's because von Willebrand's is a genetic disorder, which means that if you don't know about it, you could unwittingly pass it down to any children you bear. Plus, any surgery, even simple elective ones, may require pretreatment with DDAVP to be safe.

Expert consulted
Deborah Goodman-Gruen, M.D., Ph.D.
Assistant adjunct professor of family and
preventive medicine
University of California
San Diego

and grains, has been shown to cut cancer risk by two-thirds. Selenium is most effective when taken in the supplement form, but be careful: Taking too much can be toxic, warns Dr. Healy. Keep your daily dosage at 200 micrograms or less.

See yourself well. "Visualization helps you get in touch with the part of your body that is cancerous," says Dr. Healy. Also known as guided imagery, visualization uses the power of suggestion to create empowering images, such as a mass of cancer cells being attacked by the immune system.

Feed it back. Biofeedback helps you take an active role in your treatment. Through the placement of electrodes on your body and scalp, one of more than 10,000 biofeedback therapists in the country can teach you how to control some of your involuntary bodily functions, such as heart rate, blood pressure, and emotions. "Biofeedback is helpful for general wellness and chemotherapy-related nausea," says Dr. Cain.

Antioxidize. "For prevention of all types of cancer, taking antioxidants can be beneficial," says Claghorn. You can also get antioxidants from fruits and vegetables such as blueberries and red peppers. Stay away from antioxidants during radiation or chemotherapy, however, because they may reduce the effectiveness of the treatments.

Get some support. Psychological support is a necessary part of cancer treatment, Dr. Cain says. Information on cancer support groups is available at most hospitals.

Fight back. "I have no control over what this cancer is doing to me, but I have some control over what I'm doing to it," says Lynn. She has stayed in control of her illness by spreading the word to others. Thanks to Lynn's perseverance and some help from her daughter Nora, who works for the California Senate, a bill requiring insurance companies to cover testing for ovarian cancer is being negotiated. "I hope someone somewhere lives because my daughter loves me so much," Lynn says.

Lung Cancer

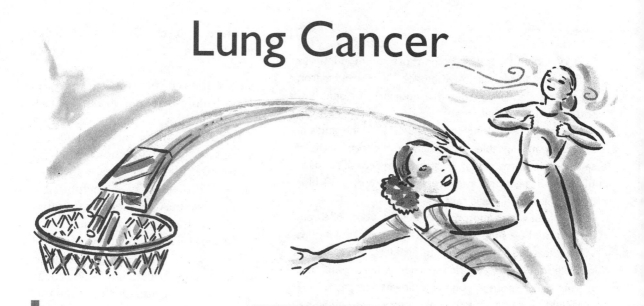

Lung cancer was a rare disease until the early 20th century. As late as 1912, there had been a total of only 374 reported cases of the disease, and the vast majority of those involved men. Although a few daring women smoked prior to World War I, we did not take up smoking in large numbers until the 1940s. Then, as lighting up became the norm rather than the exception, lung cancer rates among women skyrocketed. In 1987, lung cancer surpassed breast cancer as the leading cause of cancer deaths among women. By 1999, more than 42 percent of people who died of the disease were female. Each year in the United States, more than 77,000 women develop lung cancer, and about 68,000 die of it.

Risk Factors

Without a doubt, smoking is the number one risk factor for lung cancer. In fact, according to the Wyoming Department of Health, which has been monitoring all of Wyoming's cancer cases since 1962, the real seven warning signs of lung cancer are the cigarette-industry giants: U.S. To-

bacco, Philip Morris, R. J. Reynolds, Brown & Williamson, Lorillard, British American Tobacco, and the Liggett Group.

The tragedy is that more than 90 percent of lung cancers among women could be prevented if we did just one thing: quit smoking. Each puff you inhale contains more than 4,000 compounds and at least 60 known cancer-causing agents, including substances used to make insecticide, rat poison, toilet bowl disinfectant, and embalming fluid. Tobacco smoke even contains hydrogen cyanide, a deadly poison used in prison gas chambers. If you smoke a pack or less a day, you are 7 times more likely to die of lung cancer than women who don't. If you smoke more than a pack a day, your risk of dying of lung cancer is a staggering 15 times higher than a nonsmoker's.

"Fifty percent of women who smoke are going to die of a smoking-related illness. Fifty percent. That's like flipping a coin. The odds are not good. I can't think of anything worse for your health that you could do in your life than smoking," says Linda Ford, M.D., past president of the American Lung Association.

Granted, some women who have never taken a puff in their lives and are in the best of shape, such as Kim Perrot of the WNBA Houston Comets, do get lung cancer, but those cases are extremely rare. In most instances, nonsmokers who develop lung cancer have a long history of exposure to secondhand, or sidestream, smoke either in their workplaces or at home. Most of the chemicals that are found in mainstream smoke are also found in sidestream smoke and have the same cancer-promoting effects. In fact, each year about 3,000 people die of lung cancer as a result of breathing the smoke of other people's cigarettes.

Radon, a naturally occurring gas produced by the radioactive decay of uranium in the soil and water, has been linked to about 10,000 deaths from lung cancer annually. Statistically, it is the second most common cause of the disease. But in reality, many physicians suspect that smoking is probably a major contributor even in those cases.

"People like to blame anything else but smoking for their lung problems," Dr. Ford says. "'No, it's not the smoking I've been doing for the last 40 years that caused my cancer, it's the radon in my basement!' Very few lung cancers are caused by radon alone."

Prevention

Quit, quit, quit! Make it your mantra. Make it your obsession. Make it happen, Dr. Ford says.

"Sometimes, people have to stand up for

WOMEN ASK WHY

Why doesn't my family doctor ever recommend vitamins and herbs when I'm feeling sick?

Unfortunately, most medical training overlooks the use of vitamins and herbs to treat illness. Physicians are trained in evidence-based medicine. That means when they treat a disease, they use procedures and medications that have been rigorously studied and that have good track records of evidence showing that they are effective in treating a specific ailment.

Until recently, herbal remedies have been subjected to few scientifically rigorous studies. Although more data is available on vitamin-and-mineral therapy (such as vitamin D and calcium for osteoporosis, or zinc for a sore throat), it has yet to become part of core medical studies. Additionally, a lack of regulation of vitamins and herbal products exists. Even when your physician prescribes these therapies, she cannot ensure what these products actually contain. I believe that as more studies become available, you will quickly see vitamins and herbs finding their way into mainstream medicine.

Expert consulted
Jan I. Maby, D.O.
Medical director
Cobble Hill Health Center
Brooklyn, New York

themselves and say, 'Okay, I was foolish to start. I am addicted, but I can do something about it,'" Dr. Ford says. "You empower yourself to make that first step, which is always the hardest one. You will probably start and stop, start and stop, start and stop many times before you finally quit. That's okay. Don't feel too bad if you don't make it the first few times. Keep your eye on the goal, and the goal is quitting—living completely tobacco-free."

MY MAMA TOLD ME

Does smoking really stunt your growth?

First of all, smoking will almost certainly stunt your life expectancy. In fact, smokers live an average of 7 years less than nonsmokers. It will also very likely stunt the quality of your life as you get older, since emphysema, chronic bronchitis, and other respiratory problems associated with smoking will make doing daily chores and activities difficult. So yes, in an indirect way smoking does stunt your growth.

Smoking increases your risk of osteoporosis, a disease whose name literally means "holes in the bones." It occurs when the loss of bone tissue exceeds its replacement. A silent disease, osteoporosis robs bones of their strength over time, particularly in the years following menopause. Osteoporosis can cause the bones in your spine to crack and fracture and can make you appear as if you have lost height.

But if you stop smoking—and it is never too late to do that—and begin exercising and taking calcium and vitamin D, you actually can reverse some of the effects of this disease. So osteoporosis is yet another reason not to ever smoke if you haven't started, and to quit if you have.

Expert consulted
Jan I. Maby, D.O.
Medical director
Cobble Hill Health Center
Brooklyn, New York

body, and your ability to taste and smell will be enhanced. In 72 hours, your lung capacity will increase, and you'll breathe easier because your bronchial tubes will have relaxed. Within a week, virtually all the harmful chemicals produced by smoking will have left your body. In less than 3 months, your lung function will have improved 30 percent. Within 9 months, any residual coughing, fatigue, and shortness of breath will have dissipated. Your lungs will have increased their ability to cleanse themselves, remove excess mucus, and fend off infections.

And in just 10 years after lighting up for the last time, your risk of dying of lung cancer will be about the same as that of a woman who has never smoked.

Quitting, of course, is simple in theory—just throw your cigarettes out—but often difficult in practice. That's because nicotine, the prime ingredient in tobacco, is one of the most addictive substances known. Once you're in its grasp, it takes a determined effort to break free, particularly if you've been smoking for a number of years and you are a woman.

Women apparently metabolize nicotine more slowly than men, says Robert Klesges, Ph.D., a smoking-cessation expert at the University of Memphis and coauthor of *How Women Can Finally Stop Smoking*. This means that cigarette for cigarette, women may have higher levels of nicotine in their bodies and, therefore, may be more dependent on the drug than men are. So when a woman tries to quit, her withdrawal symptoms may be more intense.

Certainly, it may be difficult, but it is never too late to stop and allow your body to repair the harm you've done to it, says Antoinette Wozniak, M.D., a clinical oncologist at the Barbara Ann Karmanos Cancer Institute in Detroit. Within 8 hours after your last cigarette, the oxygen levels in your blood will increase and the levels of carbon monoxide will plummet. In 48 hours, the final traces of nicotine will leave your

Then, there's the weight issue. Fear of weight gain after quitting is far more common among women than among men. In fact, it is probably the single biggest difference between why women and men smoke, according to Dr. Klesges. The truth is that the average weight gain for women who quit is about 13 pounds. It isn't inevitable, however, that you will gain weight. Once you nip your smoking in the bud, you can focus on your weight. So despite the barriers, you can quit once and for all. Here's how you can get started.

Stay in sync. Timing is everything if you're a premenopausal woman trying to quit. Plan to stop smoking at the end of your period (the beginning of your menstrual cycle) because you'll experience fewer and less intense withdrawal symptoms, Dr. Klesges suggests.

Set a quit date. Women (and men, for that matter) who set a definite day to quit and stick to it are more likely to stop smoking than those who don't. Avoid picking stressful holidays like New Year's Day or Thanksgiving, and don't select a date that is weeks or months away. Odds are that your resolve to quit will evaporate by then, Dr. Klesges says.

Cut back. Since women metabolize nicotine more slowly than men do, gradually cutting down may be a better way for you to quit than going cold turkey, Dr. Klesges says. Pick situations and places where you

Pneumonia

Women who smoke more than 20 cigarettes a day are three times more likely to develop pneumonia than women who have never taken a puff.

Even if you smoke less than that, your risk of pneumonia is still greater than a nonsmoker's, says Monica Kraft, M.D., a pulmonologist and assistant professor of medicine at the National Jewish Medical and Research Center in Denver. That's because women who smoke have fewer cilia, the hairlike cells that help clear bacteria, viruses, and other invaders out of their lungs. "Cigarette smoke actually paralyzes the cilia. So you've lost an important defense mechanism right there," she says. In addition, smoking disrupts the work of macrophages, immune cells that normally surround and destroy the dangerous particles that attack your lungs.

The net result is an increased risk of pneumonia. Pneumonia develops when phlegm, fluid, and other debris clog your airways and fill the air sacs in your lungs. This accumulation interferes with your lungs' normal ability to remove carbon dioxide from your body and deliver life-giving oxygen to your blood and tissues. Viral pneumonia is more contagious but usually less severe than bacterial pneumonia. Its symptoms include gradual appetite loss, slowly rising fever, muscle soreness, and a dry, unproductive cough that can develop into a phlegm-producing cough over several days.

Bacterial pneumonia, such as Legionnaires' disease, is far more dangerous and usually causes more violent symptoms than viral pneumonia. Unlike viral pneumonia, bacterial forms of the disease can be treated with antibiotics.

The best thing that you can do to prevent pneumonia is to quit smoking, Dr. Kraft says. In addition, an annual flu shot and a pneumonia vaccine every 5 years can help keep this disease caged. If you develop chills, fever, headache, fatigue, chest pain, or a productive cough, consult your physician, Dr. Kraft urges. If you are diagnosed with pneumonia, drink plenty of fluids (at least eight 8-ounce glasses of water daily), get lots of rest, and finish any medication that your doctor prescribes for you. In addition, keep coughing—although it may be painful, it will help clear phlegm out of your lungs and speed your recovery.

PLEURISY

Some things in life just naturally go together. Spaghetti and meatballs. Pearls and basic black. Lucy and Ethel. And less pleasantly, pneumonia and pleurisy.

"Pleurisy is a common scenario with pneumonia. They tend to go together," says Monica Kraft, M.D., a pulmonologist and assistant professor of medicine at the National Jewish Medical and Research Center in Denver.

Pleurisy is an inflammation of the thin, transparent membrane called the pleura that covers your lungs and lines the inside of your chest wall. Usually caused by a viral or bacterial infection, this inflammation triggers breathing difficulties and can lead to extreme chest pain. It can precede pneumonia and is often an early warning sign of the disease, Dr. Kraft says.

Less commonly, acute bronchitis or a pulmonary embolism, which is a blood clot in your arteries leading to your lungs, can cause pleurisy.

Over-the-counter analgesics such as acetaminophen or ibuprofen, when used as directed, can help ease your chest pain, Dr. Kraft says. But remember that this is a temporary solution. Any chest pain should be evaluated by a doctor as soon as possible.

Can the cups. Women who smoke are more likely to drink coffee, tea, and other caffeinated beverages, Dr. Klesges says. Laying off tobacco increases caffeine's stimulating effects in your body. So if you are trying to quit smoking, you should cut your caffeine consumption in half. Otherwise, you may feel more jittery and start craving a smoke.

Make a pact. Team up with a friend. Research suggests that social support helps women—but not men—quit smoking. Hook up with a pal who is as committed to quitting as you are. It's a bad sign, for instance, if the person says, "Yeah, I guess I could give it a try." If you get that kind of tepid response, ask someone else to join your crusade, Dr. Klesges says. If your spouse smokes and refuses to quit when you do, frankly, it will be more difficult for you to stop. At the very least, ask him not to smoke inside your home or in your presence.

won't smoke, such as in the car, on the telephone, or in the kitchen. Or, you can try rationing your cigarettes. Carry only enough smokes with you to reach your limit for that day. If you normally smoke a pack daily, plan on cutting back to 15 cigarettes a day by the end of the first week, 10 cigarettes by the end of the second week, and none by the end of the third week.

Toss those weeds. The night before you quit, go through a quitting ritual, Dr. Klesges suggests. Throw out all of your tobacco products. Don't hold back. Lighters? Matches? Ashtrays? Pitch them. If you have any hidden stashes in places like pockets or glove compartments, toss those as well.

Stick to a plan. Once you find someone who is as committed to quitting as you are, the two of you should:

➧ Speak to each other every day. Frequent, daily contact is crucial, especially in the early stages of quitting. After you both quit, agree that you will call each other—even if it is 3 o'clock in the morning—if either of you is tempted to have a cigarette, Dr. Klesges says.

➧ Remain positive. Don't gripe or complain. Focus on the goal and how you can help each other stay on track.

➧ Support your buddy even if you are having a rough time. Don't let her down. Offer plenty of encouragement such as, "Yes, withdrawal symptoms are tough, but let's think of ways to help you past them."

♦ Think of your cravings and other withdrawal symptoms as challenges that you can overcome together.

Chew, stick, or swallow. When used as directed, over-the-counter products such as nicotine gum and patches as well as prescription medications such as bupropion (Zyban) can help lessen your urges to smoke, Dr. Klesges says. But keep in mind that these products are only a partial solution. They work best when used in conjunction with a formalized smoking-cessation program.

Keep it outside. If you are exposed to secondhand smoke on a regular basis, ask the smokers in your household to puff away outdoors. Suggest to your guests that they go outside if they wish to smoke at your house, Dr. Ford suggests. "The harder it is for a smoker to smoke, the less they will smoke—which is more healthy for them as well."

Keep radon out, too. The combination of smoking and radon exposure more than doubles your risk of developing lung cancer. So in addition to stamping out your tobacco habit, check up on the radon levels in your home, Dr. Ford suggests. Get a radon detector, available at many hardware stores, and place it in the basement or the lowest living areas of your home. Since radon levels can fluctuate daily, get a detector that will measure radon levels for at least 6 months. When the detector has completed its task, mail the device to a laboratory that analyzes the data and then sends you a report.

Radon is measured in units called picocuries per liter. If your test results are greater than 4 picocuries per liter, the highest exposure recommended by the Environmental Protection Agency, then you should consider ways to fix the problem, such as sealing large cracks in your basement with caulk, installing a venting pipe to the roof, or simply using a window fan to flush the radon out.

Get a scan. If you smoke or are a former smoker, a painless 20-second test could save your life by detecting lung cancer at an early, curable stage, says Claudia I. Henschke, M.D., Ph.D., professor of radiology and division chief of chest imaging at the New York Weill Cornell Center of New York Presbyterian Hospital in New York City.

In her study of 1,000 smokers and former smokers age 60 and older, Dr. Henschke found that low-radiation-dose computed tomography (a CT scan) can detect lung tumors long before they appear on chest x-rays. Dr. Henschke and her team found 23 early-stage lung cancers among these people. Only 4 of those tumors were visible on chest x-rays, the standard diagnostic imaging technique. Traditionally, lung cancer tumors have been about the size of oranges when they are discovered. But the CT scan found tumors that were no bigger than grains of rice.

"Lung cancer is deadly because we never had a good way to find it early. Now we do," Dr. Henschke says. "CT screening transforms the prognosis for lung cancer, just as mammography did for breast cancer. The current 5-year survival rate for lung cancer is only 14 percent. But that could soar to 80 percent if all smokers and ex-smokers received annual CT exams and early treatment." So ask your doctor about annual CT screening for lung cancer.

Signs and Symptoms

A persistent cough is the most common symptom of lung cancer.

"A lot of smokers have a nagging cough. Many pass it off as a smoker's cough. But they

SHACKLE YOUR CRAVINGS

If you are overwhelmed by a cigarette craving, you can still prevent a full-blown relapse if you follow these guidelines, says Robert Klesges, Ph.D., a smoking-cessation expert at the University of Memphis and coauthor of *How Women Can Finally Stop Smoking*.

➤ Never bum a smoke or accept a cigarette that is offered to you. Most women who relapse didn't purchase their cigarettes. They asked other smokers for them. Don't fall into this trap.

➤ Force yourself to go out and get the cigarettes yourself. If you're in a bar, for instance, don't purchase a pack from a vending machine in the lobby. Leave. Walk or drive to a convenience store or supermarket. Even then, allow 10 minutes to pass before you make your purchase. First, it will get you away from the sights, sounds, and other cues that are fueling your craving. Second, it will give you time to think about whether smoking is really what you want to do again. And third, since most cravings pass within a couple of minutes, odds are that you'll decide against the purchase.

➤ If you do purchase a pack, smoke one—in a place other than where you were originally tempted—then throw the rest of the pack away. If you want another one, repeat the process: Buy a new pack, smoke one, and throw the rest away. Most women who have cravings just want to smoke one, not an entire pack. If you keep the pack after smoking one, you'll be more tempted to smoke the rest plus a lot more.

If you do completely relapse, don't dwell on your setback. Set a new quit date right away and stick to it, Dr. Klesges urges.

ticularly if you cough up blood. In addition, be wary of the following symptoms, according to Dr. Wozniak: suddenly developing shortness of breath during routine activities, such as climbing stairs, that haven't caused breathing difficulties in the past; wheezing; hoarseness; constant chest, shoulder, or arm pain; frequent bouts of pneumonia or bronchitis; unexplained weight loss; persistent fatigue; or swelling in your face, neck, or upper chest.

Don't Panic!

Acute bronchitis also may cause a persistent cough, shortness of breath, chest pain, and bloody sputum. You also may have pneumonia or a lung abscess—a pus-laden sac of dead tissue that forms as your body fights off an infection. Or you may have a more serious condition, such as emphysema or tuberculosis.

The important thing, says Dr. Wozniak, is to see your doctor as soon as possible if you notice any of the warning signs, because the earlier a cancer is detected, the better your chances of survival.

"The worst thing that women can do is to take on the ostrich position with their heads buried in the sand," Dr. Wozniak says. "They panic, thinking that maybe these symptoms will just go away. But by the time they finally pull their heads out of the ground, it may be several months later, and they may be beyond what we can reasonably deal with."

may also tell you that it's a different kind of cough than they've ever had before. It is either more productive or constant," says Dr. Wozniak.

So see your doctor if you notice a persistent cough or any change in your smoker's hack, par-

Who Do I See?

If you experience lung discomfort, pay a visit to your family doctor first. "Most pulmonary complaints can be handled by primary-care practitioners," says Lisa Bellini, M.D., assistant professor of medicine in the pulmonary, allergy, and critical-care division at the University of Pennsylvania Medical Center in Philadelphia. If your primary-care practitioner suspects a problem, she may decide to consult a pulmonologist for a second opinion.

If an x-ray reveals a lung mass, you will probably be referred to a pulmonologist, who will evaluate whether or not the mass is cancerous. "If your primary-care physician has already made the diagnosis, you can see either a pulmonologist, who will test to see to what stage the tumor has advanced, or an oncologist," says Dr. Bellini.

What Can I Expect?

If your doctor suspects that you have lung cancer, she will likely order several tests to confirm the diagnosis. If you have a productive cough, for instance, your doctor will probably have your sputum screened for cancer cells. Your doctor also may order a chest x-ray or a CT scan. In addition, she may insert a small tube called a bronchoscope through your nose or mouth, down your throat, and into your bronchial tubes. During this procedure, your doctor will likely collect a sample of lung tissue so that it can be examined under a microscope for cancer cells. A biopsy also may be done during a mediastinoscopy, a procedure in which a scope is inserted into your chest through a small incision.

If the sample is cancerous, these tests also will help your physician determine what type of lung cancer you have and how far it has spread.

"The first thing that lung cancer patients fear is dying. And when they think about the treatment, they get totally scared. They worry about getting sick from the treatment or losing their hair. They worry about the cost," says Ritsuko Komaki, M.D., a radiation oncologist at the University of Texas M. D. Anderson Cancer Center in Houston. "They often express a lot of anger. They'll think, 'So-and-so has smoked just as long as I have, and she doesn't have lung cancer. Why me?'"

Conventional Wisdom

Treatment will depend on a number of factors, including the size and location of the cancer and whether or not it has spread to your lymph nodes or other organs. According to one estimate, 5 to 10 years elapse between the development of the first lung cancer cell and diagnosis of the disease. Because lung cancer is symptomless during much of its growth, three out of every four lung tumors have spread elsewhere prior to diagnosis and can't be cured by surgery alone.

Often, treatment will include a combination of surgery, radiation therapy, and chemotherapy.

The best thing you can do for yourself after diagnosis—if you haven't done it already—is quit smoking, Dr. Komaki says. Nicotine increases your body's use of energy and literally siphons off nutrients that could help you fight the disease.

"There is plenty of evidence that if a person continues to smoke after a diagnosis of lung cancer, the outcome is much worse compared to that of a person who does quit. If you continue to smoke—even if the first lung cancer is treatable—your risk of a second lung cancer or head-and-neck cancer in the next few years is greatly increased," adds Dr. Komaki.

Great Alternatives

In her book *Herbs for Health and Healing*, Kathi Keville, director of the American Herb Association, suggests that a "withdrawal" tincture made from fresh oats can help a smoker break the habit. To try it, combine 1 teaspoon tincture (or glycerite) of fresh oat berries, ½ teaspoon each of tinctures of valerian rhizome and skullcap leaves, and ½ teaspoon each of tinctures of St. John's wort leaves and passionflower. Keep the combination in a 1- to 2-ounce amber or dark-blue glass bottle with a dropper lid, and take 2 to 5 dropperfuls each day. All of these ingredients are available at most health food stores.

While the herbs in this formula are generally considered safe, some could cause problems for certain people. If you have celiac disease (a gluten intolerance), do not use oat berries. Do not use valerian with sleep-enhancing or mood-regulating medications. It may also cause heart palpitations and nervousness—if so, discontinue use. Do not use St. John's wort with antidepressants without your doctor's approval, and avoid overexposure to direct sunlight while taking it.

Colorectal Cancer

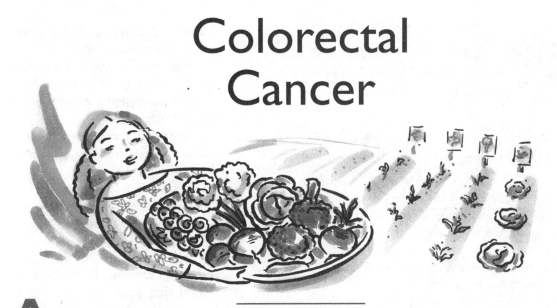

Audrey Hepburn died of cancer in 1993. You probably knew that. But do you know what type of cancer she had? Few people do, and it's no surprise. Bowel cancer isn't the sort of thing the media like to mention, especially where beautiful, elegant, and charming women like Ms. Hepburn are concerned.

"We don't talk about colon cancer; it's unmentionable," says Mary Elizabeth Roth, M.D., clinical professor at Wayne State University in Southfield, Michigan, and a member of the American Cancer Society's Committee on Colon Cancer. Nevertheless, what needs to be mentioned about bowel tumors is both deadly serious and extremely hopeful.

The facts are that cancer of the colon and rectum (colorectal cancer) will kill some 56,600 people this year—almost half of them women. It is the second leading cause of cancer death in the United States. And it is highly preventable. "This is a cancer that no one needs to have," asserts Ernestine Hambrick, M.D., founder and chairperson of the Stop Colon/Rectal Cancer Foundation in Chicago.

Risk Factors

Often silent and symptomless, colorectal tumors grow either from the colon, which is the last 5 to 6 feet of your intestine, or from the rectum, which is the last 8 inches or so of your digestive tract.

As with many cancers, there are important factors in your life that can help determine your risk for getting this disease.

Age. As years pile up, so does your likelihood of developing colorectal cancer. In fact, the incidence is six times higher among those age 65 and older than among those ages 40 to 64.

Genetics. Some people are at greater risk if one of their parents or a sibling has had colorectal cancer or polyps.

Personal history. If you've already had colon cancer, colon polyps, or inflammatory bowel disease, your risk rises.

Diet. Can't get enough red meat? If you eat too much, you may be asking for trouble. It's full of saturated fats, which some research has suggested may raise your risk for colorectal cancer.

WOMAN TO WOMAN

She Survived a Bowel Tumor through Early Detection

Professionally, she's a registered nurse working at a cancer-screening center. But Kathy Lee, 45, of Voorhees, New Jersey, had very personal reasons to take action against colon cancer. Here's her story.

When my paternal uncle died of colon cancer in 1994, I had my first colonoscopy, a test that examines the large intestine (colon) with a flexible, lighted tube and a camera. There was nothing suspicious. When my father died 2 years later from complications of a different cancer test, I had another colonoscopy. This one revealed a small, malignant polyp.

By this time, I knew my family had a strong cancer connection: Colon cancer had taken two uncles, an aunt, my paternal grandfather, and my great-uncle. Because of this family history and my relatively young age (almost 42), my surgeon wanted to remove a large section of my colon because my risk of recurrence was high.

So I spent a day taking laxatives and antibiotics to clean out my colon. Then came the operation.

Although the tumor was small (less than ¾ inch) and was caught early, it had invaded the first layer of the colon wall. I found out I have hereditary non-polyposis colorectal cancer (HNPCC). It puts me, my brother, and my sister at high risk for a number of cancers, so I pushed my siblings into cancer screenings. They both had precancerous colon polyps removed.

A few months after the surgery, I started having nightmares—even when my 6-month check for new polyps showed nothing. And I felt guilty for surviving with "just" surgery and no chemotherapy or radiation treatments. Physically, the only symptom I have from my surgery is diarrhea.

Today, I'm just glad to be alive. I spend a lot of time communicating with other cancer survivors and new patients, even sharing my experience on the Web.

I wish more people knew that if colon cancer is detected early, they can beat it. Sure, the whole process of having your colon cleaned out, examined, and operated on is embarrassing, but you can't die of embarrassment.

Lack of exercise. Being overweight raises the danger.

Hormones. There's evidence that postmenopausal women on hormone-replacement therapy enjoy a lowered risk.

Aspirin. This nonsteroidal anti-inflammatory drug (NSAID) may stave off several digestive tract cancers, including colon cancer.

Prevention

Diet, a healthy lifestyle, and screening are the three keys to minimizing your chances of getting colon cancer. "We're increasing our health consciousness about eating less fat and more fiber," observes Ana Maria Lopez, M.D., assistant professor of clinical medicine at the Arizona Cancer Center at the University of Arizona College of Medicine in Tucson. She offers these guidelines for healthy living.

Favor fruits, veggies, and fiber. Get at least five servings of fruits and vegetables daily, plus at least 25 grams of fiber per day from high-fiber foods such as whole-grain breads.

Forgo fat. Limit high-fat foods, especially red meat (try for just one serving per week).

Fortify with folic acid. Most multivitamins contain the 400 micrograms daily that may lower risk of colorectal cancer.

Go easy on the alcohol. Because it may deplete the body's folate supply, women should limit drinks to one a day.

Don't smoke. Cigarettes may promote the cell changes that lead to colon cancer.

Work it out. Just 30 minutes of physical activity (walking, jogging, playing tennis) several days a week helps cut risk.

Get some added protection. Screening tests can detect the polyps, or grapelike growths, that sometimes turn into cancers. "You find the polyps, you take 'em out, you don't get cancer; it's that simple," sums up Dr. Hambrick, a former colorectal surgeon.

"If everybody over 50 got regular screenings, we could cut the colorectal cancer death rate in half," says Dr. Lopez.

The American Cancer Society recommends the following:

Digital rectal exam. The doctor inserts a lubricated, gloved finger into the rectum to feel for irregular or abnormal areas. This is performed before a sigmoidoscopy, colonoscopy, or double-contrast barium enema.

Fecal occult blood test (FOBT). This annual test looks for hidden ("occult") blood in stool samples. You take home a test kit to collect samples from three consecutive bowel movements and return the kit to a lab for evaluation.

Sigmoidoscopy. This is a visual exam inside the rectum and lower colon. With a flexible, lighted tube called a sigmoidoscope, a doctor looks inside the rectum and lower colon for cancer or polyps. New research suggests, though, that this exam misses some cancers. A sigmoidoscopy examines only the lower one-third and left side of the colon; colon cancers show up more often on the right side of the colon. No one is quite sure why.

MY MAMA TOLD ME

Will spicy food and coffee really give me ulcers?

This myth persists because some people do have problems with spicy food and coffee, but those problems aren't ulcers.

We have a muscle called the lower esophageal sphincter that keeps stomach contents from moving back up into the esophagus. Coffee contains caffeine and acid; spicy food has capsaicin, the "hot" element in hot peppers, and all these can relax the sphincter a bit. When that happens, some of your stomach contents back up into the esophagus, and you get the burning sensation in your chest that we call heartburn.

Many people assume that this heartburn feeling is related to ulcers because it mimics the kind of pain that comes from an ulcer in either the stomach or the duodenum (the first part of the small intestine).

So the answer is no to ulcers from spicy food and coffee, but yes to heartburn.

Expert consulted
Kim E. Barrett, Ph.D.
Professor of medicine
University of California, San Diego, School of Medicine

Colonoscopy. The advantage of a colonoscopy over a sigmoidoscopy is that the colonoscopy views the entire colon. After cleaning out the colon beforehand with a special diet and laxatives, you're sedated for this procedure: With a colonoscope (like a sigmoidoscope, but longer), a doctor examines the entire colon via a video camera and display. Polyps can be removed with a wire loop passed through the tube.

Double-contrast barium enema. With this procedure, done in a hospital or clinic, x-rays of the colon are taken after barium sulfate is injected through the rectum. As with a colonoscopy, a prior cleaning out of the bowel is necessary.

WOMEN ASK WHY

Why are they giving me antibiotics instead of antacids for my stomach ulcer?

We know now that antacids treat the symptoms of stomach ulcer but not the cause. The antibiotics we give target a bacterium called *Helicobacter pylori*, or *H. pylori*, which actually causes the sore or wound of an ulcer, with subsequent pain or bleeding. Contrary to what many people still believe, stress doesn't cause ulcers. In 75 to 90 percent of ulcers involving the stomach and, often, the duodenum, or first part of the small intestine, infection from *H. pylori* is the culprit.

We have several tests available, some invasive, some not, to detect the presence of this bacteria; the basics are a blood test and simple breath test. Once you're diagnosed, you take your antibiotics and you're cured.

Men and women acquire *H. pylori* in about equal numbers, but we're unsure exactly how this bacterium is transmitted. There's some association with people in developing countries and in lower socioeconomic groups, so there may be a connection with inadequate hygiene conditions.

Unfortunately, most Americans are unaware of *H. pylori* and retain the belief that stress or poor diet causes stomach ulcers. This is a dangerous misconception because it can prevent people from getting the appropriate treatment. In addition, there's a small risk that a long-standing infection can progress to certain types of gastric cancer.

Expert consulted
Kim E. Barrett, Ph.D.
Professor of medicine
University of California, San Diego, School of
Medicine

➤ A double-contrast barium enema every 5 to 10 years

Follow the "rule of 10." For those with genetic or personal-history risk factors, more frequent screening that begins at a younger age is recommended. "Just as with breast cancer, it's important to look at your family history," advises Nancy E. Kemeny, M.D., attending physician of gastrointestinal oncology service at the Memorial Sloan-Kettering Cancer Center in New York City. If a parent had colon cancer before age 50, you should start screening when you're 10 years younger than that person's age when diagnosed. For example, if your mother had colon cancer at 40, start screening at 30.

Signs and Symptoms

The danger of this cancer is that it can appear silently, over a period of years, with no symptoms. But colorectal cancer can also announce itself in these ways, according Dr. Kemeny.

➤ Rectal bleeding
➤ Blood in the stool
➤ Change in bowel habits: constipation, diarrhea, or trouble having a complete bowel movement
➤ Cramping or stomach pain

Following an initial normal barium enema result, the American Cancer Society recommends that everyone over 50 follow one of three screening options.

➤ A fecal occult blood test every year, plus a sigmoidoscopy every 5 years
➤ A colonoscopy every 10 years

Don't Panic!

While any of colon cancer's symptoms merit prompt medical attention, they don't necessarily signal the disease. Dr. Roth details some other conditions that can mimic the symptoms of this cancer.

Hemorrhoids. These dilated veins and swollen tissue at or near the anus can produce bleeding.

Leaking blood vessel. The technical term is angiodysplasia, and it means a blood vessel in the intestine has become fragile and bleeds.

Parasites. These unwelcome visitors can cause blood in the stool.

Antibiotics. Some of these medications can produce both blood in the stool and rectal bleeding.

Other bowel diseases. Rectal bleeding can also come from ulcerative colitis, which is an inflammation of the colon that causes ulcers, and Crohn's disease, a similar ailment. Diverticulitis, an advanced condition involving small pockets ballooning out from the colon, can also cause rectal bleeding as well as abdominal pain.

Who Do I See?

For two of the basic screening tests, you probably need go no farther than your primary-care physician's office. Both the FOBT and sigmoidoscopy can be performed in a doctor's office. The more revealing colonoscopy and barium enema require a hospital or clinic.

For a colonoscopy, you'll see a gastroenterologist, a doctor with expertise in the stomach and intestines. If a malignancy requiring removal of part of an organ or other body part is found, a surgeon will be called on. At the same time, according to Dr. Kemeny, a consultation with a tumor specialist, or oncologist, may occur.

INFLAMMATORY BOWEL DISEASE

There are bumps along the road in the digestive tracts of some one million Americans, and for the half who are female, the road gets rougher every month. These are the women who have ulcerative colitis and Crohn's disease, known together as inflammatory bowel disease (IBD).

The causes of both diseases are unknown. Short of colon surgery for ulcerative colitis, there's no known cure.

Both bring ulcers, or sores, to the digestive tract. Ulcerative colitis targets just the inner lining of the colon (large intestine) and the rectum, while Crohn's disease can strike anywhere from mouth to anus. The symptoms of both chronic ailments are distressing enough, but our hormone cycles can make things even worse.

"With ulcerative colitis and Crohn's, women can have symptoms other than bloody diarrhea, abdominal pain, constipation, or weight loss," notes Sunanda V. Kane, M.D., assistant professor of medicine at the University of Chicago. The two digestive ills can also make periods irregular, she says, and research indicates that they can also aggravate premenstrual woes.

Another factor is that ibuprofen or other nonsteroidal anti-inflammatory drugs used to ease menstrual aches can worsen IBD inflammation. That's why Dr. Kane looks to alternative means to ease monthly flare-ups.

Instead of steroids, which some doctors recommend but which Dr. Kane calls "the atom bomb" of anti-inflammatories, women's IBD flare-ups may be eased by willow bark, black cohosh, ginseng tea, chamomile tea, primrose oil, and extracts from red clover or yams. (Always check with your physician before taking any herb or supplement, she cautions.)

"There's evidence that these herbs help relax the smooth muscle around the colon, easing cramping and possibly diarrhea, too," relates Dr. Kane.

Prolonged steroid use is a known factor in bone loss, so women treated with steroidal drugs for IBD may be at especially high risk for osteoporosis when menopause brings a decrease in estrogen. Here, calcium supplements can help guard against bone loss; hormone-replacement therapy, as appropriate, may also help back up bones.

What Can I Expect?

If screening tests reveal tumors, the emotional impact can be as serious as the physical. "Women are shocked to find that they have colon cancer," says Nada L. Stotland, M.D., chairperson of psychiatry at the Illinois Masonic Medical Center in Chicago and editor of the book *Psychological Aspects of Women's Healthcare*.

Fear based on ignorance is one of the biggest challenges of the disease. "The colon is kind of 'dirty' and unknown; it's supposed to just do its work and not bother you," Dr. Stotland says. To overcome that fear and ignorance, she urges these steps.

Have an appointment pal. If you get a diagnosis of cancer, request a follow-up visit to which you can bring a friend or family member. "When somebody tells you bad news like this, you don't hear anything else," informs Dr. Stotland. Your companion may be better able to absorb and retain the details.

Put pen to paper. You won't remember all your questions for the doctor, says Dr. Stotland, so write them down beforehand.

Share strength in numbers. Find a cancer support group, urges Dr. Stotland, especially one led by a counseling professional; literature indicates that it makes a positive difference.

TRACT TREK: WHAT'S BEHIND YOUR BELLYACHE

It's tough to suffer through a bout of abdominal pain when you're not sure if last night's chili is to blame. Maybe it's appendicitis? Maybe a gallstone? Use this quick guide to see what may be behind your stomachache, and see a doctor if you suspect any of the following.

Upper-Right Quadrant

- Gallbladder. Gallstones' pain is very sharp after eating, then eases.
- Liver. Dull, crampy pain could be autoimmune hepatitis or other liver ills.
- Duodenum. A burning pain after meals could be a duodenal ulcer.

Between Breasts

- Stomach. Burning, sharp pain that eases with food may be a sign of stomach ulcer.
- Pancreas. Pancreatitis inflammation causes pain, fever, and nausea.

Upper-Left Quadrant

- Nothing gastrointestinal.

Lower-Right Quadrant

- Appendix. Pain in this region is probably appendicitis; in pregnancy after 6 months, appendix moves to upper-right quadrant.
- Cecum. This is the first part of colon; it rarely gets inflamed by itself.

Belly Button

- Ileum. A dull to very sharp pain 1 to 2 hours after eating could be Crohn's disease. Commonly misidentified as the stomach, it's the small intestine.

Conventional Wisdom

On the diagnostic side, "virtual colonoscopy" may make this invasive exam less so. With the aid of computed tomography scanning, in the future, you may not have to have an instrument actually inserted into your colon, notes Dr. Hambrick.

Colon cancer treatment means basically three

Lower-Left Quadrant

❥ Colon. Crampy pain could be diverticulitis. A variety of bowel disorders often bring a change in bowel habits.

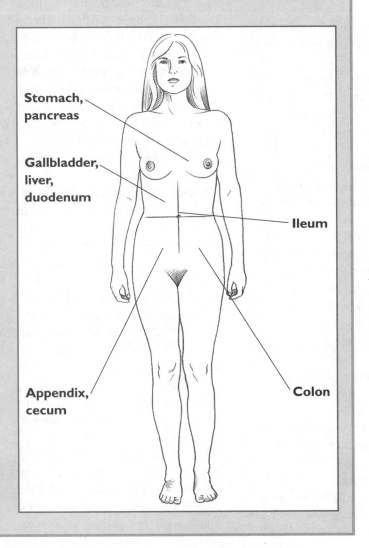

Stomach, pancreas

Gallbladder, liver, duodenum

Ileum

Appendix, cecum

Colon

they're going to get a colostomy, but that's very rare today," says Dr. Kemeny. A colostomy is an opening in the belly for eliminating body waste. Modern colon surgery removes the cancerous tumor, plus normal tissue on either side; the remaining portions of the colon are then reattached.

Often used with surgery, radiation therapy kills cancer cells with high-energy beams. Chemotherapy has traditionally concentrated on a drug called 5-FU (fluorouracil), but new companion drugs are emerging that give us a lot of new, effective options, says Dr. Kemeny.

Great Alternatives

Diet, supplements, and herbs dominate the priority treatment list, according to alternative expert Irene Catania, N.D., a naturopathic physician in Ho-Ho-Kus, New Jersey, who has studied cancer therapies extensively. Emphasizing that her work with cancer patients is considered "adjunctive therapy," that is, designed to work along with traditional approaches, Dr. Catania offers these general strategies.

Make the move to veggies. A diet shift to mostly (if not all) vegetables is Dr. Catania's prime eating advice. Consume fresh produce, grains and legumes, plus six daily glasses of fresh veggie juices.

Go organic. When buying produce, shop for organic varieties, which don't contain pesticides that may aggravate cancer, says Dr. Catania.

Dish up fish. Fish oils and flaxseed oil can help balance cancer-fighting essential fatty

things: surgery, radiation therapy, and chemotherapy. Advances in surgery and drug treatments make the future more hopeful.

"People think that if they have colon cancer,

DIVERT DIVERTICULOSIS WITH BREAKFAST

Skipping breakfast can set a place at your body's "table" for one of the most common colon problems in the country: diverticulosis. In itself, it's relatively harmless, causing almost no symptoms except rectal bleeding. But it can lead to big trouble.

Often, the disease occurs with age. By 80, half of all Americans have it, but it can hit much earlier. If people don't have enough fiber in their diets, or have extra gas or insufficient stool volume, the natural weak spots in the wall of the colon can start to sag, says Sunanda V. Kane, M.D., assistant professor of medicine at the University of Chicago. This leads to "pouching" that from the outside of the colon looks like little mushrooms sprouting, explains Dr. Kane. Over time, the pouches can attract hard-to-digest items, like seeds or corn kernels, and become infected. At that point, diverticulosis becomes diverticulitis, a potentially serious inflammatory disease that can produce an emergency infection.

Our mothers told us that breakfast is the important meal of the day for a reason, affirms Dr. Kane. "When we put food in our stomachs, this signals the colon to evacuate and make room," she says. If a woman has a busy morning routine with little time for much except coffee, this reflex starts to shut down. The result is constipation.

So breakfast is the colon's cue to clear out. But what's in the breakfast is key. "If you develop diverticulosis younger than age 60, you're probably not dispelling gas enough, or not forming solid bowel movements," Dr. Kane says. The answer is more soluble fiber. Her advice:

Go for grains. Eat whole-grain breads and cereals and anything with wheat bran for a total of 25 to 30 grams of fiber daily.

Try the soluble solution. Insoluble fiber (in some over-the-counter "fiber" preparations) can only make things worse if your colon is already irritated. Pick the preparations that contain psyllium, starting with a tablespoon dissolved in 8 ounces of water daily, Dr. Kane advises.

Welcome water. It's nature's laxative, says Dr. Kane. The optimum dosage is eight 8-ounce glasses per day.

acids; aim for a minimum of 3,000 milligrams. Don't take fish oil if you have a bleeding disorder or uncontrolled high blood pressure, if you take anticoagulants (blood thinners) or use aspirin regularly, or if you are allergic to any kind of fish. People with diabetes should not take fish oil because of its high fat content. Fish oil increases bleeding time, possibly resulting in nosebleeds and easy bruising, and may cause upset stomach. Finally, do not substitute with fish-liver oil. It is high in vitamins A and D, which are toxic in large amounts.

Send in the supplements. Studies in Europe suggest that an antioxidant called reduced glutathione helps those on chemo- or radiation therapy cope better with side effects, says Dr. Catania. Reduced glutathione is used in very high doses, so Dr. Catania recommends that you consult with your health practitioner. She also recommends a high-quality multivitamin/mineral supplement.

Popular antioxidants like vitamins E and C and zinc are also on Dr. Catania's list.

Herbal arsenal. To deliver the benefits of different herbs, Dr. Catania often prescribes combinations or sequences of different ones. These include ginkgo, echinacea, astragalus, licorice, larch (from the tree), and maitake and shiitake mushrooms, all of which may help patients strengthen their immune systems.

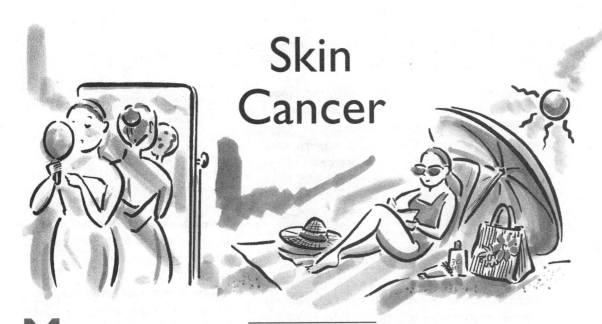

Skin Cancer

Melanoma is the seventh most common cancer among women of all ages, and it scares the dickens out of us.

Why? Because we know how dangerous a melanoma can be. It's the type of skin cancer most likely to spread to other parts of the body. It can be fast, devastating, and deadly. And it's affecting more and more women every year.

We know the major cause of it, and we think that we may know why its incidence is increasing. While sun damage has been clearly linked to melanoma risk, the thinning ozone layer in our atmosphere may be at fault for allowing higher levels of ultraviolet rays to reach people.

Unfortunately, we're not adjusting our lifestyles to counteract the increased number of ultraviolet (UV) rays. "Sunbathing and getting a 'healthy tan' are still very popular," says Mary Knapp, a state climatologist in the weather data library at Kansas State University in Manhattan. "And the use of sunblocks can lull people into a false sense of security, resulting in longer periods of sun exposure." In addition, clothing styles—from below-the-knee dresses to miniskirts and tube tops—continue to let the sun shine in to a dangerous degree. What's more, family vacations to visit highly reflective ski slopes or perpetually sunny seashores may expose our children to more sun at an earlier age than ever before.

But despite all the grim facts, the news about melanoma is actually very good. In its earliest stages, melanoma is one of the easiest cancers to prevent, spot, treat, and cure.

Risk Factors

Want to know your chances of getting melanoma? Take a look in a mirror. If you have blonde or red hair (naturally, that is), green or blue eyes (under those colored contact lenses), and a porcelain complexion sprinkled with freckles, your risk of developing melanoma is anywhere from 10 to 20 times higher than that of someone with dark or black skin.

Looks aside, melanoma, like many other types of cancer, also appears to be related to our genes. That is, if a family member—your sister, your father, or even an aunt or grandparent—has had melanoma, your risk of the disease goes up. Likewise, if you have already had a bout of melanoma,

BASAL CELL CARCINOMA

Melanoma may win the prize for most deadly skin cancer, but basal cell carcinoma is the most common. "It's actually the most common cancer in humans, period," says Tanya Humphreys, M.D., director of cutaneous surgery, laser surgery, and cosmetic dermatology in the department of dermatology at Thomas Jefferson University in Philadelphia. More than 800,000 basal cell carcinomas are diagnosed each year.

Basal cell carcinomas (BCCs) are *not* related to moles. Instead, they show up as pearly, translucent, or occasionally red-colored raised bumps, or nonhealing sores. BCCs typically occur on parts of the body that get intense, episodic sun exposure.

Most people who get basal cell skin cancers are over 40, but younger folks are not immune. Early childhood sun exposure may be responsible for the increase in basal cell carcinomas in young people, says Dr. Humphreys. "I've seen people in their late twenties and teens with this problem." Among those in their twenties and thirties, women seem to be more commonly affected, she says.

Basal cell cancers grow very slowly and rarely spread, but they can penetrate below the skin to the bone and do considerable damage where they lie. Surgery to remove the small tumors may leave little or no visible scarring, especially on the face. Some types of basal cell carcinoma are difficult to remove and may recur.

Prevention

Is melanoma preventable? Yes, it's easy to prevent it: Stay out of the sun.

It's easy, that is, if you live and work in a cave. For the rest of us, who may enjoy spending an occasional day at the park, beach, or mountains, or even puttering in our own gardens, avoiding the sun is a little trickier. Here are some ways to help reduce your melanoma risk when you can't just avoid those rays.

Use sunscreen every day. Even in incredibly sunny climes, sunscreen works. "We can see this quite clearly in Australia," says Karen Burke, M.D., Ph.D., dermatologic surgeon at Cabrini Medical Center in New York City and author of *Great Skin for Life.* "Seventy-four percent of the population regularly uses sunscreen there. And their rates of melanoma are finally leveling off for the first time in decades."

But sunscreen is effective only if you choose it with care and use it properly. According to Dr. Burke, many dermatologists recommend sunscreen that has an SPF of at least 25 and is waterproof and capable of blocking UVA as well as UVB rays. Look for ingredients that physically block the sun, such as titanium dioxide and zinc dioxide. Sunscreens containing these large molecules actually form an invisible barrier on the skin and reflect the sun away.

Apply your sunscreen early, often, and with a heavy hand. Make your first application to all exposed skin at least 15 minutes before you plan to be outdoors. Then, reapply at least every 90 minutes, more often if you're swimming or sweating (okay, perspiring) a great deal, or possibly less often

your chances of battling the beast again are higher than if you'd never had the problem at all.

In addition to pale skin and a family or personal history, other factors put you at increased risk for the cancer as well.

- Poor ability to tan
- A history of sunburns
- The presence of many (more than 50) normal moles
- The presence of unusual-looking moles
- An immune system that has been suppressed by medication or illness
- Excessive recreational or work-related sun exposure

if you're using waterproof products. And be generous.

"When sunscreens are tested in the laboratory for effectiveness, an ample amount is applied per square inch. Most women apply much too thinly to get the amount of protection listed on the label," says Dr. Burke.

Check your skin regularly. Every woman knows about the importance of doing self-exams on her breasts. You can also give your skin a monthly once-over to look for changes in its appearance, particularly changes in moles or blemishes. Here's how, based on guidelines from the American Academy of Dermatology.

- Use a mirror to examine the front and back of your unclothed torso, including your arms and shoulders. Then, raise your arms and look at your right and left sides.
- Bend your elbows and look closely at your palms, forearms, and upper arms. Be sure to check both sides.
- Turn to look at the backs of your legs, then examine your feet, including the soles and the spaces between your toes.
- Use a hand mirror to help check the back of your neck in a wall mirror. Part your hair to examine your scalp.
- Last, use a hand mirror to look at your lower back and buttocks.

Go low-fat. Research shows that eating a low-fat diet may do more than just keep our hearts healthy and our weight steady. It may reduce our risk of skin cancer as well.

SUSPECT MOLES: THE ABCs

Here are some warning signs that a mole or freckle should be seen by a doctor as soon as possible.

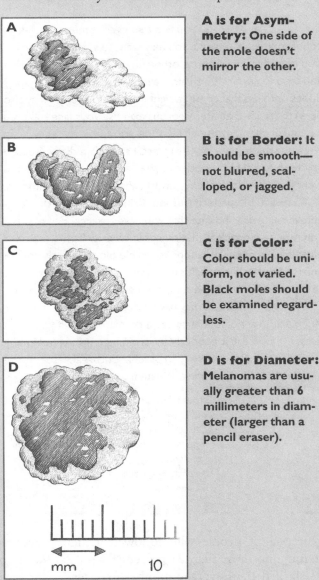

A is for Asymmetry: One side of the mole doesn't mirror the other.

B is for Border: It should be smooth—not blurred, scalloped, or jagged.

C is for Color: Color should be uniform, not varied. Black moles should be examined regardless.

D is for Diameter: Melanomas are usually greater than 6 millimeters in diameter (larger than a pencil eraser).

mm   10

One more thing to watch out for: Some melanomas may be raised, like little hills. Any mole that begins to protrude from the skin should be examined promptly.

WOMEN ASK WHY

Why does drinking alcohol make my nose turn red?

If you find that every time you drink alcohol your nose gets red, you may want to start paying attention to your facial color at other times. You may notice that you tend to flush or blush after eating certain foods, like spicy dishes or things that come straight from the oven. You may also begin to realize that after vigorous exercise your face stays red far longer than anyone else's. One good way to really keep track of what's going on is to start a symptom diary: Record any flushing that you notice as well as when it happens and what you were doing, eating, or drinking just before it came on.

A predictable pattern of food, drink, or activity that triggers flushing may indicate that you have rosacea. Rosacea is a common skin problem that ranges in severity from persistent blushing and acnelike bumps to visible blood vessels and an enlarged nose. The condition happens much more frequently to women than men and can progress rapidly if not treated.

If you think that you may have rosacea, do yourself a favor and make an appointment to see a dermatologist. If you catch it early and treat it properly by avoiding triggers (including sunlight, a major cause of rosacea outbreaks for some people), you can keep the problem from getting worse.

Expert consulted
Lynn Drake, M.D.
Editor of Rosacea Review
Professor and chairperson of the department
of dermatology
University of Oklahoma
Oklahoma City

Baylor College of Medicine in Houston.

Following a low-fat diet in order to thwart your chances of developing skin cancer makes sense, says Shari Lieberman, Ph.D., a clinical nutritionist in New York City and coauthor of *The Real Vitamin and Mineral Book.* "After all, a low-fat diet has been shown to be protective against many other kinds of cancer," she says. "Why shouldn't it work for skin cancer, too?"

Signs and Symptoms

Malignant melanoma starts out as uncontrolled growth of pigment-making skin cells. The growth builds up to form dark-colored moles or tumors. They can appear on their own, on previously unmarked skin, but they can also, and often do, develop from or near an existing, formerly normal mole. This ability for healthy moles to become malignant is why learning the location and status of your normal moles through self-exam is so very important.

Any unusual change in your skin's condition should get your attention. New moles that appear on adult women are especially suspicious. That's because we've already developed most of the moles that we'll ever have by the time we reach adulthood. Be aware of any mole that begins to itch, bleed, ooze, or cause pain. Changes in size or shape should also alert you—moles shouldn't grow, and their edges should be smooth, not jagged. Research shows that color is particularly crucial in spotting melanomas. Be concerned about moles that are

Thirty-eight people who followed a diet containing no more than 21 percent fat for 2 years slashed their average number of a certain type of precancerous skin lesion by as much as two-thirds when compared to people who ate a diet with no less than 36 percent of calories from fat, according to research at

unevenly colored, with varied shades of brown and black. And if a mole suddenly turns color, especially to black, have your dermatologist check it immediately.

Don't Panic!

If you notice a new mole, don't automatically assume that it's a melanoma. The vast majority of moles are not dangerous, says Mary Gail Mercurio, M.D., assistant professor of dermatology at the University of Rochester in New York.

Even if you find a mole that has changed shape or has taken on a new hue, there's no need for immediate alarm (though a doctor's exam *is* in order). While the presence of abnormal moles, which are called dysplastic nevi, does mean that you may be at an increased risk for melanoma, they don't all turn out to be cancerous. And, depending on your doctor's opinion, they may not even need to be removed.

Pregnancy can also make otherwise harmless moles darken. "That's not necessarily a bad sign," says Tanya Humphreys, M.D., director of cutaneous surgery, laser surgery, and cosmetic dermatology in the department of dermatology at Thomas Jefferson University in Philadelphia. "Estrogen can increase pigmentation." If you happen to notice a changing mole during pregnancy, bring it to a dermatologist's attention so that you can be monitored. But don't let it worry you unnecessarily.

Who Do I See?

Your own general practitioner or family doctor can certainly give you a routine screening for unusual spots or bumps during your yearly

---

SQUAMOUS CELL CARCINOMA

Squamous cell carcinoma is the second most common nonmelanoma cancer of the skin. This threat is also sun-exposure-related, but rather than the one-time toasting that can cause melanoma, chronic long-term sunning seems to be the problem, says Tanya Humphreys, M.D., director of cutaneous surgery, laser surgery, and cosmetic dermatology in the department of dermatology at Thomas Jefferson University in Philadelphia. The cause is day-after-day unprotected exposure, such as farmers, mail carriers, gardeners, golfers, or runners get.

Squamous cell carcinomas often appear as raised red nodules or bumps or as red crusty or scaly patches. They often arise from precancerous lesions called actinic keratoses, which are extremely common, especially as we age.

Unlike melanoma, the chance that a squamous cell cancer will spread is small. But lesions on the relatively thin tissues of the lips or ears should be examined and removed promptly just to make sure that the cancer cells don't have the opportunity to travel.

---

physical—be sure to ask if you'd like her to do so. But if you notice a new mole or a mole that's changing, you really should seek out a dermatologist, a medical doctor who specializes in the care and treatment of skin problems. "The key is in the diagnosis," says Lynn Drake, M.D., professor and chairperson of the department of dermatology at the University of Oklahoma in Oklahoma City. "Many doctors do things very well. But if you had a heart problem, you'd want a heart specialist. Likewise, with a questionable skin condition, it's best to see a skin specialist."

And don't delay. If there is a problem, early treatment is best for any skin cancer. And if it turns out that nothing is wrong after all, you will have saved yourself a lot of drawn-out worrying.

If you are diagnosed with a superficial melanoma, your dermatologist may be able to take it

MY MAMA TOLD ME

Will touching a toad really give me warts?

Quite simply, the answer is no. Touching a toad—or a frog, for that matter—may give you the willies, but never warts.

This old wives' tale probably got started because toads have warty-looking skin. Scientifically, however, the bumps you see on a toad's body are actually glands. If a toad feels threatened or in danger, these externally visible glands produce toxins that help the toad escape predators in ingenious ways. For example, if your dog picked up a toad in her mouth, the nasty-tasting toxins she'd taste would make her drool in response and drop the toad in the process.

We know that warts are produced by a specific type of virus that affects humans, and there's absolutely nothing like that located on a toad's bumpy skin.

Expert consulted
Lynnette Sievert, Ph.D.
Associate professor in the division of biological sciences
Emporia State University
Emporia, Kansas

from there by removing the lesion herself. "Dermatologists are also wonderful surgeons," says Dr. Drake. But if the melanoma is deep, a medical-team approach might be warranted. In this case, your dermatologist may choose to partner with a surgical oncologist or other specialists who can give you the best treatment possible.

What Can I Expect?

After surgery to remove a mole, you may wind up with a visible scar. But the mark that removal leaves won't necessarily be as big as you are imagining right now. "The earlier you have something removed—that is, the smaller the mole is when it's taken out—the less severe your scar will be," says Dr. Drake.

After you have been diagnosed, have been treated, and have even physically healed, you may still feel the effects of melanoma somewhere else—in your mind. Suddenly, every freckle will seem fearsome. It's natural to react this way to a brush with what is, after all, a dangerous form of cancer. "Everyone who's had a cancer of any kind becomes a little more vigilant. It's a very scary experience," says Dr. Drake.

But it helps to realize that with melanoma, we really are lucky. With regular self-exams, we can catch it early. And with prompt treatment, the majority of women with melanoma will be able to get on with their lives—sunscreen bottle in hand.

Conventional Wisdom

The most important treatment for any new or changing mole is to have it examined right away. Many dermatologists will use a specialized microscope to look closely at the mole and the surrounding skin. But in most cases, your doctor's trained eye is all that's needed to decide on the steps to take. "If a mole or other spot looks abnormal to my naked eye, I would proceed with a biopsy," says Dr. Mercurio.

Small questionable moles may be completely removed during the biopsy, and your doctor can perform this minor surgery right in her office. But if a mole is large or in an area where scarring is a concern, such as the face, she may decide to take a modest sample of skin to test before going further. All biopsied material is then sent to a pathologist, a doctor trained in detecting disease in the body's tissues, for thorough testing.

If test results show melanoma and the entire mole was already removed at biopsy, you may have no further treatment to deal with. Superficial, or shallow, melanomas have the best chance of being dealt with this way. "Removal is the key with melanoma," says Dr. Mercurio. "Often, the surgery can cure the problem as simply as that."

Otherwise, surgery to remove the entire melanoma and a "safety margin" of surrounding skin will be in order. If your melanoma was elevated or had vertical growth extending into the underlying flesh, your doctor will want to carefully examine the rest of your body, especially your lymph nodes, to be sure that the cancer hasn't spread beyond your skin.

Chemotherapy drugs that are commonly used in treating other types of cancer aren't usually useful against melanoma. But therapy using a special protein called interferon has been successfully used to help some people with cases of melanoma that have spread.

Great Alternatives

When it comes to treating an existing melanoma, conventional Western medicine remains the proven best approach. But there are new and interesting tactics developing on the front lines that may become standard treatment in the future.

WOMAN TO WOMAN

She Discovered Her Own Skin Cancer

At 36, Catherine Poole, a Glenmoore, Pennsylvania, health writer, noticed a birthmark on her leg that suddenly looked different and unusual. Because she did something about it, she's alive today to tell her story.

In January 1989, I had a miserable flu. I was caring for my 2-year-old daughter, an editorial deadline was looming, *and* I was 5 months pregnant. But with all that, I guess you could still say that I was lucky.

Had I not been resting on the couch, I wouldn't have noticed the strange mark on the back of my calf. What had once been just a small birthmark now was bigger, black, and irregular in shape.

Because of its odd shape, I rushed to the dermatologist. A biopsy confirmed that I had a risky vertical-growth melanoma. Instead of spreading over the skin's surface, the cancer was burrowing deeper into the tissue. I had an 80 percent chance of living 8 years.

I was gripped with fear. Would I lose my baby? Would my kids lose their mom?

Doctors removed the cancer surgically and patched the area with a skin graft from my hip. It was a grueling and painful ordeal. I hobbled on crutches for the rest of my pregnancy. But I didn't care. They could take my whole leg as long as my kids had a mom.

After the surgery and the birth of my healthy son, I busied myself with research and realized that I'm in the high-risk category for this type of cancer.

I now consider myself a skin-cancer-prevention advocate. I'll tell complete strangers to have suspicious-looking moles checked. My doctor and I wrote a book called *Melanoma: Prevention, Detection, and Treatment* to help others recognize melanoma. And I helped establish the Foundation for Melanoma Research in Philadelphia to provide funding for research.

Needless to say, the experience changed my attitude toward the sun. Now, I always use sunscreen on myself and my family. And I get my skin checked regularly by my doctor.

REAL-LIFE SCENARIO

She Thinks That Using Sunscreen Is More Dangerous Than Tanning

When Cindy goes to the beach, she goes prepared to protect her ivory-white skin. She wears a broad-brimmed hat, a terry-cloth robe, and wraparound sunglasses. She also takes a beach umbrella. And she never leaves the house without slathering on sunscreen with an SPF of 20. Or at least she didn't until recently, when Cindy heard a news story claiming that sunscreen does more harm than good—that using it may actually promote cancer. Now she's confused. She loves the beach, but if she can't venture out from under her umbrella feeling secure that her skin is protected, she feels she may as well stay home. Should she?

If there's one thing Cindy *should* do, it's continue to use sunscreen. The controversy over whether or not sunscreens can actually increase the risk of skin cancer came about because of a presentation of misunderstood data that happened to catch the public eye. That said, there are a few reasons why it might be tempting to mistakenly think that sunscreen use leads to skin cancer, even though it probably does not.

For starters, people who use sunscreen the most religiously, usually very fair-skinned people who know that they burn easily, are also the ones genetically most likely to develop skin cancer in the first place. Next, once someone puts on sunscreen, she may tend to feel safe in the sun and stay out longer than she should. Finally, when people do use sunscreen, not many use it correctly.

Cindy is right to wear a hat and use an umbrella—these are great ways to protect herself from the sun whenever she's outdoors. But she would be even better off going one step further by using, every day, sunscreen with an SPF of 25 that protects against both UVA and UVB rays.

Expert consulted
Karen Burke, M.D., Ph.D.
Dermatologic surgeon
Cabrini Medical Center
New York City
Author of Great Skin for Life

Keep an eye on the vaccine. New melanoma vaccines appear to have lifesaving potential. Custom-made for each patient from a sample of her own skin cancer cells, the vaccine augments her own immune system's ability to fight the cancer. Ongoing trials are only examining use in very advanced melanoma. And although the vaccine looks very promising, says Dr. Humphreys, there's still a long way to go.

Ask your doctor about B_6. A certain vitamin may also play a role in treating skin cancer. According to Dr. Lieberman, vitamin B_6 shows promise in inhibiting the growth of malignant melanoma cells. There are many other benefits for women who get enough of this B vitamin, including anemia prevention, better immune function, and possibly reduced PMS symptoms.

While the Daily Value for vitamin B_6 is only 2 milligrams, even that small amount is difficult to garner from food sources alone, says Dr. Lieberman. Some cancer specialists suggest that those at risk for melanoma as well as those being treated for or who have had melanoma in the past take 100 to 300 milligrams of vitamin B_6 a day. This amount of B_6 should be taken along with a complete B-complex since B vitamins work synergistically, Dr. Lieberman adds.

But don't take this dosage without your doctor's approval. Excess vitamin B_6 can cause pain, numbness, and weakness in the limbs.

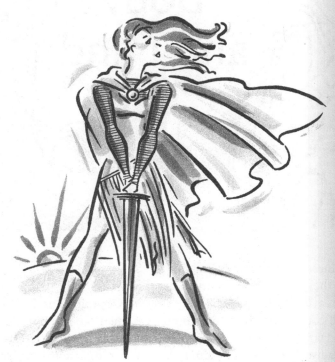

PART SIX

Recovery from Illness

Nurture Your Body and Mind

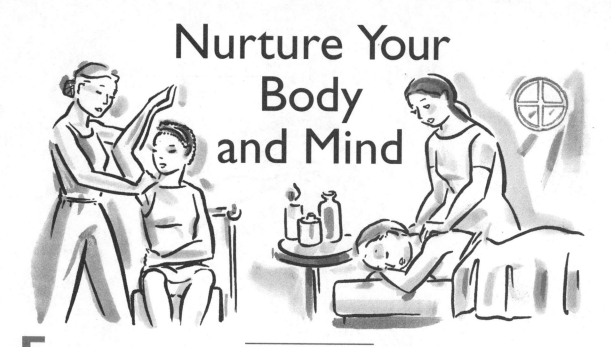

Fighting off an illness is difficult, exhausting work. And when the job is done, your body needs to rest and recover. It needs a vacation, so to speak. So if you could take your body anywhere, where would you go?

To a tropical paradise, lying under a palm tree and drinking chilled coconut milk from the husk, as aquamarine water laps quietly at the sand around your feet? To a mountain retreat in the deep stillness of the woods, where the only sounds are the chirping of birds and the occasional rustling of leaves as squirrels play among the branches? Or maybe to a spa, where the most taxing thing that happens all day is an hour-long massage followed by a visit to the sauna and Jacuzzi?

Makes you feel better just thinking about it.

And that's the point. You don't need an island or a mountain or a spa. You can help your body recover after an illness through the medium of your mind, using techniques like meditation, guided visualization, or yoga. They're all part of complementary medicine, a branch of healing that often uses the mind-body approach to assist in the healing done by conventional medicine.

Good Complements

"Complementary medicine is a place where women can reconnect and reclaim their bodies. It really empowers a woman to reawaken her ability to care for herself," says Cynthia Knorr-Mulder, a licensed nurse practitioner and manager of the complementary medicine program at the Center for Health and Healing at Hackensack University Medical Center in New Jersey.

Here's a sampling of the many complementary therapies that can help you reclaim your body after a serious illness or accident.

Sit calmly. Meditation can help you reclaim your body and possibly speed healing after an illness or injury, Knorr-Mulder says. "Meditation relieves stress and decreases blood pressure, heart rate, and your perception of acute pain, while it increases your perception of health. Cumulatively, all of those things put you in a better position for healing," she adds.

Meditation has been shown to reduce high blood pressure, headaches, and chronic pain. In addition, studies have shown that it boosts the immune system. Some practitioners, such as Knorr-Mulder, also use it to help women cope with cancer and heart disease.

You can try a simple meditation technique yourself. Find a quiet spot and sit in a comfortable position. Take a few slow, deep breaths. As you breathe out, ask yourself, "Who am I?" Notice the associations that sprout in your mind: "I'm a wife," "I'm a mother," "I'm angry." Allow these thoughts to flow through your consciousness—enter and exit your brain—without judging them. If you find yourself thinking, "I'm a cancer survivor" and begin worrying about a recurrence or ways that the disease has affected your family, let those thoughts go and refocus your mind on the fundamental question, "Who am I?"

Try to practice this meditation twice daily for 15 to 20 minutes each session.

See yourself healthy. Your imagination can help you reclaim your body even after a major trauma, says Barbara Dossey, R.N., director of Holistic Nursing Consultants in Santa Fe, New Mexico, and author of *Florence Nightingale: Mystic, Visionary Healer*.

Imagery is the language that your mind uses to communicate with your body. Each day, thousands of thoughts, images, and sensations flit through your brain. At least half of these thoughts are negative even when you're healthy. If you've had a serious accident or illness, these negative thoughts may alter your

WOMAN TO WOMAN

She Used Physical Therapy to Recuperate after Her Cancer

An experienced oncology nurse, Marcy Fish, 43, of Wyncote, Pennsylvania, had spent much of her career caring for women with breast cancer. After she was diagnosed in 1998 with ductal carcinoma in situ (an early, noninvasive form of cancer) in her left breast, she had a mastectomy and breast reconstructive surgery. Her recovery from the surgeries went smoothly except for some range-of-motion problems in her left shoulder. Concerned, she consulted complementary-care specialists at Fox Chase Cancer Center in Philadelphia. Here's her story.

During reconstructive surgery, the plastic surgeon removes fat and muscle from the abdomen and uses it to form the new breast. So after the surgery, my breast area and underarm region had things attached where things didn't used to be attached. Plus, scar tissue formed from my lower abdomen all the way up to my left underarm. I received 2 months of physical therapy at the Complementary Care Center at Fox Chase, and they got me back to full range of motion. They were able to teach me stretches that would give me maximum benefit without any harm. A lot of it was a matter of regaining confidence in my body. I wanted to get on with my life, but I didn't want to hurt myself doing it.

After I finished physical therapy, I began taking dance classes that the center was offering to its patients. It is a way of continuing the exercises necessary to maintain your muscles' full range of motion but in a nonthreatening, noncompetitive way. We're not out there dancing to *Twist and Shout*. These dances are actually just very gentle movements set to music and specifically geared for people who have just undergone surgery.

I think physical therapy and dance have helped in a couple of ways. It's accomplishment without competition. I'm able to say, "Hey, I did that today." And there is the camaraderie that comes from people who are in the same situation. It's almost like a support group of sorts because all the women in the room know that all the others have been through a similar situation.

physiology, complicate your recovery, and possibly make you more susceptible to ongoing physical problems, such as arthritis or urinary tract infections.

On the other hand, if you harness positive images in your mind, you can help your body heal itself. In essence, your brain and body react to an imagined sensation as if it were a real one.

Here's how you might use guided imagery to help you reclaim your body after a heart attack, says Dossey. Set aside 20 minutes several times a day to practice. Resting in a comfortable position, take several deep breaths. Imagine that somewhere deep inside of you a brilliant light begins to shine. Allow the light to grow brighter and more intense. The light is powerful and penetrating. Notice that a beam begins to grow out of it. This beam shines into your body as you prepare to nurture your heart. Travel on this beam of light to your heart and just watch it for a few moments. As you observe your heart, clearly see all of its structures interacting in a coordinated, rhythmic dance. Listen to your heart beat. Hear it going stronger and stronger.

Next, imagine running your hands along the muscular walls of your heart, feeling the strength in them. If you've had a heart attack, spend some time observing the area of scar tissue. Notice how smooth and strong the scar is. See the new collateral blood vessels starting to form. Watch as these vessels bring blood, proteins, oxygen, and other substances to the healed area.

Spend a few moments seeing how you will look when your heart is completely healed. Imagine looking at yourself in a mirror. See yourself as strong, straight, and healthy. Visu-

REAL-LIFE SCENARIO

She's Afraid to Exercise Now That She Has Had a Silent Heart Attack

At 52, Fran was feeling great. She had her own small house-cleaning business, she was taking an aerobics class at night, and she had planned a cross-country trip with her husband. In fact, the only time she could remember being ill over the past year was on Super Bowl Sunday, when she had felt a little light-headed and had an upset stomach. During a routine physical, her family doctor told her that her blood pressure was too high and her heartbeat sounded a little irregular. He gave her an electrocardiogram. The result floored her. Apparently, she'd had a silent heart attack at some point and hadn't even realized it. The information so frightened her that her entire life went on hold. She quit her job, figuring it was too strenuous. She decided to postpone her trip because she didn't want to be on the road if an emergency occurred. And she decided to give up exercising altogether. Now, she does little more than sit at home, worry, and scan the Internet for information about cardiovascular disease. Does her life have to change so drastically?

Women tend to become depressed, withdrawn, and sedentary after heart attacks. In fact, after heart attacks, more women than men do not return to pre—heart attack levels of activity, particularly sexual activity, be-

alize yourself playing with friends or your family. Feel the strength returning to your lungs and your legs. Picture yourself being able to walk as far as you want, breathing easily and feeling robust.

When you have finished this guided imagery, take a few slow breaths as you regain awareness of your surroundings. Know that you are doing your best to help your body heal.

Yoga your way, I'll go mine. Yoga, a system of precise posture and breathing, can reduce levels of stress, relieve pain, promote wound healing, and improve your stamina and sense of well-being, whether you have a chronic illness, such as diabetes, or you're recovering from an

cause they are afraid of triggering additional cardiovascular events. So Fran's reaction is quite typical.

But no, she doesn't need to alter her lifestyle to such a great extent. She should ask her doctor for further testing such as a stress echocardiogram, an ultrasonic record of heart activity, in order to determine how well her cardiovascular system is working. Then, after being thoroughly evaluated by her cardiologist and receiving his approval, she should immediately enroll in a supervised cardiac-rehabilitation program. She should be encouraged to exercise and lead a normal life. With proper care, she should be able to lead a completely active life. In fact, Fran might have a better life than she led before because a heart attack, rather than limiting your life, often can serve as a wake-up call to make choices, such as dietary changes, that can enhance your whole being.

Expert consulted
Marianne Legato, M.D.
Founder and director
Partnership for Women's Health
Columbia University College of Physicians and
  Surgeons
New York City

acute condition, such as a heart attack, says Cynthia Geesey, a Kripalu yoga instructor at the complementary medicine program of Fox Chase Cancer Center in Philadelphia.

Practitioners believe that moving your body into different poses forces blood out of vital organs, allowing fresh blood to take its place. This not only cleanses your organs but also provides more nutrients, making your organs stronger and more resistant to disease.

This ancient Indian practice has been used successfully in many cardiac-rehabilitation and cancer-treatment programs. "It's a gentle, compassionate modality that is able to work with the limits of your body at a given point in time. So if you have heart disease or have just undergone quadruple-bypass surgery, you can still do yoga," Geesey says.

And you can do it without twisting yourself into a pretzel, she says. To try it, stand as straight as possible with your back against a wall and your feet shoulder-width apart. Let your arms dangle at your sides. Inhale for a slow count of 10. As you do this, slowly raise your arms out to your sides and over your head. Then, exhale—again for a slow count of 10—and lower your arms back to your sides. Do this for 2 to 3 minutes twice daily.

There are many types of yoga, and it may take you some time to find a form that you feel comfortable doing. Phone around and talk to a number of instructors before committing to any classes, Geesey suggests. Talk to your doctor before starting a yoga program, and be up-front with instructors about any medical conditions.

Stretch your limits. Though they're often overlooked, occupational and physical therapies are potent allies that can help you reclaim your body when you have—or have had—cancer or heart disease, says Karen Mohr, a physical therapist and research director at the Kerlan-Jobe Orthopaedic Clinic in Los Angeles. If you feel fatigued as a result of your disease or treatment for your disease, a physical or occupational therapist can teach you energy-conservation techniques that will help you do household chores or other activities. If you have had extensive surgery that has left you with limited motion in your joints, weak muscles, or decreased endurance, a physical therapist can help you improve your range of motion and increase your strength and endurance. If you suspect that

THERAPEUTIC MASSAGE

Therapeutic massage is a terrific addition and complement to regular medical care that offers many benefits. It has been known to improve circulation and lymph flow, increase relaxation, and decrease stress and tension, says Caron M. Hunter, a licensed massage therapist and associate director of integrative pain medicine at ProHealth Care Associates in Lake Success, New York. Massage, when done by a medical professional, may help to promote recovery from the muscle fatigue and soreness that can result from exercise.

Many physicians now recommend using it on patients with acute or chronic pain because massage helps rid the muscles of lactic acid, a substance that can lead to body aches. Massage may also be used as a modality in heart disease because it reduces stress that can cause the blood vessels to narrow and the heart to work faster. If you are recovering from one of these diseases, however, you should discuss this option with your physician before receiving therapeutic massage. Other medical conditions, such as asthma, arthritis, sports injuries, gastrointestinal disorders, and muscle spasms, can be helped by frequent massage therapy.

You might wonder how getting a back rub is different from undergoing therapeutic massage. Many states have strict criteria and education requirements for training as a massage therapist. Massage therapists who graduate from accredited schools are medical professionals, and in many states they sit for licensing exams. They are trained in all aspects of the physical anatomy and have a deep understanding of appropriate application and proper technique for a variety of medical conditions. So while a back rub from a friend may be soothing and feel good, a treatment from a licensed professional will incorporate educated and proficient massage that not only soothes but also heals.

If you would like to find a reputable massage therapist in your area, write to the American Massage Therapy Association, 820 Davis Street, Suite 100, Evanston, IL 60201-4464.

you might benefit from either of these therapies, discuss them with your doctor.

Note: Your state or insurer may or may not require a referral from a doctor for you to see a physical or occupational therapist.

Feed Your Recovery

Making dietary changes is one of the most important things that you can do to reclaim your body after heart problems or cancer, says Nicole Napolitano, R.D., a certified dietitian-nutritionist and senior nutrition consultant at ProHealth Care Associates in Lake Success, New York. Here are some ways that you can use diet to help you regain your health.

Skip the fat. Of the eight controllable risk factors for heart disease, including elevated cholesterol and excessive weight, five have been linked to high-fat eating. Dietary fat may also have a role in 60 percent of cancers that affect women. Unfortunately, a typical American woman eats enough fat each week to equal six sticks of butter.

To keep your body healthy after you recover, start by limiting your fat consumption to no more than 25 percent of your total caloric intake, says Napolitano. The easiest way to control fat consumption is to count grams because that's how fats are measured on nutrition labels. So if you eat 1,500 calories a day, for instance, and want to keep your fat intake below 25 percent, multiply

1,500 by 25 percent. That's 375 calories. Then, divide that by 9, which is the number of fat calories in 1 gram of fat. Rounding off, you get 42, the number of grams—from all the foods that you eat in one day—that you can allocate for fat.

In particular, eat no more than 10 grams of saturated fat—usually found in red meats and other animal products—or products like mayonnaise and margarine that contain hydrogenated oils, says Napolitano. These fats increase the amount of the bad low-density lipoprotein (LDL) cholesterol and triglycerides in your arteries. One way to ensure that you stay on track is to eat no more than one palm-size, 3-ounce serving of lean animal protein daily. Experiment with miso, tofu, and other soy products. These alternatives are terrific substitutes for meat in your diet, and they contain substances that may lower your risk of recurrent cancer or heart disease.

Give three cheers for the superfoods. Eat at least eight servings of fruits and vegetables daily, Napolitano urges. Keep in mind that a serving can be as simple as eight baby carrots, ½ cup of cooked vegetables, or half of a banana. Make sure that your mix includes spinach, chard, romaine lettuce, and other green leafy vegetables. These foods provide plenty of folate and beta-carotene, which are loaded with an-tioxidants that help fend off recurrences of heart disease and cancer.

Fruits and vegetables are also a source of fiber, which may help speed foods through your body so that fewer carcinogens can be absorbed by your digestive tract. In addition, dietary fiber may help lower blood cholesterol.

In general, you should eat four bites of fruits, vegetables, and whole grains for every bite of meat you take, says Napolitano.

Pitch a safety net. Supplements such as vitamins C and E and beta-carotene can promote recovery and reduce your risk of recurrence of heart disease or cancer, Napolitano says. These antioxidants prevent the formation of free radicals, rogue cells that can damage arteries and promote dangerous cellular mutations. Take 250 to 500 milligrams of vitamin C, 100 to 400 IU of vitamin E, and up to 6 milligrams of beta-carotene daily.

Go nuts. Some varieties of nuts and seeds are excellent sources of vitamin E, Napolitano says. They also contain the heart-healthy, good kind of fat, monounsaturated fat. But keep in mind that they are chock-full of calories and should be used sparingly. Try adding a tablespoon of sunflower seeds to a salad or six almonds to a scoop of nonfat frozen yogurt.

Draw On Your Inner Strength

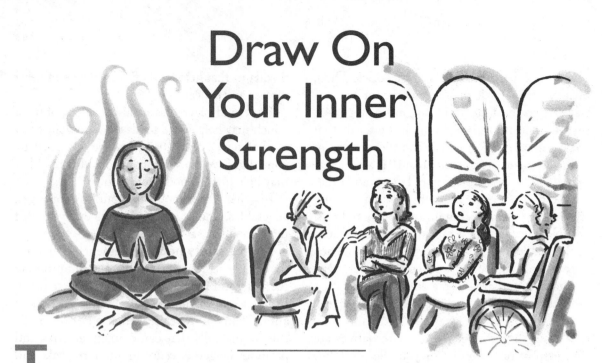

The medications are gone. The treatments are finished. The illness is cured. And life continues. Except that living will never be quite the same now because you'll always know that catastrophe can strike again at any time, any place. You feel fragile, uneasy, and vulnerable. Surviving doesn't feel like a victory.

"Survivorship just means that you're alive. You're breathing," says Wendy S. Harpham, M.D., author of *After Cancer*. "It tells you nothing about the quality of your life or how you've integrated the disease experience into your outlook on life. People rid of their disease but paralyzed by untamed fear and anxiety or trapped by an inability to accept the loss of a body part or function are not healthy survivors."

Healthy survivorship after cancer, stroke, heart disease, and virtually every other catastrophic illness or injury depends as much on your mind-set, on your attitude, as it does on your medical care, Dr. Harpham says. And she should know. She has survived seven recurrences of non-Hodgkin's lymphoma in a decade.

Regaining a Healthy Mind-set

Certainly, there are limits to what your mind can do for you. All the positive thinking in the world probably won't prevent a recurrence of cancer or another heart attack if your body harbors health-threatening changes. But the mind is a good place to start your quest for healthy survivorship, Dr. Harpham says. Because if you believe that you can make a difference, you're more likely to get the best medical treatments available, eat well, get regular exercise, and do other health-promoting activities. At the same time, regaining your mental vibrancy will help to quiet worries, douse fears and anxiety, and resist denial, all of which can prevent you from living a rewarding life.

"How do people become healthy survivors? By obtaining sound knowledge, finding and nourishing realistic hope, and acting effectively," Dr. Harpham says. Here are a few ways that you can tweak your mental outlook and become a healthy survivor.

Make knowledge your best friend. Healthy survivors realize that ignorance is not bliss, Dr. Harpham says. Learning all you can about your disease and its consequences may initially add to your anxiety. In the long term, however, basic medical knowledge tames fears and helps people regain a sense of control over their world. So gather all the information you can about your illness (or have a friend or family member do it if you can't for some reason). It will lessen your fears and at the same time allow you to recognize problems early, when they are most treatable.

Return to sender. Write a letter expressing how you feel about what has happened to you, suggests Anne Coscarelli, Ph.D., a psychologist and director of the Rhonda Fleming Mann Resource Center for Women with Cancer at UCLA Jonsson Cancer Center in Los Angeles. It can be cathartic. "Writing a letter gives you the freedom to express whatever it is you feel. And expressing those feelings—whether of anger or anxiety—helps you grieve, let go, and move forward," Dr. Coscarelli says. "You can write whatever you want as long as it embodies what you feel. Expressing yourself is an important part of the process."

Keep up the correspondence. Once you've completed that first letter, take out another sheet of paper or open a new file on your computer. Write a new letter to yourself that embraces who you are now. Don't be afraid to express love for yourself and to reaffirm that you're still the same wonderful person that you've always been. Write these letters to

MY MAMA TOLD ME
If I cross my eyes, can they really get stuck?

Of course not. Muscles surrounding your eyes allow you to move them in toward your nose to the crossed position. But they certainly won't get stuck there any more than bending at the elbow will cause your arm to get stuck in one position.

Normally, eye movement is coordinated so that both eyes look at a person or object at the same time. Eyes that cross involuntarily occur when this ability is disrupted for some reason. In most cases, crossed eyes result in double vision and should be immediately brought to your doctor's attention. In adults, crossed eyes can be triggered by diabetes, high blood pressure, brain injury, stroke, thyroid disease, or myasthenia gravis or other disorders of the muscles or nerves surrounding the eyes. Special glasses or surgery may be required to correct this problem in adults.

Infants under 3 months old may occasionally cross their eyes, and it is no cause for alarm because they are still learning how to coordinate their eye movements. But if it persists—and it is very important to be watchful for crossed eyes or lazy eye among young children—the lazy eye can weaken and lead to impaired vision.

The real myth is that a child with crossed eyes will outgrow it. This is a dangerous misconception. If a child is treated from ages 7 to 9, crossed eyes can usually be corrected without lingering problems. After that age, vision impairment becomes permanent. The earlier the detection of a possible disorder, the better.

Expert consulted
Sheri Rowen, M.D.
Assistant clinical professor of ophthalmology
University of Maryland School of Medicine
Baltimore

yourself as often as needed. You don't need to show them to anyone. If you wish, you can throw them away after each session or keep them as a reminder of your journey.

Bust a gut. Hilarity—sidesplitting laughter—can help you cope with your anxieties and fears during a major illness, Dr. Coscarelli says. It allows you to look at scary situations, such as checkups, in funny or sarcastic ways. Humor also is a distraction from the loss and suffering.

"Humor is life-affirming and life-giving," Dr. Coscarelli says. "When you laugh, you breathe deeply. So the harder you laugh, the more deeply you breathe, and the more you will relax."

Rejoice! Celebrate each year of survival as you would any important anniversary, Dr. Coscarelli suggests. It will help turn negative memories into positive ones.

"Make a point of letting others know that you're a survivor. Celebrate what you've accomplished in the past year and what you intend to do in the upcoming 365 days," she adds. Host a party, plan an adventurous trip, or simply invite a few friends over to share how wonderful it is to be alive. Your appreciation for life may teach others about living.

"Having people around you for these moments can be very helpful. It will allow you to talk about what you've gone through, acknowledge any sadness you may feel, and share a sense of pride in having survived. All of those things can be very comforting after a serious illness," Dr. Coscarelli says.

Cling to others. Many women participate in survivor groups after their disease, Dr. Coscarelli says.

"Once treatment stops, for any disease, you can suddenly feel alone in the big, scary world. There is a sense of isolation, of being detached. So who understands and can share the feelings

REAL-LIFE SCENARIO

She Became a Real Hypochondriac after Having a Mole Removed

Jeanine, 41, never thought much about her freckles. As far as she could remember, she'd always had them. Then, something happened. After a sunburn one summer, a dark brown freckle on top of her foot became very black and looked almost perfectly round, almost like a burnt match head. She paid it no mind until she heard a dermatologist talking about black moles and melanomas on a television talk show. That pricked her attention. She immediately made an appointment to see a doctor and, within a few days, had the mole removed for tests. She almost went crazy with anxiety waiting for the results. Fortunately, the tests were negative. But the doctor told her that the mole was a "precancerous, dysplastic nevus" and that she would have to keep an eye on her moles from then on. Without meaning to, he had badly frightened her. From that day on, she found herself checking her moles so diligently that she spent most of her time in front of mirrors or using a magnifying glass. And she goes back to the doctor almost monthly to question him about something on her skin. She can't go on living this way. What should she do?

Jeanine does have an increased risk for melanoma because of her light, freckled skin and history of dysplastic nevus. She will always have a higher risk of developing melanoma than the average person. But her overall risk is still quite low. Jeanine can influence her overall chance of developing skin cancer, too. First of all, her risk of developing melanoma can be decreased if she avoids sun exposure, uses sunscreen every time she goes into the sunlight,

you have about the changes that have occurred in your life? People who have been through the experience. That's why survivor groups can be so helpful. They bridge the gap," Dr. Coscarelli says. Ask your medical team about survivor groups in your area.

Don't fear the Reaper. At some time, you may hear or read that someone you know has

and wears clothing that protects her skin when she is outdoors (such as wearing a T-shirt over her bathing suit when she is not swimming).

She can also decrease her risk of death from melanoma through appropriate screening, including regular, but not obsessive, head-to-toe inspections of her skin as well as an examination by a dermatologist every 3 to 6 months, or as often as her doctor recommends. Jeanine would probably benefit emotionally from regular visits because of her anxiety. If she does see something suspicious during one of those checks, certainly she should notify her doctor right away and not wait for her routine scheduled visit.

If Jeanine is examining herself regularly and has good checkups with her doctor, continued fearfulness is counterproductive. It isn't decreasing her risk of cancer. It's simply taking away from her quality of life. She needs to tame that fear. A good starting point would be for her to realize that she can still protect herself from this cancer without obsessing about it. She should understand that the chances of her developing a life-threatening melanoma in a month or two are almost zero. She should continue to do skin self-exams every 1 to 2 months (or however often her dermatologist recommends). If she doesn't find anything during her skin exam, she has to trust that she is fine. Also, she has to trust that because she is being diligent, if she should develop melanoma, she will probably pick it up early, when it has a good chance of being curable.

Expert consulted
Wendy S. Harpham, M.D.
Author of After Cancer

died of the same disease you had. It can be frightening and sad. You may feel a shiver down your spine because it rattles your sense of being safe from death, Dr. Harpham says.

You can rein in your fears if you remember that the other person's death has no effect whatsoever on what will happen to you. Keep in mind that there are many factors that affect any individual's chances of long-term survival from an injury or disease. Look for ways in which your disease's course differs from that of the person who has passed away, suggests Dr. Coscarelli.

Dr. Harpham suggests reaching out to others and talking about your feelings. It's okay to cry and feel sorrowful. Paradoxically, this grieving can actually affirm your will to live, help you embrace a positive attitude, and enhance the quality of your life.

If reading obituaries disturbs you, skip that page of the newspaper. If you find yourself dwelling on obituaries and you cannot stop thinking about death, seek professional help to sort out your fears and feelings, Dr. Harpham suggests.

Watch your mouth. Language is powerful. Wordplay is not trivial mental gymnastics, it is one of the forces that shapes our perception of reality, Dr. Harpham says.

"I did an interview on a national news program a few years ago that identified me as 'Wendy Harpham, cancer victim.' I cringe when I hear those words," she says. "Victims, by definition, feel helpless and hopeless. Survivors have succeeded against a challenge or threat. I have always considered myself a cancer survivor. Sometimes, I'm a cancer patient. But I have never been a cancer victim. Cancer victims and cancer survivors are in the same situation, but they have different frames of mind."

So whenever you catch yourself using negative language, stop and change your thinking. If necessary, jot down a new, more positive phrase. Dr.

books for both children and adults about coping with cancer.

Stop your mind from wandering. If you frequently find yourself ruminating on how you might deal with your disease if it recurs, stop. It probably won't help you. Set limits. If you find yourself drifting into an ugly scenario, do whatever you can to distract yourself. Be grateful for today and let go of worries about tomorrow.

"If a recurrence happens, I'll deal with it then," Dr. Harpham says. "I don't want to deal with it twice—now in imagination and again when it really happens."

Shrink it down to size. Don't be afraid to seek professional assistance, particularly if you have any of the following symptoms.

- You have a sad, worried, or empty feeling that never goes away.
- You think of suicide.
- You can't sleep, you're sleeping too much, or you're waking too early in the morning.
- You have trouble concentrating or making decisions.
- You feel as if you can't get back into the swing of life, even though your illness has long since passed.

"Just because you seek professional assistance doesn't mean that there is something terribly wrong with you," Dr. Coscarelli says. "It's just part of the experience, and it may be helpful to talk to someone who can help you sort these feelings out and build an effective emotional toolbox that will make it easier for you to cope with them in the future."

Harpham, for instance, never thinks of her cancer as incurable, even though there are no known cures for it today. Instead, she describes her disease as one of the types of cancer for which scientists are still looking for a cure.

Chart a new course. Instead of letting an emotion such as anger or anxiety fester, use it as a positive force to change other lives. Some women have created Web sites on the Internet that are loaded with information about their diseases. Others become advocates, fund-raisers, or volunteers. Dr. Harpham has written several

Renew
Your Spirit

You shake a fist at God and ask, "Why me?"

That's how many of us react to getting sick. Finding meaning and nobility in your situation is probably the furthest thing from your mind, at least initially. But meaning and nobility are there.

After living with illness for a while, many women, out of necessity, slow down and take stock of their lives, says Rabbi Nancy Flam of Northampton, Massachusetts, director of the spirituality institute Metivta, based in Los Angeles. "They make priorities in terms of what's most important, and often that turns out to be love and wisdom. They might have preferred to come to those decisions in a more pleasant fashion, but people can certainly change their lives for the better because of serious illness."

That's not to say that suffering is a good thing, of course. "I have known only a handful of people who would claim that they wouldn't have traded their cancer for good health because of what they learned and how they grew as a result of having it," Rabbi Flam adds. "But I've met many, many more who felt that

they would rather have remained healthy and shallow.'"

The point is to make the best out of a less-than-wonderful situation. With some effort, you can turn sickness into an opportunity for real spiritual renewal.

What Does It All Mean?

Pain and adversity can make you bitter, or they can make you better. It's your choice, says Freda Crew, D. Min. (doctor of ministry), director of Truth for Living Ministries in Spartanburg, South Carolina, and author of *Get Off Your Own Back*. "I tell people, 'It's here, it's a reality, you can't deny it. So let's get everything we can out of it.'" Here are some ways in which you can begin to do that.

Change the "Why me?" to "What am I going to learn from this?" It can take some time, but you can change from feeling like a helpless victim to regaining a sense of control in your life. Just ask yourself, "If this is part of my life's journey and lesson, what am I going to get out of it?" says Rabbi Judith Abrams, Ph.D., coauthor of *Illness and Health in the Jewish Tradition*. "This is more useful than wallowing in your situation."

Seek the truth. "Very often, pain and adversity will cause a sincere person to start yearning for answers," says Dr. Crew. "But the truth doesn't usually end up laid on our doorsteps. The best way to find answers is to become a searcher, a seeker after truth and reality, and then to deal with things as they really are."

For instance, Dr. Crew says, you're kidding yourself if you think that by trying to please God you'll avoid pain or suffering during your lifetime. "The Bible, which we turn to for our truth, never says such a thing. We have conjured this up ourselves," she says. Realizing that God is not to blame, that you are not to blame, that you are not being punished, and that suffering is pretty much a fact of life for everyone can make a big difference in helping you cope with your illness.

Turn to prayer. Most religions have prayers that you can say when faced with anxiety, such as "The Lord is my shepherd" (Psalm 23). And many have prayers for the morning and evening. "These are natural times in the day when one realizes that one is living on a globe, spinning through the cosmos, affected by the sun and gravitational pull," Rabbi Flam says. "When the light changes, it is really an opening and awakening of our awareness. It's also a time when one realizes that everything changes, that everything is fleeting, transient, momentary, and so it is really a time for becoming aware of the moment and its blessings."

Instead of asking, listen. "I strongly believe that prayer is about listening and waiting for a

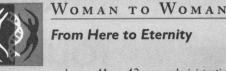

WOMAN TO WOMAN
From Here to Eternity

Joann May, 43, an administrative assistant from Philadelphia, had never considered herself a particularly religious person. Then one evening, when she was 37, her heart stopped during an asthma attack. Before the night was over, she would forever change her concept of God, heaven, and life on Earth. Here's her story.

I was at home, folding laundry, not feeling so great, when my chest started to tighten, and I knew I was in trouble. I took some of my usual inhaler, but it didn't work. My last resort, which I had never used before, was an EpiPen, a shot of epinephrine, which is a hormone sometimes called adrenaline. That didn't kick in either, so I called my dad, who lived a few blocks away, and told him I needed to go to the hospital. I remember going down the first five steps to the car, and that's it. I collapsed out in the street, and the paramedics worked on me there for close to an hour. My heart stopped once in the ambulance and twice more in the hospital, so I was pretty much going in and out of it for about 5 hours before I woke up on a respirator in the hospital.

It's very hard to explain what happened to me during that time, because it was like a dream, a beautiful dream. I was very disappointed that it started to fade so quickly after I woke up.

I did move through a tunnel toward a point of light, which I

response—not asking for a response the way I want it, but listening for what is the right thing to do, which may be something I never even thought about," says Sister Felicia Petruziello, a licensed professional clinical counselor at St. Joseph Wellness Center in Cleveland. "Part of prayer is learning to listen to my own heart, my own gut." People do better in adversity if they realize that they do have some control in the matter. "So they need to recognize that there are answers for their situations but that the answers

learned is common during near-death experiences. I had a spiritual guide who gave me a tour of the universe, and that was a sense of the vastness of the universe, of being there at its creation, of being a part of the universe from its beginnings. I had no sense of self; I was everything and everything was me, including God. It was a very reassuring feeling, and I felt very safe and protected. I felt unconditional love and joy and peace.

I didn't want to go back into my body. I started arguing with God, and God said that I needed to go back because my mission here wasn't complete. I was told that I hadn't loved enough and that part of my mission was to spread the message to love one another.

I never had much of a sense of God, but now I know that he is not some guy with a beard who sits on a throne and says who's in and who's out.

My sense now of "heaven," of the afterlife, is that what happens to you when you die is your choice. You can choose to exist in a state of unconditional love, or not, and it all comes from how you forgive yourself for the blunders that you made in your life. You totally judge yourself. You feel the pain that you created during your life, and it all comes back to you as its creator. When you forgive yourself, you experience the love, joy, and peace to move on.

I am not afraid of death now—no way. But I don't do anything to risk my life. I know that's not the way to get back there. I was told that I wouldn't be going back there any time soon.

might not be immediate or apparent. There are answers if we wait and listen," she says.

The Most Important Job You'll Ever Have

Illness often motivates women to start looking for the places where their lives have gone off course. "Just realizing where you need to do some work and then starting in on it can help resolve a lot of unhealthy stress," Dr. Crew says. Here are some ways you can do that.

Explore where your life may be out of balance spiritually. Now is your chance to restore that balance. Are you working too hard? Feeling sorry for yourself? Unable to accept others' comfort? Unable to experience joy or wonder? Carrying around feelings of fear, guilt, anger, or shame?

"We need to take an inventory of our lives, to take a journey into our very thoughts, motives, relationships, and behavior," Dr. Crew says. "Are there those we have failed to forgive, or do we have unresolved conflicts with people? Are we breaking God's law and unwilling to stop?"

Count your blessings. Learning to shift your attention from what is gone or painful to what you have and enjoy can help you cultivate a more positive attitude, says Sister Felicia. Some easy ways to cultivate a sense of gratitude are to say thank you to people and to God and say grace over meals. Take time to do things that you enjoy, to be a part of nature, and to realize that you are a part of something greater than yourself. Keep reminders of love and beauty around you—photos of loved ones, mementos of good times, a rock from a beautiful lake, flowers from your garden.

Pick up a Good Book. Words can convey hope and provide guidance, says Sister Felicia. "I frequently refer people to the Psalms because they are about feelings. I tell people that, often, when they are angry or distressed, that is their prayer. Sometimes, just yelling at God or crying out to God is your prayer, and the Psalms are very much that."

THE POWER OF PRAYER

If you think that praying is something you do out of helplessness when there's nothing else you can do, that you're simply humoring yourself, then you're underestimating its power. Studies, some of them controlled enough to qualify as scientific, suggest that prayer can have an impact on the course of an illness.

In one landmark study, patients in a cardiac-care unit were randomly divided into two groups. The members of one group were remembered in what's called intercessory prayer, prayers offered to help others, while the other patients were not prayed for. Neither the patients nor the hospital staff knew which patients belonged to which group.

The people doing the praying did it outside the hospital, using only the patient's first name, diagnosis, and general condition. They prayed for the patient's rapid recovery and freedom from complications.

Those patients who were prayed for had less congestive heart failure (8 versus 20), needed less antibiotic therapy (3 versus 17), had fewer episodes of pneumonia (3 versus 13), and had fewer cardiac arrests (3 versus 14). Twenty-seven of those in the group of patients who were prayed for did poorly while 44 of the others had a poor recovery.

A similar, more recent study, done with AIDS patients, found that healing messages sent from healers of both religious and secular traditions lessened the severity of the patients' illnesses and improved one measure of mood.

As for meditation, it's surprisingly well-documented for its ability to reduce blood pressure, relieve pain, and lower anxiety. In one study of people treated at the University of Massachusetts Medical Center in Amherst, those who meditated were able to use less pain medication and said that their pain was much less likely to stop them from doing things than people did who did not meditate. The meditators also reported less anxiety and depression.

In another study, psoriasis patients who meditated while undergoing ultraviolet light treatment had their skin clear up significantly faster than did nonmeditators.

The Book of Job also does a good job of presenting anguish and introspection in the face of adversity, Dr. Crew says.

Ask others to pray for you, and listen to what they say. A powerful feeling of being loved can come from knowing that people are praying for you. "I have a real sense that I am being covered in prayer, and as I gain strength, I realize that people's prayers are being answered," Dr. Crew says.

Most religions have special prayers for healing body and soul. In Catholicism, it's the Anointing of the Sick; in Judaism, it's the Mi Shebarakh.

"Praying publicly for someone who is sick has a double effect," Rabbi Flam says. "There is the prayer one offers up or within, which provides hope of healing body and soul. And there is the connection that the community makes around the person who is ill. The person's name is said and everyone is informed, so there are also visits and food and offers to help."

Make meditation a habit. Meditation has proven abilities to calm and center you, to slow your breathing, and to lower your blood pressure. To do a simple meditation, just close your eyes and pay attention to your breathing, Rabbi Abrams suggests. Focus on a short phrase, perhaps a verse from the Bible or a spiritual picture or scene. "Just focus and allow yourself to stay in that state for a while," she says. "It doesn't have to be hours. Even if all you do is a minute, you will feel yourself calm down, and pretty soon all it takes for you to begin is to focus on your breathing and the calming will start. You develop a reflex."

Start treating your body like the temple that it is. Whether it's overeating, drugs, or alcohol, if you are having trouble overcoming bad habits and addictions that are contributing to your health problems, pray for help, Sister Felicia advises. "If we ask for anything in our religion, it is for strength. And even though we believe that God is always with us, there is something comforting about the request."

Seek spiritual companionship and renewal. Lots of people start reattending church or synagogue, even after an absence of many years, because of sickness or some other crisis. And that's nothing to feel ashamed or embarrassed about, Dr. Crew says. Studies show that people who attend religious services regularly are healthier and live longer.

"In fact, you might want to look for a church that ministers to people in need, to people who are hurting," she says. "Check out what kind of support system they have for people who are going through crisis. Who is there to assure them that they are loved and cared for? Are people encouraged to reach out to others? Are others often willing to help if they know about a situation or are asked to help?"

Take the disheartened into your heart. "People who help others always seem to say, 'I

MY MAMA TOLD ME

Will sitting too close to the television really wreck my eyesight?

Scientific research has proven Mom wrong on this one. Studies that look at the number of hours children spend watching TV have been unable to find any link with vision problems. It's true that long hours of close vision work, such as reading, are associated with nearsightedness. But nearsightedness has never been linked with TV viewing. You can sit right on top of the TV, and it doesn't seem to matter.

On the other hand, a fair number of people develop eyestrain—fatigue or aching around and above the eyes—from viewing a computer screen for long hours. And they may be more likely to have such problems as they get older and need bifocals. The solution is a special pair of glasses designed just for computer work. The lens targets your "middle vision" at about 24 inches. In the old days, we used to call these piano glasses. They were prescribed for ladies who played the piano and needed to be able to read the music.

Expert consulted
Karla Zadnik, O.D., Ph.D.
Associate professor in the College of
*   Optometry*
Ohio State University
Columbus

get more out of this than the people I am helping,' and I feel that way myself," Sister Felicia says. "I am amazed at what people can get through, and I believe we gain strength from going outside of ourselves to help others."

"People feel a deep impulse to redeem some of their suffering by helping other people," Rabbi Flam adds. "Instead of letting their suffering be an event of disillusion and destruction, they salvage their experience and make meaning and build up the world again by providing a comfort and a sense of compassion and wisdom and guidance for others."

Say the "D" Word

It's the elephant in the middle of the room that nobody talks about. While we fear pain and suffering, we also mourn the eventuality of our own deaths. Instead of ignoring it, it's better to ponder it and come to some terms with it, spiritual leaders say.

Confront your mortality. Are you afraid of dying? Most people are, and they resist thinking about it, Dr. Crew says. "But I don't know of anything that makes us face mortality more

quickly than a serious illness or accident. People have to start thinking about what they believe, and they start working through the grief of their own death."

Create your own immortality. Whatever your sense of life after death, there are ways that you can leave an impression of yourself here, Rabbi Abrams says. "Whether you're a car mechanic or a college professor, strive from your heart to pass on your special knowledge, and you'll make the most of the gift you have been given. Give to your family, friends, your community, to anyone to whom you can act as a parent. Do good deeds, and know that your good deeds live on after you, that the world is a better place for your having been here."

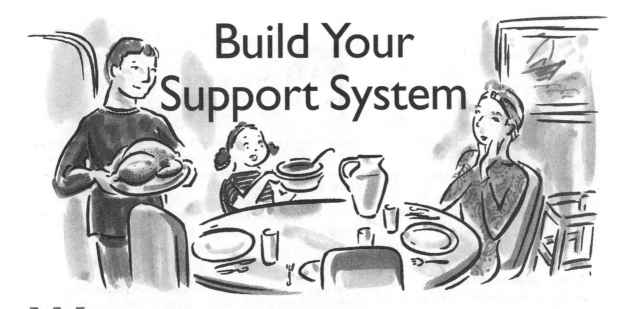

Build Your Support System

When Linda McCartney phoned her husband to tell him that she'd been diagnosed with breast cancer, he dropped everything and rushed home to be with her. For the next 2½ years, as they fought her disease, he gave her unstinting support and devotion. Even in her final moments, he was at her side whispering love and encouragement to her.

It's a beautiful story, and we all hope that, should we ever get sick, our loved ones will be as loyal and caring as Paul McCartney was. Unfortunately, we know that life—and people—don't always turn out as we'd hoped.

Illness sometimes brings out the best in people, but not always. "It can really draw people closer together, but it also has the potential to blow a relationship apart," says Catherine Classen, Ph.D., a clinical psychologist at Stanford University School of Medicine.

Being sick can make us very needy, and the constant challenge of meeting our needs can leave our partners feeling resentful and inadequate. A husband accustomed to being waited on at home, for example, may suddenly find his new role as caregiver too much to handle.

"Illness can be the stress that finally ends a troubled relationship," says Mary K. Hughes, R.N., a psychiatric clinical nurse specialist at the University of Texas M. D. Anderson Cancer Center in Houston. "Husbands *do* leave—not always, of course, but often enough that it isn't a rare occurrence. And when it happens, it's devastating to a woman."

On the other hand, a couple that survives an illness often uses the challenge to put trivial problems into perspective and to come to appreciate and value each other more than ever. "It's about both sides being gentle with each other and knowing that illness, acute or chronic, is really hard to process into a relationship," says Susan Brace, R.N., Ph.D., a clinical psychologist practicing in Los Angeles. "Both people are likely to feel as if life is being changed and it isn't fair—life *is* being changed, and it *isn't* fair."

When Opportunity Knocks

What may seem especially unfair is that, even when she's ill, a woman often remains the emotional caretaker of her family, if only because no one else will assume the role. But what at first looks like a burden can turn into an opportunity to strengthen the relationships she cares about most, if she takes a few simple steps.

Give the gift of time. Head off resentment by encouraging family members to take some time for themselves, Dr. Classen says. "I'm not saying that they need your permission, but they feel less guilty if you tell them something like 'I'm okay here for a while. Why don't you go to a movie or take some time to yourself?'"

Show appreciation. Don't take your family for granted. Every day, let each of them know how much they are appreciated and valued, says Mary Cerreto, Ph.D., an industry consultant and specialist in relationships and illness in Natick, Massachusetts. "We forget to praise or reward the little things we have come to expect, and the people who do the most get the least thanks sometimes." Don't assume that those who are helping you know you're grateful for what they do. Tell them.

Be explicit. The more clearly you can express your needs, the more likely you are to have those needs met, Dr. Classen says. "A lot of women say how disappointed they are in a particular family member's response. Often, these women have a wish that they can't bring themselves to ask for explicitly. But if they don't ask, they don't get. So they need to state their wants and needs very clearly."

Deal with feelings. To keep the lines of communication open and your relationships strong, you need to discuss whatever emotions you and your family may be going through concerning your illness. But don't stop there. "Recognizing feelings without moving ahead is

REAL-LIFE SCENARIO
She's a Real Do-It-Yourselfer

April, 45, would call herself a self-reliant woman. She cooks, she cleans, she repairs her house, and she has raised four kids on her own—her husband, a merchant marine, has been at sea most of the time. When she became a widow 6 years ago, she went out and got herself a job cashiering at a local drugstore and worked weekends cleaning offices for a local transportation company. Then, this breast thing happened. It started with a lump in her right breast, and before she knew it, she was in the hospital recuperating from a mastectomy. Her sons and daughters instantly showed up to help, offering to cook and clean for her and to help her financially, but she's finding it difficult to accept their kindness. She somehow feels ashamed of being off her feet for a while, and, as a result, she's been irritable and cranky with everyone. As much as her kids want to help her, they're starting to resent the way she treats them—and she knows it. But she just can't help herself. What should she do?

At some emotional level, April is probably convinced that she doesn't deserve any help, and she doesn't want to be a burden to others. In fact, if she hasn't been so nice to be around lately, there's a good chance that it's because she feels guilty about accepting help.

But why should she feel unworthy or guilty? After all, April has almost certainly given her children lots of care whenever they've needed it in the past, and now they're

useless," says Dr. Cerreto. "At some point, you have to say, 'Okay, now what do we do about these feelings?'"

For a son who is feeling neglected, for instance, you might say something like, "Now that Dad can't take you to baseball games as much as he used to, I've noticed that you've been getting angry at me more often. I can understand why. My being sick has really made some big changes in your life. What can we do about it?"

Or for a husband who has shut down and stopped communicating, you could say, "You've

eager to help her in return. By turning them away, she's robbing them of the opportunity to show her in concrete ways that they care about her and appreciate what she has given to them over the years. She may not realize how much doing things herself isolates her from her family.

April surely has chores or errands that other people could do to make her life easier right now: running for sundries, cutting the grass, cleaning the house, even doing some of the cooking. And by giving her children specific suggestions, she'll remain in control so that they don't go overboard and start trying to run her life.

As for financial help, if her pride won't let her accept money outright, her children can make the situation easier by offering to do things like fill her gas tank or pay for her groceries. If she still says no, they should be sensitive enough to accept her answer at face value.

April could benefit from easing up on herself. There may be days when the pain or stress of illness makes her irritable. On those days, it would help if she just let her children know that. A generous thank-you would make both April and those who care about her feel a lot better.

Expert consulted
Mary Cerreto, Ph.D.
Industry consultant and specialist in relationships and illness
Natick, Massachusetts

been so quiet lately that I don't know what you're thinking. I can't tell if you're worried, but I know you're sad. I'm sad, too. What can we do to start talking about it? I want to help you understand what I'm feeling and going through with this illness so that you don't worry so much and so that we can handle it together."

Bring Friends into the Fold

Friends react to illness as they do to any other difficult situation. "Some will be a wonderful ex-ample of what it means to be a friend, and others will feel helpless and not want to be there," says Dr. Brace. Close friends may have more presence of mind than even family members about what needs to be done and how you're feeling. Others will want to help but may be uncomfortable and unsure of how to go about it. Here are some ways you can help your friends support you.

Reach out and touch someone. Friends don't call for a variety of reasons. Your illness may have struck too close to home for them, they may lack confidence in their worth as companions during this time, or they may prefer to say nothing rather than risk saying the wrong thing. Their absence does not necessarily mean that they no longer care about you. You, too, may have withdrawn during part of your illness to protect your own feelings. But you can't draw comfort from an empty room.

If you really don't want to lose someone's friendship and you believe discomfort rather than fear is keeping a particular friend away, try a phone call to dissolve the barrier, Hughes says. And try using humor to break through the initial awkwardness. Tell a joke, laugh together, then say something like, "It feels so good to laugh. I haven't laughed in a while."

If you've been withdrawn because you were depressed, your closest friends should know. Your honesty will promote intimacy. But you don't need to tell everyone you know. To acquaintances, you might just say, "I wasn't feeling well," and leave it at that.

Help friends to help. Believe it or not, most people are grateful if there is something concrete that they can do to show their continuing

MY MAMA TOLD ME

Will swimming too soon after eating really give me cramps?

It's true that you are more likely to develop a side stitch, a muscle cramp in your diaphragm, if you do any kind of vigorous exercise soon after eating a large meal. And a cramp may make it difficult to swim since you're likely to want to curl up in a ball. But it's more uncomfortable than dangerous.

The cramp occurs because blood-rich oxygen is being diverted away from your muscles to your intestines to aid in digestion. Oxygen-deprived muscles can cramp up.

So that old "mom's rule" of waiting an hour after you eat before you swim laps isn't such a bad idea. Wait until you feel comfortable, until your stomach is no longer full. But feel free to get into the pool to just cool off or swim slowly. That shouldn't cause cramps, even with a full belly.

Expert consulted
Jane Katz, Ed.D.
Professor of health and physical education
City University of New York, John Jay College
*   of Criminal Justice*
World masters swimming champion
Author of Swimming for Total Fitness

friendship. So if a friend says, "Is there anything I can do?" take her literally. If you could use it, ask for simple assistance—to run an errand, to prepare a meal, or simply to come and visit. "These small acts bring friends back into contact and help them feel useful and needed," Hughes says. "You have done them and yourself a favor."

Assign a point person. Sometimes, one close friend can become the go-between for you and other friends, setting up visits from people, getting old friends back in the room, and calling people to tell them how you're doing, Dr. Brace says.

Use friends as rehab helpers. Use their visits to structure your day. For instance, if your doctor wants you to start walking to rebuild your strength, have a friend take a walk with you, Dr. Brace says. Don't just rely upon going to physical therapy three times a week.

Learn to share. One of your best immediate resources is someone who has the same condition as you do and is doing well, Dr. Cerreto says. You may be able to find such a person in a support group, which can provide understanding, support, and companionship for both you and your family. Ask your doctor about local support groups, or contact American Self-Help Clearinghouse, St. Clare's Hospital, 25 Pocono Road, Denville, NJ 07834-2995. They will provide, free of charge, information on a support group nearest you. Or look in your local library for a copy of the book *The Self-Help Sourcebook*, 6th edition, which includes contacts for hundreds of groups. As you recover, sharing your experiences with others can help you regain strength and courage.

Work Things Out at Work

When you return to work, coworkers, like friends, will respond in a variety of ways. So you may need to deal with people individually. Some won't even know about your illness, and that's just as well, Dr. Cerreto says. "If you don't want to tell them, just say, 'I was sick. I was in the hospital, but now I'm feeling fine.'" But in some cases, it's good to have one cool, calm person around who knows what you have and who can help you if you need it.

If your illness has left you permanently disabled, you should contact your company's personnel office when you return to work. By federal law, the Americans with Disabilities Act requires employers of a workforce of 15 or more to make reasonable changes in your work site that will allow you to do your job, such as giving you a wheelchair-accessible work area.

If you're worried about not being able to get back up to speed right away, your employer may need to make some accommodations for you. Here again, you have legal rights.

On the other hand, if you're being coddled at home, returning to a situation where others do not think of you as sick may be the greatest therapy yet devised.

The Gift of Wisdom

When God said to Solomon, "Ask what I shall give thee," Solomon begged for wisdom. If you've recovered from an illness, or if you're still sick but you've learned how to cope successfully, you've received the very same gift, whether or not you realize it.

How so? From your own experience, you now know things about weathering illness that you never before realized. You know about the needs, the fears, and the wishes that being sick can create. You can use your newfound wisdom in

---

WOMEN ASK WHY

Why were people afraid to touch me when I was sick, even though I wasn't contagious?

Lots of people worry about getting or giving germs when they're around someone who is sick, even when the chances of transmission are slim. They know that some germs can be transmitted through touch, but they don't know enough to know when that's not likely to happen. And some people may worry about how touching might be received. They don't want to do something that might be taken the wrong way or that might cause pain.

What's more, people often don't realize how beneficial a caring touch is to someone who is sick. The love and comfort that is conveyed through touching often has benefits that outweigh the risks.

When you are visiting a sick friend, wash your hands before you have direct contact with her, especially if you are in a hospital and have been touching handrails and doorknobs. Then, try gently squeezing her hand during a conversation or laying your hand on her shoulder. If your friend squeezes back, smiles, or lays her hand over yours, your touch is welcome.

Expert consulted
Charlotte Eliopoulos, R.N., Ph.D.
Specialist in holistic geriatric and chronic-care
*   nursing*
Author of Integrating Conventional and
*   Alternative Therapies*

---

your day-to-day dealings with anyone who may be facing a challenge to her health. Here are some examples.

State the obvious. People who are sick or who have recently been sick often have trouble talking about what is going on with them, Dr. Classen says. "They may be afraid and kind of deny it," she says. "Or they may not want to burden another with their own concerns. They may find that when they do try to talk about their worries, they don't get the response they want, and that's very painful, so they shut down." If someone is depressed, she may isolate herself all the more.

To break the ice, approach her directly. Just say, "What's going on today? You look sad," suggests Hughes. "That person is just waiting for someone to notice that she is different, that something is wrong."

People who have been seriously ill are often fearful of dying, of always feeling bad, of never getting well, of not knowing what's next. "Just getting these feelings out in the open and talking about them takes away some of their power,"

Hughes says. Someone who is depressed, however, may also need medication to be able to shake some of the oppressive feelings.

Be absolutely honest. Sick people just know things about their state of health whether the doctor tells them or not, Dr. Brace says. "Some people will say they're afraid that, if they're honest, they're going to hurt someone's feelings. But if you're honest, you at least have a real solid bridge to the other person, and if it hurts her feelings, you can apologize. If you're not honest, you have no bridge. And sick people feel most isolated not having those bridges. What makes the sick person feel most isolated is pretense, by the doctor or by the family. Sick people don't want to be lied to."

Index

Underscored page references indicate boxed text. **Boldfaced** references indicate illustrations.

A

Abdominal pain, 346–47, **347**
Acetaminophen, 336
Acidity (pH), 10, 88
Acne, 79
Actonel, 297
Acupuncture, for arthritis, 267
Acyclovir, 241, 308, 310
Adventure, sense of, 140–41
Advil, 222
Aerobic exercise. *See also* Workouts, exercises
  active lifestyle and, 50–51
  aging and, 59
  energy and, 47
  health benefits of, 46–48
  metabolism and, 46–47
  muscles and, 46
  for preventing and treating
    arthritis, 49
    cancer, 48–49
    depression, 49
    diabetes, 49
    disease, 48–49
    heart disease, 48
    menstrual cramps, 47
    osteoporosis, 49, 291–92
    stroke, 49
  sex and, 47
  skin and, 47–48
  sleep and, 47
  for stress management, 47
Age
  breast cancer and, 312–13
  colon cancer and, 341
  diabetes and, 270
  osteoporosis and, 289
  reproductive cancer and, 324
Age-related macular degeneration (ARMD), 16,
    148–49
Age spots, 59

Aging
  aerobic exercise and, 59
  alpha-lipoic acid and, 24
  attitude and, 6–7, 136–37
  of baby boomers, 2–3
  bioflavonoids and, 25
  clothing styles and, 126, 129–33, **130–32**
  coenzyme Q_{10} and, 26–27
  diet and, 5, 8–10
  disease and, 4–5
  education and, 7
  exercise and, 5
  flaxseed oil and, 28
  genetics and, 58–59
  "gifts" of, 3
  ginkgo and, 29
  hearing and, 146
  height and, 293
  joints and, 261
  longevity and, 3–4, 9, 12
  melatonin and, 30
  memory and, 151–52
  menopause and, 5
  phosphatidylserine and, 31
  physical features and, 105
    eyes, 79–81, **80–81**, 80–81, 105
    hair, 113, 116
    skin, 72
  Pycnogenol and, 30–31
  resistance training and, 56, 57, 64
  sex and, 5–6, 166–67, 168, 171–72
  skin care products and, 82, 85
  sleep and, 173, 176
  soy foods and, 19
  sweets and, 4
  teeth and, 111
  vision and, 148–50, 148–49
  vitamin C and, 31–32
  vitamin E and, 17, 32
  vocabulary as sign of, 137
  weight and, 38

F